D0401273

table of contents

Also available from the
American Academy of Pediatrics

Common Conditions

ADHD: What Every Parent Needs to Know

Allergies and Asthma: What Every Parent Needs to Know

My Child Is Sick! Expert Advice for Managing Common Illnesses and Injuries

Waking Up Dry: A Guide to Help Children Overcome Bedwetting

Developmental, Behavioral, and Psychosocial Information

CyberSafe: Protecting and Empowering Kids in the Digital World of Texting, Gaming, and Social Media

Mental Health, Naturally: The Family Guide to Holistic Care for a Healthy Mind and Body

The Wonder Years: Helping Your Baby and Young Child Successfully Negotiate the Major Developmental Milestones

Immunization Information

Immunizations & Infectious Diseases: An Informed Parent's Guide

Newborns, Infants, and Toddlers

Baby & Child Health: The Essential Guide From Birth to 11 Years

Caring for Your Baby and Young Child: Birth to Age 5*

Guide to Toilet Training*

Heading Home With Your Newborn: From Birth to Reality

Mommy Calls: Dr. Tanya Answers Parents' Top 101 Questions About Babies and Toddlers

New Mother's Guide to Breastfeeding*

Newborn Intensive Care: What Every Parent Needs to Know

Raising Twins: From Pregnancy to Preschool

Your Baby's First Year*

Nutrition and Fitness

Food Fights: Winning the Nutritional Challenges of Parenthood Armed With Insight, Humor, and a Bottle of Ketchup

Nutrition: What Every Parent Needs to Know

A Parent's Guide to Childhood Obesity: A Road Map to Health

Sports Success R_x! Your Child's Prescription for the Best Experience

School-aged Children and Adolescents

Building Resilience in Children and Teens: Giving Kids Roots and Wings

Caring for Your School-Age Child: Ages 5 to 12

Caring for Your Teenager

Less Stress, More Success: A New Approach to Guiding Your Teen Through College Admissions and Beyond

For more information, please visit the official AAP Web site for parents, www.HealthyChildren.org/bookstore.

*This book is also available in Spanish.

DAD to DAD
Parenting Like a Pro

Expert Advice, Guidance, and Insight From a Pediatrician-Dad

David L. Hill, MD, FAAP

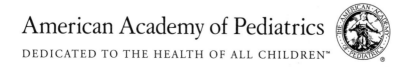

American Academy of Pediatrics
DEDICATED TO THE HEALTH OF ALL CHILDREN™

American Academy of Pediatrics Department of Marketing and Publications Staff

Director, Department of Marketing and Publications
Maureen DeRosa, MPA

Director, Division of Product Development
Mark Grimes

Manager, Consumer Publishing
Carolyn Kolbaba

Coordinator, Division of Product Development
Holly Kaminski

Director, Division of Publishing and Production Services
Sandi King, MS

Editorial Specialist
Jason Crase

Print Production Specialist
Shannan Martin

Manager, Art Direction and Production
Linda Diamond

Director, Division of Marketing and Sales
Kevin Tuley

Manager, Consumer Marketing and Sales
Kathleen Juhl

Manager, Consumer Product Marketing
Maryjo Reynolds

Published by the American Academy of Pediatrics
141 Northwest Point Blvd, Elk Grove Village, IL 60007-1019
847/434-4000
Fax: 847/434-8000
www.aap.org

Cover design by R. Scott Rattray
Book design by Linda Diamond
Illustrations by Anthony Alex LeTourneau

Library of Congress Control Number: 2011940120
ISBN: 978-1-58110-650-3

The recommendations in this publication do not indicate an exclusive course of treatment or serve as a standard of medical care. Variations, taking into account individual circumstances, may be appropriate.

Statements and opinions expressed are those of the author and not necessarily those of the American Academy of Pediatrics.

Products and Web sites are mentioned for informational purposes only. Inclusion in this publication does not imply endorsement by the American Academy of Pediatrics. The American Academy of Pediatrics is not responsible for the content of the resources mentioned in this publication. Web site addresses are as current as possible but may change at any time.

CB0069
9-316

1 2 3 4 5 6 7 8 9 10

what people are saying

You'd expect a book on parenting from someone with Dr Hill's credentials to be highly informative and well written. What might surprise you is that it's also really quite funny, as well as chock-full of practical "do this; don't do that" advice guys especially will appreciate. Becoming a new father can be terrifying, but *Dad to Dad: Parenting Like a Pro* will make the journey seem not only manageable but actually kind of fun. I predict this book will become as essential to new dads as *What to Expect When You're Expecting* is to new moms (and a lot more fun to read). And when it does, I hope David will cut me in on the royalties. A man can dream, can't he? I wish I'd read this book before my children were born—and more importantly, so do my wife and kids.

Dan Tynan
Contributing editor, *Family Circle;* author; journalist; and father of 2

Dad to Dad is the best book I've ever read on having and raising healthy children. Armed with abundant humor and warmth, Dr David L. Hill is the perfect pediatrician to guide nervous first-time parents through a variety of dilemmas, real and imagined. The best part? His writing style is never stodgy or technical but rather completely approachable and understandable. Every parent should own this book. It's like having a doctor in the house!

Celia Rivenbark
Best-selling author of *Stop Dressing Your Six-Year-Old Like a Skank*

Anyone can be a father, but to be a *good* father requires more than intuition and good intentions. It requires an expert guide for the well-trodden road ahead—and there are few better than Dr Hill, an expert in his field and a down-to-earth dad. He shows new fathers everything from the lay of the land to the details they'll need to thrive.

Dr David Eagleman
Neuroscientist, Baylor College of Medicine, and best-selling author of *Incognito: The Secret Lives of the Brain*

We live in a mom-eat-mom parenting world, so where do dads fit in? Dr Hill provides a fresh, candid, and expert voice to being not only a very present father but one who is ecstatic and ready for the challenge of raising children. From sex after childbirth to starting baby food, and from bed-wetting to attending PTA meetings, Dr Hill lends a helpful, clear, and hilarious voice for fathers. Let *Dad to Dad* accompany you on your journey through fatherhood. It's a perfect gift for any new dad.

Wendy Sue Swanson, MD, MBE, FAAP
Mother, pediatrician, and @SeattleMamaDoc blogger for Seattle Children's Hospital

To Abby, Sellers, and Julian;
I give all 3 of you permission to laugh hysterically
if you ever hear your dad referred to as a
"parenting expert."

acknowledgments

Given the subject of this book, I obviously have to start by thanking my dad, but even that task is not simple. John R. Hill III, MD, FAAP, is the man I've called Dad since he married my mother and adopted me. He inspired me to read Tolkien, practice typing on an old Olympus, enter the citywide high school poetry contest, attend medical school, and become not just a pediatrician, but a good one. I strive daily to be the best father I can be in an attempt to live up to his example. He also taught me to knot a bow tie, a skill I use almost every day.

I also must thank Lloyd E. Ramsey, my father of birth. He showed me how to look under logs and rocks without risking snakebite. He took me scrambling up cliff faces to discover fossils secreted in their layers and clambering down caves to seek stalactites studded with bats. From him I learned an insatiable curiosity about the world and a willingness not only to look at nature but touch it, smell it, and taste it, or at least the parts of it that are not poisonous.

I have to thank some fathers who, while not my own dad, behaved at times as if they were. Andy Andrews, husband of my mom's best friend, spent the summers of my boyhood teaching me to tool leather belts, crimp shotgun shells, scuba dive in lakes, and four-wheel over stumps. None of that stuff is easy to do while holding a copy of *The Hobbit* and wearing a bow tie.

More recently, my partner at Cape Fear Pediatrics, Tom Blackstone, MD, FAAP, has proven to me that a pediatrician can not only survive in private practice but thrive by following his conscience and showing every patient the love he or she deserves. I still haven't learned how to perform his famous disappearing-ball trick without having 4-year-olds call me out on my sleight of hand.

My children's grandfather, Francis S. Collins, MD, PhD, continues to inspire me as a doctor, an author, and a father. Through all our family's challenges his love and support have never wavered, and I am deeply grateful to him, although I may never again agree to risk my life on the back of his Harley-Davidson Road King.

Fathers who read and contributed ideas to this book include my own dad, as well as my partner at Cape Fear Pediatrics, Hoke W. Pollock, MD, FAAP; vaccine pioneer and author Paul Offit, MD, FAAP; adolescent medicine expert and author Victor Strasburger, MD, FAAP; developmental expert and author William L. Coleman, MD, FAAP; fatherhood expert and author Kyle Pruett, MD; and fatherhood expert Craig Garfield, MD, FAAP. Honestly, it's amazing the world-class authorities who will lend their expertise to a project if you'll just promise to bake them cookies.

Without mothers there would be no fathers, nor would there be this book. My own mother, Anne F. Hill, was my first editor, and she continues to provide unvarnished observations with the eye of a voracious reader. Mom did not teach me to tie a bow tie, catch snakes, or shoot cans off a fence post, but she did teach me to write and bake some wicked chocolate-chip cookies.

The mother of my children, Margaret B. Collins, MD, FASH, works every day to prove that co-parenting is more than a nice idea. Her devotion to ensuring our 3 children enjoy a stable and loving environment wherever they go proves that parenting and friendship can thrive even when a marriage does not. Without what we have been through and continue to face together, this book never would have come to be. Come to think of it, the same holds true of our family.

Christy Eakins, PA-C, lent not only her love and support to this effort but her critical eye as a reader, mother, and pediatric practitioner. In the midst of momentous life transitions she made time to inspire me, listen to me go on about this book forever, and bring me protein shakes so I wouldn't have to leave my computer. Literally and figuratively, she has helped me write the next chapter.

Other mothers who contributed to this book include my sister, Elizabeth Anne Edlund; parenting expert and author Tanya Remer Altmann, MD, FAAP; media/social networking expert and author Gwenn Shurgin O'Keeffe, MD, FAAP; parenting expert and author Laura A. Jana, MD, FAAP; and media expert Kathleen Clarke-Pearson, MD, FAAP. They didn't even know about the cookies!

I have to thank my children, not only for inspiring everything I do but for being extraordinarily patient as I worked on this book. "Just one more minute" stretched into hours and days. They entertained themselves creatively while causing only minor property damage, for which I and my homeowner's insurance company are eternally grateful.

Finally, I must thank Carolyn Kolbaba of the American Academy of Pediatrics Department of Marketing and Publications for believing in this project and shepherding it through from conception to completion. To say that I could not have done this without her is no less true for being self-evident. Carolyn, I hope it's not too late to ask: Do you like cookies?

foreword

According to the 2010 US Census, nearly 68 million men in the United States are fathers. If you were to include the range of men playing key roles in children's lives today, that number would be even higher and include grandfathers, foster fathers, fathers in same-sex couples, and men who simply play father-figure roles.

Yet today's father is not our father's father for at least 4 reasons. First, as William L. Coleman, MD, FAAP, and I wrote in 2004 in the American Academy of Pediatrics clinical report, "Fathers and Pediatricians: Enhancing Men's Role in the Care and Development of Their Children," the term *father* has evolved to mean more than just wage earner or bread-winner and now encompasses caregiver, sharer of responsibilities, and co-parent. Second, our father's fathers typically married younger and had children earlier in their relationships. Becoming a father today in the United States is not necessarily preceded by being married, with about one-third of children born today to unmarried couples. Third, educational and economic shifts have resulted in more women entering the work force. In fact, by the middle of this decade, more women are expected to receive graduate-level degrees than men, a step that may open more doors to a higher job status for women and a resulting increase in salary. Once these women (many of whom will become mothers) achieve equal pay compared with men in the workplace, we are bound to see young families decide to send mothers to work for higher pay and ask fathers to increase their involvement at home. Finally, expectant fathers' own expectations have changed. Many men on the verge of becoming a father anxiously await the opportunity to be engaged, involved, and equal parents.

However, are fathers comfortable and ready to take care of their children? After all, it was not long ago that many young boys were discouraged from playing "mother" with baby dolls and encouraged to play more active, outdoor, and sports-focused games. Now faced with a baby of their own making and having missed being exposed to modeling how to provide care and practice parenting in their own childhood, many men are looking for guidance on what to do and how to do it.

Thankfully, fathering is not simply mothering without a dress. Fathers bring their own talents, sensibilities, and perspectives to being a parent. As a result, fathers have their own unique effects on their children. For example, positive fathering results in children enjoying a long list of benefits, including improved cognitive development, advanced language development, greater academic achievement, decreased delinquent behaviors and behavioral problems, and improved social competence.

This book will help start expectant fathers down the parenting path on the right foot. It respects fathers and their intelligence and desire to do right by their children and family. It nicely covers all the basics a new father needs to know to optimize the health of his baby and infant—from early child development to feeding to common illnesses and immunizations. It also tackles what we call in pediatrics anticipatory guidance, or letting parents know what is likely to happen next with their child so they can plan accordingly. This book is terrific as a go-to resource for those parents who wish they could spend unlimited time with their child's doctor to answer all their questions.

Welcome to fatherhood—jump right in!

Craig F. Garfield, MD, FAAP
Northwestern University Feinberg School of Medicine
Departments of Pediatrics and Medical Social Sciences
Chicago, IL

1

welcome to the club

like many expectant fathers, there was little else I could talk about in the months leading up to my daughter's birth. Someone might say, "Looks like we're about to get some rain," and then I'd say, "Yep. I hope it's not raining in 5 weeks when my first child is due."

When I told people I was going to be a father, I got a lot of different reactions, but the most predictable came from those who were already parents. They would cock their heads knowingly, smile a little, and say, "Your life is going to change."

"Ya think?" I wanted to ask. "Did you all get together and rehearse this answer? Will you invite me to practice it with you once I'm a dad, and if so, will there be beer? I sort of figured my life would change, what with the baby and all. You want to be a little more specific?"

And then it happened. As a medical student I'd helped deliver plenty of babies, but this one was mine. It was her water that splashed on the floor, her purple face suddenly visible, her tiny hands and feet waving in the air. There she was, my little girl! My life had changed.

The first call I made was to my mom to apologize for how much I must have frightened her. I never knew I could love someone as much as this baby, which means I never knew how scared I could be that something would happen to her. Would she keep breathing? Would she have a happy childhood? Would she be accepted into a good graduate school? OK, too soon for that last one. Better to just start with the breathing part.

Over the next week I spent hours holding the wondrous being that was my daughter. Everything she did fascinated me. I was enthralled at the way she slept, the way she sucked on her hand, even the way she pooped. And pooped again. And again. OK, the hand-sucking was more interesting.

By her second week of life my new daughter could lift her head and sort of squirm around my chest. She'd squirm, drop her head, and wiggle her face back and forth, then she'd squirm a little farther and repeat the process, almost like she was looking for something; food, maybe. When she did this to her mommy she'd soon be happy, but with me it was an exercise in futility. As her rooting became more frantic and she began to whimper, I could almost hear her thoughts: "This isn't getting me anywhere! Dad, what are good you for?"

As I gazed down at her little scrunched-up nose I whispered gently to her, "Oh, precious girl, one day you will know what I'm good for. There will come a day, sooner than you or I can imagine, a day when you will really badly want to open a pickle jar. When that day comes, there I will be, to hand that jar to your mom, along with that jar-opening gadget someone gave us as a wedding present."

I don't know a father alive who has not wondered what his role is in his child's life and whether he's doing a good enough job of it. (OK, there is this one guy I met, but seriously, he's a complete jerk.) As a father it's common to feel some ambiguity about your role in nurturing your child. After all, she didn't grow inside your body, and you can't nurse her, at least not without the sorts of secret, experimental steroids available only to certain major league batters and Tour de France contenders.

dads: who are we, and what are we good for?

The answers to these questions are not, as you might imagine, straight-forward. The US Census Bureau counted 70.1 million fathers in 2011, meaning the 85.4 million mothers outnumber us (one of many good reasons not to upset them). Of those fathers, 25.3 million (well under half) live as members of a married couple in a house with their children. Another 1.8 million are single fathers, accounting for around 15% of all single parents.

In 2010 about 154,000 married fathers stayed home for at least 1 year to care for their children while their wives worked. They were busy—collectively these dads watched 287,000 kids. But you don't have to be a stay-at-home dad to provide primary care for a child. In 2006 fathers cared for a total of 2.7 million preschoolers while their mothers worked. That number represents nearly a quarter of all children in that age group.

Families are growing more complex, and fathers include many people whom the Census Bureau might not have counted. They may be step-fathers, foster fathers, uncles, grandfathers, mothers' romantic partners, or 2 male partners who share in the primary care of a child. If you're the main guy on whom a child depends for security, guidance, and love, congratulations, you're a dad!

Dads, as it turns out, are good for a lot, and our positive effect spans the life of the child. Premature babies gain weight better if their dads are involved in their care. Those same preemies score better on developmental and psychological tests over a year later as a result of dad's involvement. Mothers are more likely to successfully breastfeed their babies when dads help. Children with involved fathers have better language skills, make better grades, enjoy better self-esteem, and suffer substantially less psychiatric disease, including depression and anxiety. Positive paternal involvement can even reduce conflict among siblings. Children whose fathers are involved in their care are less likely to wind up in jail, use drugs and alcohol, or become pregnant in their teen years.

Dads are not good for kids just because we do the same stuff moms do. That's not to say doing that stuff isn't important; it's critical! Mothers and fathers have a similar effect on their children's moral development, social competence, school performance, and mental health. There is a reason, after all, it takes 2 parents to make a baby, and not just because it's more fun that way.

Probably the most accurate generalization about dads versus moms is that fathers play more. In the first 4 years of a child's life we tend to focus on activities that involve touch and stimulation, like tickling, wrestling, and playing airplane. It's our job, in other words, to get kids all wound up so they won't go to bed, to make them laugh until they pee on themselves. (*Note:* If this happens, be a good sport and help with the clothing change; after all, it is your fault.) During middle childhood, we're more likely than mothers to get out and do stuff, like take walks, go fishing, or see a ball game. Are you surprised? No, you are not. You already knew that from watching sitcoms.

You might not have guessed, however, that dads also engage in a lot of private talks, and not just the Big Talk. We also have a major effect on our children's sense of their gender roles, both sons and daughters. (What this means in practical terms is that you may at times have to wear a dress, especially if your son is wearing one.) We tend to focus more than mothers on risk-taking and problem-solving. (Wearing the dress can provide an opportunity to model both behaviors.)

The realm of discipline holds another surprise: while fathers and mothers often choose different discipline roles in a given family, the differences are not broad enough to generalize. It seems that for every mother who says, "You just wait until your father comes home," there is a father somewhere saying, "Just wait until your mother hears about this!"

your life is going to change

I am not allowed to reveal the secret location where we parents practice saying this line to soon-to-be parents, but I can tell you this: someone often brings beer. That said, I can be specific about some other stuff. Presumably if you're a dad or you're going to be a dad, at some point in your relationship you've had sex. This is one part of your life that will change, but you also knew that from watching sitcoms.

Pregnancy and sex are not incompatible, but they don't always go together well, either. Many women experience levels of fatigue and nausea in the first trimester of pregnancy that put them in a mood, just not *the* mood. By the second trimester of pregnancy some women start feeling better, and changes in their hormones and blood flow may actually renew their interest in sex. Then again, they may not, so prepare to be understanding. In the third trimester sex is still often fine, although between weight gain and back pain, finding a comfortable position may require a level of creativity usually reserved for yoga instructors. Look for positions that give the woman a lot of control over the depth and frequency of penetration in case she experiences unexpected discomfort.

Sexual activity is generally safe during pregnancy, but there are some exceptions. Most critical is the presence of sexually transmitted infections (STIs). HIV, hepatitis B and C, syphilis, and herpes are all transmissible during pregnancy and childbirth, and any of those diseases can be lethal to the baby. Chlamydia and gonorrhea can cause severe eye infections and even blindness if the baby gets them during birth, and chlamydia can also cause dangerous pneumonia. The mom's doctor will test her for some STIs, but that doesn't mean she cannot contract them after testing. If you are not in a monogamous relationship with the mother of your baby, it is critical you wear a condom whenever you have sex. You should also visit your own doctor to find out if you carry one of these diseases.

Remember, people transmit STIs all the time without having any symptoms whatsoever.

There are other special circumstances where the mother's doctor might advise her to avoid sexual intercourse. If she is at risk of preterm labor, if she has unexplained vaginal bleeding, if she is leaking amniotic fluid, if her cervix is opening too early, or if the placenta is covering the cervix, it may not be safe for her to have sex.

One danger of sexual activity during pregnancy and the first several weeks following birth is so bizarre it sounds like an urban legend. If you blow air into the mom's vagina during oral sex you run a small risk of the air blocking an artery in her body, which can be deadly. I told you it was weird—but seriously, don't do that. You don't want to explain that one. The other alternative sexual activity to avoid during pregnancy is anal sex. I'm not saying you'd do that, but just be aware it can introduce bacteria into the vagina that may infect the baby at birth.

For 4 to 6 weeks after delivery sex is pretty much off limits. Whether she delivers vaginally or by cesarean delivery, the mother's uterus, cervix, and vagina have undergone profound physiologic changes and they need some time to recover. In most cases her doctor will want to examine her and clear her before she resumes sexual intercourse.

This is also a period when you're both probably exhausted and stressed, and intimacy is likely to suffer. The hormonal changes associated with pregnancy, childbirth, and nursing are not always conducive to the libido, so don't be too concerned that the sort of activity that got you this baby is slow to resume. That said, there may not be any more important time to practice communication and to enjoy intimate contact that does not necessarily involve sexual intercourse. Many people find their sensual lives grow deeper and more stimulating as they explore novel ways to make each other happy. Even if that's not necessarily your experience, be patient. When your sex life does return it will carry with it a deeper bond than ever before.

dads can get postpartum depression—really

It's hard to overstate the difference a child makes in your relationship. No detail of your lives remains untouched. There are the obvious things—you can't sleep when you want, you can't leave the house without a truckload of stuff, you can't even watch a ball game without interruptions during the best parts (why is it babies never cry during commercials?). There's also the laundry that piles up, the dishwasher crowded with bottles or breast pump parts, and the danger of lacerating your face trying to shave while holding a baby.

Then there's the really big stuff: you have to spend more money, but you also have more demands on your time. Your partner may feel differently about her body now. You may feel guilty about having made her pregnant, or you may feel jealous of the affection she shows the baby. Most importantly, there is now a whole new human being who is incredibly important to both of you, who literally redefines the meaning of the word love. Should it surprise you, then, that this time can be a little stressful?

Doctors are now paying more attention to postpartum depression in mothers and fathers. While it's normal for mothers to become emotional in the week or two following birth, these symptoms should clear up pretty quickly, usually by the end of the first month. Some women, however, don't recover. They may actually feel worse over time. About 12% to 20% of women develop depression or anxiety following a delivery, and up to 10% of fathers suffer depression as well. Parental depression affects children profoundly, causing developmental delays, social problems, and behavioral issues. Depressed fathers are much more likely to spank their children than fathers without depression, and they are less likely to play games, sing songs, or read to their children. On the other hand, for children whose mother is depressed, having an involved and nurturing father protects them from some of the negative effects of mom's depression.

The most widely used tool to screen mothers for postpartum depression is called the Edinburgh Postnatal Depression Scale. Recently doctors have begun using the same questionnaire to evaluate dads (see next page for a sample of the scale).

when to call the doctor
Postpartum depression often responds well to treatment; untreated it can pose a profound hazard, not only to the person suffering from the disease but to the baby as well.

Edinburgh Postnatal Depression Scale (EPDS)

As you have recently had a baby, we would like to know how you are feeling now. Please <u>underline</u> the answer which best describes how you have felt in the past 7 days, not just how you feel today. Here is an example, already completed:

I have felt happy:
  Yes, most the time
  <u>Yes, some of the time</u>
  No, not very often
  No, not at all

This would mean: "I have felt happy some of the time during the past week". Please complete the other questions in the same way.

In the past 7 days:

1. I have been able to laugh and see the funny side of things:
  As much as I always could
  Not quite so much now
  Definitely not so much now
  Not at all

2. I have looked forward with enjoyment to things:
  As much as I ever did
  Rather less than I used to
  Definitely less than I used to
  Hardly at all

*3. I have blamed myself unnecessarily when things went wrong:
  Yes, most of the time
  Yes, some of the time
  Not very often
  No, never

4. I have been anxious or worried for no good reason:
  No, not at all
  Hardly ever
  Yes, sometimes
  Yes, very often

*5. I have felt scared or panicky for no very good reason:
  Yes, quite a lot
  Yes, sometimes
  No, not much
  No, not at all

*6. Things have been getting on top of me:
  Yes, most of the time I haven't been able to cope at all
  Yes, sometimes I haven't been coping as well as usual
  No, most of the time I have coped quite well
  No, I have been coping as well as ever

*7. I have been so unhappy that I have had difficulty sleeping:
  Yes, most of the time
  Yes, sometimes
  Not very often
  No, not at all

*8. I have felt sad or miserable:
  Yes, most of the time
  Yes, quite often
  Not very often
  No, not at all

*9. I have been so unhappy that I have been crying:
  Yes, most of the time
  Yes, quite often
  Only occasionally
  No, never

*10. The thought of harming myself has occurred to me:
  Yes, quite often
  Sometimes
  Hardly ever
  Never

Translations of the scale, and guidance as to its use, may be found in Cox, J.L. & Holden, J. (2003) *Perinatal Mental Health: A Guide to the Edinburgh Postnatal Depression Scale*. London: Gaskell.

become an emotional genius in 3 easy steps

Until you have a baby you may not even be aware of some of your own assumptions about parenting. You might fall back on whatever skills you learned from your own parents, even if time has proven those practices ineffective. On the flip side, you may be so determined not to repeat your own parents' mistakes that you overcompensate. Regardless, you'll almost certainly find your partner has some different ideas than you do, setting the stage for conflict. How the 2 of you resolve those differences will have a profound effect on your child's well-being and also on the future of your relationship. Having 2 parents who cooperate well is one of the strongest factors ensuring children's healthy development, even when those parents are separated or divorced.

The first step is to have a conversation. Men are not always known for their conversational skills, but even if you're not much of a talker, now is a good time to try it out. Start with a question; sometimes you'll find the answer reassuring, and sometimes you'll find it upsetting, but either way at least you'll know where you're starting.

Begin with something open-ended: "How are you feeling right now?" Most women are pretty good at answering this one, but get ready, because they might ask you the same thing. It's OK to ask for some time to figure out how you're feeling before you answer. We're guys; this kind of thing may not come naturally to us.

The next step is even harder for most men than describing our feelings— acknowledge your partner's emotions. This is the kind of thing they teach preschoolers on television, but you'll be amazed at the response you get if you do it as a grown man. Try, "I can tell you're really upset," or, "I'm sorry I made you angry." For men, the bar for emotional IQ is so low that just making these statements will amaze your partner, even if you did learn them from Elmo.

Now it's time to score a hat trick. Assuming you've identified a problem, you will feel an overwhelming need to propose a solution. This is because you have a Y chromosome. I cannot emphasize the following statement enough: *don't do it!* Instead, try a question along these lines: "Is there something you'd like to see change?" You are now a super-genius, the kind of guy whose partner brags about him when he's not even around to hear. (*Note:* if she's already asked you to change something, skip this step.)

In some cases your partner doesn't want you to do anything. She may just want you to know how she feels and to comfort her. (If that's the case, do so now.) In other cases she may indeed want something to change, and now you can decide how you feel about that change. Hopefully you can start working toward a solution.

Just because a conversation is easy to start doesn't mean finding a solution will be simple. Child care issues produce some of the strongest emotions in any relationship. As you work your way through these challenges, remember 2 words: *prioritize* and *compromise*. Some things are important; others are not. Not spanking a child is important. Choosing between spinach and beans is not. There are a few absolute rights and wrongs in child care, but a lot of stuff falls in the middle. If you're unsure how important something is, you can use this book and others like it to help you prioritize, and when a question comes up feel free to ask your child's doctor. That's what doctors are there for.

Compromise is tricky; to compromise, you first have to prioritize. You may not want to compromise on issues that are critical to your child's health and development. But you may start thinking about some things and realize you're just doing them the way that seems familiar, and there might be another approach that's just as good. If the 2 of you reach an impasse, feel free to seek out a doctor, counselor, spiritual leader, or other trusted third party who might be able to help you through it. Your child's doctor should be able to help you find resources in your community.

You've heard this one before, but really, do try to find time to nurture your relationship with your partner. Children who grow up in a home with 2 supportive parents enjoy better outcomes in almost any realm you care to measure, from school performance to mental health to drug use and teen pregnancy. Child care can easily take over your life, and without making time to nurture each other and build your new relationship, you can all-too-easily find yourself sharing a home with someone you don't feel you know any more. Extended family, babysitters, even friends can help the 2 of you find time to find each other. You'll hear variations on this advice over and over again, but don't ignore it just because it's obvious. Don't forget the little things, either—compliment mom frequently; remember her birthday, your anniversary, or any other meaningful occasion; and show her affection frequently. These things may seem little, but the difference they make is enormous!

and you must be dad!

Since 1965 married fathers have increased the time they spend on direct child care from an average of 2.5 hours a week to nearly 7 hours a week. (The number for married mothers is 12.9 hours.) Figures for non-married fathers are harder to find; when the Current Population Survey began in 1965 they weren't on most people's radar. Despite the massive shifts in family dynamics occurring in our society, there are many places that can feel unwelcoming to a dad, starting in the home.

You might think the child's mother would want you to do absolutely anything to help out, but fathers can find their offers of assistance turned down, a situation that can easily cause hurt feelings. Some mothers feel they'll do a given job better or faster than dad, a fact they learned from watching sitcoms. If the 2 of you are fighting, she might restrict your involvement in child care as an act of hostility.

She may have other reasons, however, that you might even find complimentary. She may feel you already do enough, or she may not want to bother you. She might even come to the relationship with different cultural beliefs about men's and women's roles that neither of you has addressed.

Before jumping to conclusions, try starting a conversation along the lines of, "I feel like you never want me to change the baby's diaper. That upsets me because I would like to help more." That opener may get you a big hug, or it may get a container of premoistened wipes thrown at your head, but either way it's likely to start a dialogue. Often the more mom feels you support her, the more supportive she will be of your involvement with your child.

Some people might still call this a man's world, but the corners of it devoted to child care can sometimes feel downright unfriendly to fathers. I recall times when, taking my young children to the playground, moms actually got up from a park bench where they had been talking and moved over to the next swing set. It's possible they were just following the shade, but I couldn't help looking around to see if my picture was stapled to a nearby utility pole.

As an involved father you might expect everyone you encounter to smile and praise you or tell you how impressed they are at what you're doing. At times you will get this reaction. Some people seem amazed I can get my kids out of the house wearing 2 matched shoes. In fact, one of my pet peeves is when the children's clothes clash and someone says, "Daddy must have dressed you today." I want to look that person dead in the eye and say, "You don't know me very well, do you? My daughter here left the house in a perfect little outfit, but she threw up on that one, and this is what was in the trunk of the car. Now stand back—she's looking a little pale."

I have sat awkwardly as the only dad in dentists' waiting rooms, pediatricians' offices, school field trips, PTA meetings, and any number of children's birthday parties. Be aware of subtle biases that may make you feel uncomfortable, like pink, flowery wallpaper in a waiting room, or a magazine selection that runs the gamut from *Women's Day* to *Martha Stewart Living*. Also know that your presence may be altering the all-female dynamic, just like if, say, your mom showed up to your poker night. The important thing is not to let the fact that you're a dad keep you from being appropriately involved in your child's care. If your child's pediatrician or teacher seems to be directing all the questions to mom, you might have to speak up. There's no need to become adversarial, but at the same time, some people involved in child care don't expect you to be interested, and when you are it may surprise them.

when you're not there

What if you're not living with your child full time? Do you still matter? There's no question you do. While the statistics for children of divorce can be daunting, there is good evidence that a strong relationship with a nurturing father improves these outcomes. In some cases divorce might even improve children's well-being, if it helps resolve conflict between parents. There are no studies to compare, but it's a fair guess that living with 2 happy parents apart is better than living with 2 parents who are in the same house but miserable.

Separation and divorce can also pose your biggest challenge. Children of divorced parents fare better when the parents work well together. Given the anger and pain so often associated with these situations, you may never want to see mom again, much less work with her. But how the 2 of you handle this situation will make a difference in your children's lives, so making it work will pay off in the long term.

Remember too that quantity of time matters, but the quality of your time with your children is equally important. If your time with them is limited, it can also be focused, allowing you to really slow down and learn who they are. Not every day has to be a trip to the zoo. Just reading a book, playing a game, or walking in the backyard provides you an opportunity to listen to their thoughts, show them stuff, and play. Chances are the things they will remember about your time together will not be those grand, elaborate events you worked so hard to plan, but instead they will be small moments that you may not have even registered.

Of course, if you're already a dad, you probably knew that stuff. Your life, after all, has changed. But you knew it would. You've watched sitcoms.

2

when can he play ball?
infant and child development

wow! i mean wow! There he is, your newborn baby! Holding him is the most amazing sensation you've ever felt, really. You can't believe the fullness in your chest as you gaze down at that sweet, vulnerable face; feel those tiny, perfect hands grasp your index fingers; and hear his strawberry lips pucker. Amazing, isn't it? You whip out your camera to shoot some video, and then it strikes you—he's heartbreakingly sweet, but he doesn't do much. So when will he make good footage, and can you speed the process along?

the first month

The transition from life in the womb to life on the outside is pretty dramatic. There are some new skills to master like, say, breathing and eating. Your newborn may be small, but in the first month you'll already see him make enormous strides in his development.

Your baby's sensory world starts with touch. He will enjoy skin-to-skin contact immediately after birth. This form of touch, known as kangaroo care, helps stabilize his heart rate, breathing, and sleep patterns. Many

14

2. When Can He Play Ball? Infant and Child Development

hospitals try to get the baby on mom's chest as soon as possible after birth, but your chest will work, too, at least until he gets hungry.

Infant behavior in the first couple of weeks seems simple enough. Your baby is probably sleeping around 20 hours a day. In the remaining time he will nurse or bottle-feed, suck on his hand, sneeze, hiccup, cry a little, pee, poop, and repeat. You'll see his arms shoot out when he's startled, and they may quiver at times. You'll notice his hands are almost always balled into fists. Go ahead and pretend he's a prize fighter. We all do.

He may be able to pick his head up enough to turn it from one side to the other, but when you're holding him, make sure you have a hand cupped under his head; prize fighter or no, he needs time to build those neck muscles. He will gaze around, but any eye contact is probably a coincidence. It doesn't look like much is happening, but his brain is growing fast, and in just 2 to 4 weeks you'll already notice some dramatic new behaviors.

Among the most exciting moments in fatherhood is when you can tell your baby is really looking at you. Sometime before the end of the first month your baby will develop the ability to make out faces at a distance of about 8 to 12 inches, roughly the distance from your chest to your face. When he's not watching you, strong patterns in black and white will attract his attention. You may see his eyes wander and cross sometimes; don't worry, that's normal for now. In addition to your face, he's learning the sound of your voice, and he may already turn toward you when he hears you. Smell and taste play huge roles in the baby's sensory world. By 1 month, newborns can already distinguish the smell of their own mother's milk!

At first your baby won't say much, but even in the first few days of life you'll start learning his different cries for hunger, fatigue, and discomfort. (Impress your friends; when your infant pipes up, casually toss off the words, "Wet diaper." Then go change it, with extra points if you make the free throw.) Within the first month he'll start cooing, a sound you'll want to record on your cell phone and listen to if you're having a bad day.

So how can you encourage development at this age? First of all, don't listen to anyone who tells you not to hold your baby because you'll spoil him. There may be times you have to put him down to help him learn to sleep or so you can grab a snack, but your baby is learning about the world and about you through all the sensations that come from being close to your body, so go ahead and pick the little guy up! Talk to him, rub his back, let him suck on your finger, get in his face. You're getting to know each other, and this time is precious for both of you.

the second and third months

It's possible you're the kind of guy who goes around making silly faces and talking goofy all the time. (If you are—stop, dude, you're creeping people out!) But if that hasn't been you up until now, brace yourself— you're about to meet the most powerful force known to human interaction: the responsive smile. Sometime in the second month of life, your infant is going to see you smile, and he'll smile back. This won't be that weird, "Maybe I have gas" kind of smile that drifts across his face sometimes when he's sleeping. This is the, "Hey, Dad, you're smiling!" grin that will make you grin back even bigger to see if it will happen again (*Spoiler alert:* it will). This tells you not only that your infant can now see your face well enough to interpret your expression but that he is building an emotional world, a world in which your face plays a huge role.

You'll notice your infant imitates more than your smile. He will also mirror alarm, surprise, and other emotions, and as he does he will start learning how to feel about things going on around him. He'll want to play with you, and he may become upset if something interrupts your interactions. You'll also see his eyes start working together better. He'll be able to see objects at a greater distance and follow a toy or your face from one side to the other without losing track of it.

Your infant is also engaging his ears and his voice more. You may notice he smiles as soon as he hears you talking, and he will turn more reliably to look at you when you speak. His cooing will develop into more of a babble, and he will start imitating sounds he hears.

Your little prize fighter is now developing a stance—when you place his feet on a surface, he'll extend his legs like he's trying to stand. It's fine to hold him up in this position; standing at this age will not cause bowed legs. Don't invest in boxing gloves just yet, though, because his fists will actually relax. Now is a good time to get out those cute rattles he wouldn't play with before. Your infant will be able to bat at objects that interest him, and he'll be able to grasp and shake toys and to let them go when he's done. You'll see your baby's neck strength has grown dramatically. When he's on his tummy you'll see him lifting his head and some of his chest in a pose yogis call the cobra. This will develop into more of an upward-facing dog by 4 months.

16

2. When Can He Play Ball? Infant and Child Development

Stimulating development at this age consists largely of following your instincts. You'll find yourself close to your baby's face making exaggerated facial expressions repeatedly; talking in singsong, drawn-out syllables; and expressing surprise at the existence of mundane things like, say, toes. You'll hand him rattles, blankets, and anything else a baby can grasp and explore, and you'll find yourself fascinated with the expressions that flit across his face as he responds to different sensations. Don't let self-consciousness get in your way. If other people could see what an adorable baby you have, they would be right there next to you making those faces.

months 4 to 7

All of childhood development is amazing, especially when it's your child doing the developing. That said, the middle of the first year of life begins a time when you're almost afraid to look away for fear you'll miss something. It's like when you finally get up to pee during the game, and you hear everyone yelling, "Oh my gosh! Did you see that?!" The good news is you don't have to miss a moment; many commercially available infant carriers can go pretty much anywhere.

Your baby's vision will improve dramatically by the seventh month of life. In addition to your basic black, white, and red, your baby will now perceive colors only an interior decorator could love, like puce. Infants may even prefer some colors over others at this age. Distance vision improves dramatically; your baby's eyes will now light up when he sees you from across the room! He will follow even relatively fast movements (test this if you want by dashing back and forth a few times). More complex patterns no longer lose your baby's attention but give him some visual interest in his world. By age 6 months you really should never see one eye turn inward or outward; if you do, be sure and alert his doctor.

Your infant is using his hearing and voice in new ways, too. He will giggle, babble, and make other sounds to express joy or displeasure. At the same time, he is learning to interpret the sounds you make to express your own joy or displeasure (although it will still be months before he can curse). He is already starting to understand one very important word: "No."

Your baby's muscles are growing as well, and his brain is gaining more control over what they do. He won't sit up immediately but will progress from being propped in a seated position to leaning forward on his hands (tripod position). Stable, independent sitting usually comes around

7 months of age. He will also learn to roll over, usually from front to back around 4 months of age, then from back to front a month or two later. Your infant's body will be in near-constant motion when he is awake, rocking, rolling back and forth, kicking, and "swimming" with his legs.

You'll notice your baby getting more talented with his hands as well. Instead of batting or swiping at objects he'll reach out and grab whatever interests him, often with some force (remember this if you wear hoop earrings or have a large, sensitive nose). He will be able to grab smaller objects using a raking grasp that involves the whole hand. When he gets hold of something you'll see him explore it with one hand, then another, passing it back and forth. Whatever winds up in his hands will be in his mouth very shortly, so keep his environment clear of anything small enough to choke on or gross enough that he shouldn't taste it.

Among the things your infant will get hold of is his own body. He will use his newfound motor skills to take inventory, smacking his legs, putting his toes in his mouth, grabbing his ears and hair, and figuring out what's going on under his diaper. His movements will appear rough at times, but don't worry—I've never seen an infant injure himself checking out his parts. Letting go is a skill that comes later, however, and this is an age where babies sometimes grab their own hair and pull it until they cry. In these cases you should gently help your baby release his hair while laughing to yourself sympathetically.

Putting all these skills together, your infant will start exploring the concept of cause and effect, an exploration which really will never end. Does banging a toy make a particularly interesting noise? Do objects fall when dropped? Will Daddy pick them up? Will he do it every time, or just sometimes? If I laugh at Daddy, will he laugh back? Will he pick that thing up one more time? Your baby is just beginning to figure out the laws that govern the universe and human behavior, and his every act is an experiment. In his world you play the roles of laboratory assistant and research subject.

There are tons of things you can do to promote your infant's development at this age. Take him places and name all the things you see, pointing them out as you go. He may find a mobile visually stimulating, but be sure it's mounted in such a way that he can't reach it and become entangled. A mirror provides fascination to an extent that won't occur again until the teen years. Toy stores have entire sections devoted to infant-safe

18

2. When Can He Play Ball? Infant and Child Development

toys abounding with colors, textures, and sounds, but plenty of household items work well, too. Just be sure they are large enough not to fit in his mouth and don't have sharp points, breakable parts, or lead paint.

months 8 to 12

Countless amazing things happen in this developmental period, but 3 always strike me as most wondrous and surprising. The first is when you put your baby down and suddenly he's not where you left him. After months of spreading a blanket out on the floor and assuming your baby would stay on it, you're bound to look up at some point and find he's half-way across the room. (If this happens, try not to let anyone see the look of panic on your face.) If you hadn't taken baby-proofing seriously before, this is your wake-up call. Your grandmother's collection of glass animals, your older child's Lego-people heads, your display of antique straight razors…it's time to put them all in storage. Also, if you've been waiting to install those stair gates, your wait is over! If you need motivation, reward yourself with a new set of drill bits. Mobility is here, and life will not be the same again until the little guy grows up and gets his own place.

Your baby is now really working his way toward walking. This process has been going on the whole time, but now you can see he's going to succeed. Baby walkers, by the way, slow down the normal development of balance and pre-walking skills, in addition to being seriously hazardous. If someone gives you one as a gift, just say thank you, then exchange it for a full set of drawer and cabinet latches. One useful item to have is a play yard where your baby can hang out safely and explore while you do important dad things like shaving.

Long before he walks you'll notice your baby getting to a seated position without anyone's help. He may launch himself forward and begin to move by pulling with his arm and pushing with his legs. The classic hands-and-knees crawl is a step some babies skip entirely, choosing instead to roll or scoot around the house, but many infants will get pretty fast on all fours. Around this time you'll also see your baby pulling up on his crib railing, the sofa, and the coffee table, first just holding on and bouncing, then working his way along the edge. This is your clue to adjust the crib mattress to its lowest setting. You don't want to wait for the second clue: the sound of your baby tumbling to the floor.

Next he will try letting go, which will result in a diaper-cushioned thud for a while. Then he'll stay up, and soon he'll try taking a step or two. Many parents fear that if their baby has not started walking by his first birthday there is something wrong with him. Walking, however, often develops a month or so later. In the meantime, just because his little cousin started walking at 9 months does not mean that his cousin will be a running back for the Steelers, so just smile and congratulate his parents when they act smug about it.

The second amazing development is the first time you shake your head at your baby and he shakes his back at you. You try it again. He does it again. Soon you're both giggling and dizzy. He's ready to play: he's in there, and he knows you're in there too! Go ahead at this point and try the old raspberry. You'll both end up covered in spit, but indulge, you've been waiting for this! You can expand this imitative play to include patty-cake, peek-a-boo, and other games that don't require a napkin when you're done.

Your baby's social and emotional interactions are growing more complex by the moment. Where in the past he may have never met a stranger, he may now show some very strong preferences, particularly in favor of his parents. This behavior can cause hurt feelings, especially if grandparents come for a visit and find their grandbaby screams as soon as they make eye contact. Reassure them that he does this with everyone he doesn't know, which is probably true. Your baby has now figured out not every-one has his best intentions at heart, and he is likely to be quite fearful of people he does not know well. He also may fear being alone, having grasped the idea that you are an important person in his life and com-bined it with the concept that even though you're not in the room, you must be around somewhere and may come back if beckoned. This is a time many babies will deal with anxiety by adopting a particular toy or blanket as a transition object to comfort themselves. You can only hope whatever he chooses can be easily washed. I also recommend equipping the transition object with a GPS tracking device in case of loss.

The third development is when you say, "No," and your baby stops what he's doing. You may think it's random chance the first time, but on repe-tition you'll find he really understands the word. (Don't be disappointed if he responds only some of the time. This will be the case for the rest of your lives together.) You will soon find he responds to other simple commands like, "Put that down," and "Come here."

20

2. When Can He Play Ball? Infant and Child Development

Your infant's vocalizations are growing increasingly complex now and even resolving themselves into words. By his first birthday these will probably include "Mama" and "Dada." (Dada usually comes first, but don't gloat. It's poor form.) He's likely to add 1 or 2 more words, like "Uh-oh" or "Bye-bye," in addition to dozens of sounds that convey meaning through their inflections if not their syllables. He may not yet say, "No," but he is likely to shake his head with unmistakable meaning.

Less dramatic but equally important are the new things your infant is doing with his hands. He is now learning to use his thumb and forefinger to pick up even very small objects (remember those Lego heads?). He will pick up a toy in each hand and bang them together, which often has the added benefit of making a lot of noise. He can drop an object into a container, take it out, and repeat. He is getting better at letting go of the things he grabs, unless they're your glasses, in which case—good luck! He will poke at small items with his index finger, and he may even imitate you scribbling on paper (or walls, clothes, pets; whatever is in reach).

Your baby will integrate all these new skills to tirelessly explore his world. He knows what common objects are for—he will put the phone to his ear, roll cars along the floor, and hug his teddy bear. He will also shake objects, bang them, throw them, and drop them, all in an effort to confirm the basic tenets of Newtonian physics. How does he know gravity is reliable, after all, if he doesn't test it multiple times?

Your baby will imitate gestures and sounds, and he will start probing your responses to his actions. What will you do if he refuses to eat? If he bangs the table? If he throws his cup? Will the same action get the same reaction from you each time? There's only one way to find out. This is the beginning of discipline, a time when you can start demonstrating that certain actions he takes will not have desirable consequences. Sometimes the consequences simply result from the actions: if he throws his milk, it spills and it's gone. Sometimes you create the consequences: if he hits the dog, you put the dog in another room. The good news is that most of the things your baby is doing at this age have wonderful consequences: giggles, gasps, and spittle on both of your chins.

your 1-year-old

They say that with great power comes great responsibility. That is pretty much the theme of the second year of life. It's hard to overstate the magnitude of the tasks your toddler will now master: walking, running, talking, and eating table food top the list, which gives you an idea of what's ahead. Of course this year is full of the sorts of firsts that inspire men to tears. Your toddler will clomp around in your shoes, dance, maybe even say, "I love you."

If your child hasn't already started walking, he probably will by around 13 months of age. By 15 months he will be able to bend down, pick up an object, and stand up again without falling down, at least most of the time. He'll also be able to work his way up stairs. Remember that baby-proofing? It's time to reconsider what you think is in reach. He'll soon be using chairs or stools to reach countertops, and drawers and cabinets are all fair game! By 18 months your child will be running, although it may not be pretty at first. As you might imagine, falls are nearly constant at this age. Don't worry; toddlers are built low to the ground, and they rarely get up enough momentum to seriously hurt themselves. Children learn to kick a ball and walk on tiptoes at this age, but sadly neither soccer teams nor dance studios will usually enroll kids until they're out of diapers.

Your child's manual dexterity will progress rapidly in the second year of life. No longer will he be restricted to picking up only those things that stay put; he'll pounce on objects in motion, like rolling balls. He will use his hands to cover and uncover objects, twist and turn items, and build towers of up to 6 blocks, which he can then knock down with a satisfying crash. In quieter moments he will practice turning the pages of books, scribbling, and even painting. Putting things together, sticking pegs in holes, and shaping modeling clay will all keep his hands and brain busy. You might notice by the end of the second year that your child prefers using one hand over the other, but it's OK if he doesn't; not all children have a strong handedness. There's no promise your child will be a switch-hitter, but you can always hope.

Your toddler's language skills will blossom in the second year of life. His understanding of what you say will far outpace his own ability to speak for quite some time. By 15 months of age he'll be able to follow a wide variety of simple commands even though he may still only use a handful of words. You can test his comprehension by asking him to retrieve an object from another room; if he brings back the right thing, you know that's yet another word in his vocabulary! You'll soon find yourself spelling out words or using code around your toddler when you don't want him to know what you're planning ("B-E-D time?"). He won't just understand nouns and verbs, either. Words that describe relationships in space, like on, under, and on top of, will all click into place.

22

2. When Can He Play Ball? Infant and Child Development

While talking lags behind understanding speech, your toddler will start to surprise you with the things he can say. Toddlers have difficulty making some sounds, and it's common at this age for children to use words only their immediate family members understand. Especially in the early part of the second year your child will talk in what's called fluent babble. This babble has all the inflection of normal speech, and while it seems your child knows perfectly well what he's trying to say, it simply doesn't make any sense. With time, words will bubble up out of this soup, and by the end of the second year your toddler will have a vocabulary of around 50 words, maybe more.

At around 18 months of age he will say his own name. By age 2 he will link words together to form sentences of 3 or more words, many of them expressing rather strong opinions. He will also start to use pronouns like me and you, adding a whole new level of meaning to his speech. Remember as he tries to talk to you that this whole speech thing is new territory. It may take your toddler quite some time to get out the words he wants, but if you can be patient, you'll find out what he's thinking, and that is something worth waiting for!

For some reason it seems language is a skill that's especially tempting for parents to compare among different children, perhaps because it seems easy to quantify. It's important to remember that every child develops at his own pace, and also that when it comes to language, girls seem to talk earlier on average than boys. Your child's doctor can tell you at each wellness visit whether your child's speech development is normal for his age. If your child is not reciting Shakespeare by age 2, just remember, plenty of "late talkers" have gone on to have very successful careers in politics.

Socially and emotionally, the second year of life is tremendously challenging for your toddler. For one thing, he spends much of this year in a one-sided conversation where you are able to say much more than he can. Second, he has yet to develop a sense that other people have feelings and desires that may differ from his own. He will assume that when he is hungry you will somehow know and you will want to give him food. The world will therefore often fail to meet his expectations. Third, he is integrating a vast new set of skills and concepts, which means his universe is changing around him all the time. Yesterday he couldn't reach the countertop; today he can. It's no surprise he'll have to test the limits of his world often; they keep moving!

There's no better environment in which to appreciate a 1-year-old's social development than a playdate. (Of course, if your child has siblings, every day is a playdate—a really, really long one.) Your toddler may acknowledge another child but more in the way he would acknowledge a toy, continuing to do his own thing. This behavior is called parallel play. He may hit his "friend," poke her, or pull her hair in an effort to figure her out. He might even appear to offer her a toy or a bite of food, but don't be surprised if he gets upset when his offer is accepted; sharing is an unnatural concept at this age. There's nothing wrong with trying to help your child learn to share, but remember, he's not sure when he gives something away that he'll ever get it back. You should make sure there are plenty of toys for everyone, and you might save a few of his most prized possessions somewhere else. When you do help him hand something over, reassure him that he'll be getting it back soon.

You'll spend a lot of time at this age teaching your toddler not to hit or bite. In his mind, other people don't feel pain, so he will be confused about why these activities upset everyone so. Remind him firmly, "We don't hit [bite, pinch, smack, kick, poke, etc]," and remove him from play for a couple of minutes. Inevitably someone will advise you to bite him back yourself, but when you think about your child's understanding of the world it becomes clear how silly that advice really is, not to mention mean. You have a luxury he does not—you can behave like an adult.

As your child struggles to figure out what he can and cannot do, you'll notice him deciding between independence and dependence, often within a matter of seconds. For example, he might find strangers very interesting at a distance of a yard or two, especially when viewed from your arms. But the same nice lady who set off a flurry of giggling and babbling from 3 feet away may find your child clinging to you and crying when she tries to come closer. This fear of strangers is a sign of normal development and should reassure you. You may be tempted at the sitter's or at child care to sneak away while your child is distracted to avoid what's likely to be a period of fearful crying. Imagine, though, how frightening it is for a child when a parent disappears randomly for unpredictable periods. The crying can be hard to handle, but your toddler will feel more secure watching you leave with the reassurance that you will return.

The second year is a time when your child will begin trying to do some things for himself and even for you. By 18 months he may help take off and put on his clothes, although not always in appropriate situations.

24

2. When Can He Play Ball? Infant and Child Development

He will want a role in self-care, such as bathing and brushing his hair and teeth. Although he may be eager to grab the toothbrush, remember to give him a little help getting to all tooth surfaces that need cleaning. You can make a game out of this; let him brush for a count of 5, then it's your turn to help him. You'll even see him check himself out in the mirror, now fully aware the image he's looking at is his own. He will also imitate your household chores. He may not be very good yet at polishing table-tops, but he will be thrilled to grab a rag and feel like he's helping. (His pleasures in this may wear off over the next 12 years or so.)

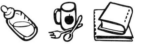

what you can do

There are tons of things you can do in this second year of life to help your child master his growing world. Start by talking to him, a lot. Use clear, simple language, not baby talk. The more words he hears, the more he will understand and say back. The television (TV) is your enemy here. No study of TV viewing before age 2 has shown that it helps development, but studies do show that it can slow down learning. Even when the TV is just on in the background, parents tend to speak many fewer words each hour, which means children are hearing fewer words and learning less. Children who don't seem to be paying attention to what's on still interrupt their play more frequently, hampering with their ability to pay attention to tasks for extended periods.

As for toys, your toddler will enjoy things he can take apart and put back together. Peg boards and simple building sets give him tons of material to practice with, but a stack of plastic cups will work well, too. (*Safety tip:* Poke holes in the cups so he can't suck them over his nose and mouth.) Modeling compound is great fun, too, and you can make it yourself with a little flour, salt, and water.

The terrible 2s get bad press, but the 1s can be just as trying. You'll probably have more opportunity than you want to model appropriate behavior, using your words to express simple ideas like, "Don't hit Daddy, that hurts," or, "I'm going to pick you up now so the other shoppers can get by." This is a good age to start short time-out periods when your child's behavior becomes dangerous, painful, or disruptive of the peace. Two minutes in a boring place is usually enough; after that he will have forgotten why he was there in the first place.

your 2-year-old

Remember those terrible 2s? Congratulations, they're here! This is a year of new and very real challenges, but it is also a year of magical developments. Your child will zoom down slides, prepare gourmet mud pies, read stories in your lap, and draw you pictures. Your job will be to stand back and let him go, then when he's gone far enough, step in and slow him down. Sounds simple, right?

Your child is now learning to grasp some really huge concepts, like time. The words before and after, previously just filler between more important words like cookie and nap, take on real significance. Ordinal numbers start to make sense, at least the numbers 1 and 2. Simple puzzles and shape-sorters will interest him as he figures out the ways objects can relate to each other. Cause and effect are huge—"If I flick this switch, the light comes on!" he thinks. When your kitchen has the strobe lighting of a disco, you'll know he's testing this concept.

His attention span is longer as well; you'll see this play out in his imaginary activities. Instead of just feeding his teddy bear, he'll feed the bear, brush his teeth, tuck him in, and pretend to read him a story. He will imitate you with impressive detail, down to your words, your inflection, and your body language. You may find this imitation charming, or you may hear something that makes you rethink the way you handle certain situations!

At this age your child is still figuring out what can and cannot happen in the real world. Having learned that he can affect his environment, your child will assume he causes everything to happen, from the spilled water cup to the thunderstorm outside to his great grandfather's hospitalization. You may need to anticipate his sense of guilt and reassure him about events that clearly have nothing to do with him. Likewise, fantasy and reality have almost no meaning to your 2-year-old. This means when you say something we understand as simple hyperbole, like, "You'll burn up out there," he is likely to take it quite literally, imagining himself in flames. As far as he knows you mean absolutely everything you say.

26

2. When Can He Play Ball? Infant and Child Development

And speaking of what you say, he now understands almost all of it. Your child may use around 50 words when he celebrates his second birthday, but his vocabulary is poised for a massive growth spurt. You'll also notice the complexity of his speech increasing. At the beginning of this year he may say sentences of 3 words. By the end of the year 8-word statements are not uncommon. Another huge leap in language is the addition of pronouns such as I, you, me, we, and they. You may not realize just how important pronouns are to meaning until your child starts to use them properly. There's a big difference between, "You go potty," and, "I go potty." He will also understand and use the word mine. As you might imagine, you'll be hearing this one quite often.

Two-year-olds are not known for their senses of shame. If, for example, there are certain words you use that you think perhaps children shouldn't say, be prepared to hear your child say them, usually while enjoying Sunday supper with his grandparents. Expect him to ask complete strangers about their body parts or to let the whole grocery store know he has some bodily function to attend to. Practice your guilty smile and be glad the people who hear him will have something to talk about when they get home.

Grammar is also critical to meaning, another point you'll appreciate as your child's language abilities grow. He will now be able to follow a story and will remember characters, plots, and facts from books you read together. That said, 2-year-olds are still working on patience, so don't be surprised if he slides out of your lap when he feels like a book is getting too long. As your child approaches his third birthday, he'll have a good enough grasp on language to enjoy wordplay. He may take great pleasure in rhymes, puns, and jokes that center on different meanings of a word. If you know a knock-knock joke, now is the time to tell it; it may never be this funny again.

If you watch your 2-year-old walk, you'll see the wide-based gait of the last year tightening up into a much more adult-type stance. As his strength and balance improve, your child will become capable of new movements such as running smoothly, making quick turns, and walking backwards. Now that he doesn't have to use all his concentration to stay upright he will be able to move around the house while talking and kicking a ball. He will grow adept at climbing and descending stairs so long as he has something or someone to hold on to. You might even see him standing on one foot!

Along with these new skills comes a boundless supply of energy. Sometimes it seems like 2-year-olds are all accelerator, no brake. You'll also notice their actions are not exactly predictable. Where an adult walking in a particular direction is likely to keep going that way, a 2-year-old will swerve, veer, backtrack, and serpentine his way through the world. While this sort of movement is useful when, say, evading a predator, it can be quite dangerous in parking lots or crowded stores. Add to this the fact that 2-year-olds are very poor judges of risk, and you start to understand why their parents are a jumpy lot. You are likely to interrupt a lot of conversations this year dashing off to save your child from pending disasters. You may be amazed to learn that almost all 2-year-olds go on to become 3-year-olds.

As your child is growing faster on his feet, he is also becoming more adept with his hands. He is now able to manipulate small objects with ease. He can turn the pages of a book, work a zipper, and unwrap a piece of candy. He is mastering twisting motions, opening up a wondrous new world of doorknobs, jar lids, and windup toys. This newfound dexterity also allows him to grasp a crayon or marker between his thumb and forefinger. Instead of simply scribbling or marking on paper he can make loops, curves, and circles. You are now in the position of deciding what is art and what is recycling.

A 2-year-old's model of the universe still puts him at its center. Among the concepts he has yet to learn is that other people have feelings that may differ from his own. This means the line of reasoning we use to test our own actions, "How would you feel if someone did that to you?" has little meaning to your child. In his mind someone would not do that to him because he wouldn't want them to. Long discussions about the Golden Rule, therefore, are not likely to alter his behavior nearly as much as a 2- to 3-minute time-out. But take heart—as your child imitates you and others around him, he is working on the concepts that one day will become empathy.

Remember, too, that controlling impulses is a skill that has to develop, just like talking in sentences or kicking a ball. Enforcing consistent consequences every time he displays violent or dangerous behavior will help your child build this skill. Deciding when to step in and when to let situations play themselves out will take trial and error on your part. Ideally you'd like to let your child work things out himself, intervening just before someone gets hurt. With time you'll get better at seeing the warning signs.

28

2. When Can He Play Ball? Infant and Child Development

You'll find your 2-year-old's emotions all over the map. One moment he's running around, giggling uncontrollably. The next moment he dissolves into tears. His inner life is at the mercy of powerful forces: excitement, hunger, thirst, fatigue, frustration. Your child is building new emotional tools, which means you'll be developing new ways to respond. When other people tell you what an angel your child is when you're not around, they're not just messing with you. He is more likely to test limits with you, knowing you can be relied on to keep him from really endangering himself.

Even though your child might behave better for other caregivers, he still is not likely to let you leave him without protest. Even when he has grown comfortable with some other people, you may find times when he responds to your departure by crying or clinging to you. Know that this is normal behavior, and reassure him you're coming back. Be sure to say good-bye even if you know it will leave you wiping snot off your knees. Looking up to find you've disappeared without warning is a lot more upsetting to your child, even if it seems less traumatic to you.

When you establish limits your child doesn't like, don't be surprised when he reacts with kicking, screaming, hitting, even biting. It's up to you to model adult behavior, ensuring he can regain control of himself in a safe setting. At the same time, be on the lookout for positive behaviors and be sure to lavish praise on your child when you see him share a toy, comfort a playmate, or put away his toys. Your approval has enormous power, and those moments when you can express how proud you are of him are times you'll both treasure.

what you can do

This year offers all sorts of opportunities to help your child develop. Toys that involve cause and effect, like those with lots of lights and buttons, will delight your child even as they drive you crazy. He will want to explore how things fit together using shape-sorters and building sets with large, interlocking pieces. The more you talk and read to your child, the more language he will acquire. Remember, he lives in a literal world, so avoid "joking" with him by telling him things that are untrue. You know a beanstalk won't grow out of his mouth when he eats peas, but he may spend weeks looking for leaves.

This is a great age to run outdoors, to explore toddler-friendly playgrounds, to give horseback and piggyback rides. Your child has an insatiable drive to run, jump, climb, and challenge his budding balance skills. In quieter moments he will want to draw, color, paint, and flip through books. Stocking your house with plenty of books and art supplies is a good way to ensure that he has some of those quieter moments.

Playing with other children may frustrate your child at times, but the more practice he gets around others, the better playmate he will become. Do your best to stand back and let him learn how other children respond to his actions, but be ready to step in when he lashes out in frustration. Make sure he has simple, predictable limits to his behavior by enforcing consistent consequences. The first 67 times you put him in time-out for hitting might feel fruitless, but the 68th time you may see him use his words, not his hands, to solve a problem. That's a moment too satisfying to miss!

your 3-year-old

The world of the 3-year-old is a lot like Disneyland. Reality and fantasy mix effortlessly. Adventures abound, but people are on hand to keep you safe. Playing with other others is fun, except when they get cranky. There are lots of rules to follow. Sometimes you have to wait too long for things. Candlesticks and teapots start dancing for no apparent reason. Wait, that last one actually was Disneyland, but when you're 3 that kind of thing can totally happen.

By this age, children have grasped the basic rules of the world—things fall when you drop them, it gets light then dark again every day, parents get upset when you throw food. They are now ready to tackle more advanced concepts. Time, for example, gains more meaning as your child begins to look forward to daily rituals, like breakfast, a walk, or the arrival of the mail. Events that occur less frequently are still confusing. Why, for example, are some days weekends and others workdays? He understands that birthdays only come once a year, although the concept of a year is beyond him.

Descriptive concepts like numbers and colors become clearer; he may enjoy counting items or naming their hues. The ideas of same and different also come into focus, allowing for endless comparisons. Your 3-year-old will be able to hold a sequence of events in his head, allowing him to

30

2. When Can He Play Ball? Infant and Child Development

follow 3-part commands ("Go to your room, get the book, and come sit with me"). The same skill will help him remember events in stories.

You'll notice your 3-year-old is insatiably curious. Don't be surprised if he peppers you all day with questions, mainly starting with the word why. Your child has determined everything in the world has a cause or an origin, and he's in a hurry to catalogue them all. It's OK if you don't know the answers; it's also OK if you do know the answer but just need to gloss it. When your child asks, "Why does the sun shine?" he's not really primed for a lesson in the physics of hydrogen fusion. That said, every question he asks is serious, and each one deserves the best answer you can come up with while simultaneously merging onto the freeway and juggling a cup of coffee.

As your child's understanding of the world continues to evolve, so will his use of words to describe it. He now has the basics of grammar down, and he is probably speaking in sentences of at least 5 to 6 words. He may still have trouble making certain sounds; r may become w, so that you "wide in a wed caw." Even so, most of what your child says now makes sense to people outside the family. You no longer find yourself serving as a translator whenever he speaks. Three-year-olds love to tell stories, although their narratives can be prolonged by their difficulty finding the words they want. You might hear your child begin the same sentence 3 or 4 times in a row, stopping each time until he figures out how to express himself. You may also see him use his body to express and understand words. If you're talking about dogs, for example, he might be on all fours, barking.

Building on the strength and skills he learned as a 2-year-old, your child now finds controlling his body increasingly effortless. Walking, running, and riding a tricycle are second nature. He can get up and down stairs without support, stand on one foot for up to 5 seconds, and even hop. He will catch a large ball in 2 hands, throw a smaller ball overhand, and kick a ball forward reliably. He is still full of energy and movement, but that activity is no longer random. It is now directed toward more concentrated efforts, such as playing in the sandbox or sliding down the slide for periods of several minutes or more.

Your child will be able to play on his own in a safe place like his room without your constant supervision. That said, when he is outdoors or with friends, you'll still want to keep a close watch. Three-year-olds are lousy at judging the speed and direction of things like cars, bicycles, and pedestrians, so parking lots, streets, and even malls require your constant vigilance. Even in the safety of your own home you'll get that parent instinct for reassuring noise, like a cowboy in an old Western: "It's quiet. Too quiet."

Your 3-year-old will take delight in the cool new things he can do with his hands. Rather than using all 4 fingers together as a unit, he can now move each one at will. As his coordination increases he will be able to build a tower of 9 cubes (which make an incredible sound when he knocks them down!), pour water from a pitcher into a cup, use a fork to eat with only a little spillage, and unbutton clothing.

Your child's artistic talents will flourish now that he can grasp a crayon easily between his thumb and forefinger. He will be able to copy a circle, make a square, cut paper with scissors, mold clay, and paint. He will move from abstract to representational art, making figures of people with 2 to 4 body parts. In the past he might have created a scribble or series of curves and lines and decided it looked like something; now he will start choosing ahead of time what to draw, which means there's a good chance he will draw you. If these early portraits don't look much like you, don't worry; he'll get better with time. If they do resemble you, dude, join a gym!

Socially, your 3-year-old is achieving a milestone that seems difficult for some adults—he is recognizing that other people have thoughts and feelings of their own. This realization enables him to grow much less selfish and dependent. At the same time he can now develop a sense of himself as a person distinct from others. He will envision himself as a whole person, seeing his body, mind, and feelings as all part of him, separate from other people. He will use his new skills of comparison to see how people are like him in some ways and unlike him in others. He will make friends, perhaps even a best friend, and he will probably decide there are some children he doesn't enjoy playing with.

Instead of playing side-by-side with other children and occasionally grappling over toys, your child will now play by interacting. He can share toys, take turns, and ask for what he wants politely, skills that enable cooperative play. You may see him use his words to solve problems that arise. Don't miss a chance to praise him for this behavior, unless of course you'll ruin the game by butting in.

32

2. When Can He Play Ball? Infant and Child Development

Of course things will not always go so smoothly. There will still be times when your child's frustration spills over into aggression. At those times you may need to pull him out of the situation, explaining he needs to use his words. You might have to help him name his feelings: "It made you angry when your friend took your toy." Naturally you'll have to lead by example, using your own words when his actions frustrate or embarrass you. Don't be surprised if the arrival of a friend brings out a rude streak in your child. He may not want his friend to see him being deferential to you. You may have to remind him quietly but firmly that all the same rules apply whether or not he has someone over.

One way your 3-year-old will learn about interactions is through a vivid fantasy life. Remember, this is a kid who just grasped the concept of gravity, so anything he sees or hears or even makes up could be true. Three-year-olds live in a world where everything has an inner life. Not only are his stuffed animals and dolls alive, but the lamp, chair, and tissue box all have feelings too. He will not distinguish between stories and real life, cartoons and documentaries, jokes and serious admonitions. Your child assumes whatever you say is true, even if it seems outlandish to you. Don't threaten, for example, to leave him behind in the store when he's throwing a fit. You're not really going to leave him behind (even though you may feel like it at the moment), and he may spend the rest of the day fearing that you'll abandon him.

Your child will use his imagination to explore all sorts of ways people might relate in various situations. By pretending to be mommy, he can imagine how mommy might feel if he gives her a hug or if he hits her. He can inhabit the lives of a superhero, a dog, and his baby sister, all in rapid succession. He is likely to have an imaginary friend, perhaps several of them. These "people" are handy for him to practice elements of relationships with when real playmates are not around.

Joining your child in play can give you a delightful insight into what's going on in his world. Don't get carried away just because you don't usually get to play superhero. Let your child tell you who you are and what you're doing, and ask lots of questions. His answers will tell you a ton about the way he thinks the world works.

All this understanding of differences between people naturally leads children to become curious about the differences between boys and girls. Three-year-olds can reliably tell you their gender, and they express great interest in what it means to be a boy or girl. While the biological differences between boys and girls do lead to some differences in behavior, much of what we think of as masculine and feminine is transmitted through the cultural messages children receive simply being part of society. Children may respond to sex roles by doing everything they can to conform. Three-year-old girls often embrace what's become known as the princess culture, dressing up in tulle and satin, with or without fairy wings. Boys may carry trucks or robots with them or insist on wearing a cape and mask everywhere they go.

At the same time, they will be curious about what is involved in being the opposite sex. Your son may clomp around in high heels, makeup, and a Cinderella dress; your daughter might pretend she's driving a monster truck to her job as a lumberjack. These activities are all part of the way children use their imaginations to test out ideas of identity. Sexual orientation and identity are deeply ingrained mental properties, and no doll, dress, or truck has the power to budge them. Respond by asking your child about the role he's playing, and feel free to join in; that is, if you can find a fetching enough ball gown.

Your child is using his growing analytic skills to build a sense of morality for the first time. His moral world, however, is simplified. The abstractions of good and bad behavior are still beyond him. At this age he just knows that some actions lead to desirable consequences, others to undesirable ones. He will therefore feel guilty any time an action has a "bad" consequence, regardless of his intention. You'll want to point out that some things are accidents. Throwing a vase on the floor in anger deserves a time-out. Bumping a vase to the floor when it was too close to the edge of the bookshelf wants reassurance.

Three-year-olds are eager to please their parents, and your child will interpret your anger at his actions as a rejection of him personally. It's therefore critical that you use language to distinguish between your child's actions and the child himself; "I love you, but I'm upset about what you did," is a very different statement than, "You were bad." A child may behave horrendously at times, but he is still a good child. Remember again, 3-year-olds believe what you tell them. So if you tell a child, "You're bad," what will he think about himself?

One way to help your child develop confidence is to give him tasks you know he can do. He can pick up his stuffed animals and trucks, he can

34

2. When Can He Play Ball? Infant and Child Development

bring his cup to the sink, he can hand you a screwdriver. Just watch the look on his face when you praise him for doing these things! You'll feel like you really deserve that "#1 Dad" coffee mug.

If your child has older siblings, this is an age where he desperately wants to follow them around and do what they're doing. Not all older siblings understand what a great honor this is, and fights can erupt. You're going to want the kids to love each other and be best friends all the time, but forcing siblings to share and play together can sometimes lead to more resentment. You'll have to walk a fine line between encouraging the older kids to include the younger one and guaranteeing them some autonomy and freedom from intrusions.

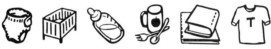

what you can do

There are tons of things you can do to promote your 3-year-old's development without necessarily turning your house into Disneyland (don't laugh, I've seen it). Building sets can become more complex, allowing your child to create his own worlds. Simple jigsaw puzzles, pegboards, and stringing beads promote problem-solving skills and finger coordination. Dolls or activity boards with buttons, zippers, and other fasteners will build a skill set that soon results in your saying, "Go get dressed!" Ample art supplies, including large sheets of cheap paper, encourage creativity and may supply much of your interior decor. A sheet and a card table can turn any room in your house into the Magic Kingdom.

Outside there are playgrounds to explore, balls to throw and catch, and water containers to pour from and into. Sandboxes are especially fun at this age, as are small swings and slides. This is a great age for kids to engage in work as play. If there is a screwdriver or lightweight hammer your child can use alongside you, or if he can stir batter or put plates in the dishwasher, he will glow with pride.

Your 3-year-old will need plenty of time with peers to sort out the mysteries of social interactions. Some children come by this time naturally in child care, extended families, or houses of worship. In other cases you may have to take the initiative to find playgroups or other group activities where your child can bounce off lots of other children.

At this age you have the luxury of giving your child choices about all sorts of things. Does he want the white shirt or the blue? Broccoli or peas? Buzz or Woody? You'll want to pare down the list to 2 or 3 items at most, lest he feel overwhelmed. The people behind you in line will thank you.

your 4-year-old

Yes, your child is a prodigy. At age 4 he is doing something absolutely amazing, something you don't know any other 4-year-old can do. He will go pro, he will be a star, and the camera will pan to your face in the audience, beaming with pride. The words at the bottom of the screen will read, "#1 Dad." But before you retain an agent, let's look at what kids this age are normally doing.

Four-year-olds are insatiable learners, driven by a growing understanding that the world is governed by systems and processes that, if they can just decode them, will deliver the keys to independence. Your child's concept of time has grown to include cyclical occurrences like morning, afternoon, and night as well as seasons of the year. By age 5 he will grasp minutes, hours, and weeks. Size relationships, geometric shapes, numbers, and even letters will all assume meaning, arming him with the intellectual tools to more fully explore his world and describe what he discovers.

As his intellect grows, the size and complexity of his questions will grow as well. Common subjects include life and death, the origin of the universe, where babies come from, and the nature of God. Fortunately for those of us who are not all-knowing, the world is full of museums, zoos, libraries, and Web sites dedicated to helping children at various ages understand the answers to these questions. "Let's go look it up," is a great answer to almost anything. You can make stuff up, but do you really want your child calling you from college going, "You remember when I was 4 and I asked you about volcanoes…?"

The answer to the title question of this chapter, "When can he play ball?" is…now! As this year progresses, your child's coordination and balance will come to resemble an adult's. He will scamper up and down stairs, stand on his tiptoes, pump a swing, and turn somersaults. There are plenty of skills that may still take practice to master, such as riding a

36

2. When Can He Play Ball? Infant and Child Development

bicycle without training wheels, hitting a baseball, and making a layup, but these skills are now all within reach, given time.

Your child's sometimes amazing motor skills may lull you into a false sense of security about his safety, but remember that your 4-year-old's judgment is still quite immature. He cannot accurately gauge the speed of an approaching car, the risk of a fall, or the friendliness of the neighbor's dog. Even if your child has taken swimming lessons, water remains a tremendous hazard. It's not enough to just be in the pool with him; you must focus like a lifeguard on his safety. Children may drown silently in the time it takes to compose a text message.

Your child is also using his hands in near-adult ways. He can dress and undress with minimal help, especially if he has those shoes with the Velcro fasteners. He can brush his teeth, too, although you may want to help make sure he gets all the surfaces. He can use a spoon or fork with ease and even serve himself from a larger bowl or platter.

Using his growing dexterity, your child will make more elaborate art projects. Drawings of people will include eyes, a nose, a mouth, and usually arms and legs. The body may be missing at first, giving his figures the appearance of humanoid puffer fish, but with time they'll evolve. He will use paint, clay, paper, scissors, and glue to make increasingly complex designs, some of which may pass for expensive works of modern art. The docent at your local museum will still be unamused if you stare at a display and exclaim, "My 4-year-old paints better than that!" even if it is true.

Your 4-year-old's language development is now beyond the basics of words and grammar and beginning the long climb toward literacy. He will address adults with more confidence. He may be learning various letters and the sounds they make. He will enjoy reading with you, and he may memorize favorite books and "read" them to you. You can help your child learn to read by reading with him as often as possible, running your finger under the words as you do. Enjoy the pictures and have fun making up voices and sounds for the characters. Stop and answer any questions he may have, and if he wants to try reading himself, be patient and help him out when he gets stuck. The more fun the experience, the more he's going to want to read.

Some children really do learn to read before their fifth birthdays. You may find yourself panicking because your sister's 4-year-old is reading *Ulysses,* or you may be contemplating letting your own young genius skip kinder-garten and instead apply to college. Recognize in either case that these early skills, while exciting, don't predict much about a child's ultimate academic success. You or your sister may indeed have a savant on your hands, but chances are you have a normal kid who learned to read a little earlier or later than other kids his age.

Your 4-year-old's social and emotional development is evolving in more complex ways. He will build on the empathy he learned at age 3, becoming even more interested in how other people feel. He will show sympathy and concern if others are hurt or sad, offering a hug or even kissing a boo-boo when needed. He will be proud of himself when he makes other people happy. Reinforcing these behaviors with praise spreads the joy even more.

Your child will still engage in lots of fantasy play, but he will have a better idea of what things might not happen in the real world. He will be able to tell you that his games are "just pretend." Some parents get alarmed when games involve pretend violence or killing, but remember that the concept of death holds little meaning to your child at this point. Guns are just another way to project power and move the plot along. You'll see that no one in his games stays dead for long.

Four-year-olds become more interested in the concept of sexuality, their own and others'. This interest is innocent and should be handled casually. Your child is likely to ask questions about various body parts and what they're for. Keep your answers short, limiting them to precisely the ques-tion asked. He'll come back with new questions as he thinks of them. Use proper anatomic language rather than slang or invented words for body parts. Do not pull down your textbook from the human sexuality class you took in college. He'll find that on his own in several years.

As part of this process, children discover their own sexual organs and may masturbate or explore themselves. When this happens, you may have to overcome an instinct to freak out. Instead, let the child know this behavior is normal but strictly private. This is also a good time to remind him that no one else should touch his private parts unless it's a health care provider examining him or a parent bathing him or checking out something that hurts. A key part of this conversation is reminding him to tell you if such a thing ever happens. Child sexual abuse is not usually perpetrated by strangers but by people the child already knows and trusts. Abusers tell their victims to keep what they do a secret, and children, being obedient, usually do.

38

2. When Can He Play Ball? Infant and Child Development

Athletic teams will often sign up 4-year-olds, and it can be tremendous fun for your child to learn the rudiments of a sport with other children. The hazard at this age is that some children do some things so well you start envisioning a career for them. While it's exciting to see your child excel at anything, remember that every experience is new and he needs time to explore. Your child may indeed be the next Tiger Woods or Lang Lang, but for now he has something much better—he has you for a dad.

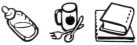

what you can do

Encouraging your 4-year-old's development involves opening up as many opportunities as possible and letting him run with them. Having books around encourages reading and learning and has been shown to improve school performance later in life. As your child's artistic skills improve, you'll want to make sure there are plenty of media he can work with when inspiration strikes. This is a wondrous age to explore museums, zoos, aquariums, and the outdoors, all of which take on a magical element when viewed through the eyes of a 4-year-old.

assessing developmental delays

Parents often get concerned when a child doesn't do something by the age he's "supposed to." It's even worse when a friend or relative is telling you all the amazing things his child is doing that yours is not. Your child should be getting regular wellness examinations to check not only his health but also his growth and development. At those examinations his doctor should be performing a more formal evaluation of his development, looking not just at 1 or 2 skills but at whole clusters of developmental milestones. There are tools like the Ages and Stages Questionnaire, Modified Checklist for Autism in Toddlers, and others designed to identify children at risk for developmental delays. When problems are identified, your child's doctor can refer him to specialists who can determine whether your child might benefit from developmental services. As long as those periodic evaluations are normal, you can rest assured that your child is developing normally and should be fine.

Among the greatest joys of parenthood is watching your child develop and learn new skills. As a father you're teaching your child constantly, whether or not you're even trying. He is watching your every move, and over time his speech, walk, even facial expressions will come to mirror yours. All the while, he's teaching you, helping you become a more responsive dad and eventually bringing you facts, music, adventures, and philosophies you would never have encountered without him. As the umpire says, "Play ball!"

3

infant feeding for the mammary-challenged: what your baby will eat and when

ok, i'll admit it. There is one thing a mom can do that a dad simply cannot. You may have guessed, "Attend the Mommy and Me yoga class," and you'd be right, but the answer I was looking for was, "Breastfeeding." As soon as possible after being born, your baby should be laid skin-to-skin on her mother's chest. If mom is not able to hold her because of a delivery complication, you can volunteer; otherwise, don't worry, your turn is coming soon.

Many babies will immediately begin what's known as rooting, or instinctively seeking the breast. You'll notice whenever your newborn's cheek touches skin that she automatically turns her head to that side and opens her mouth. You may even see her gradually inch her way around, seeking food. Infants also have a reflexive need to suck for comfort, and you can satisfy this need by offering her one of your (clean) fingertips to suck on. Unlike a pacifier, a fingertip will not interfere with her learning to nurse, and it will make you both feel better. Within the first hour, however, she's going to want a meal. Now begins a process that can be intensely reward-ing or intensely frustrating, often a little of both. By educating yourself about baby feeding you can make the process as pleasant as possible for your baby, her mom, and yourself.

what's the big deal about breastfeeding?

Not having breasts ourselves, we dads have to walk a fine line when it comes to helping choose a method of feeding our babies. On one hand, it's easy to leave the decision entirely to mom, figuring it would be unfair for us to suggest what she should or should not do with her own body. On the flip side, we run the risk of seeming too directing at a time when mom is stressed, exhausted, and emotional. That said, there are some real advan-tages of nursing over formula-feeding, and one of the best predictors of successful nursing is whether the baby's father is supportive.

What makes human milk different from commercially available infant formulas? Both, after all, provide calories in the form of fats, sugars, and proteins. Both include a variety of micronutrients and vitamins, and now many infant formulas add docosahexaenoic acid (DHA), arachidonic acid (AA or ARA), linoleic acid, prebiotics, and probiotics, all in an effort to be more like human milk. There are, however, many elements of mom's milk that can never be sold in the grocery store.

Many unique components of human milk protect newborns from infec-tions. Breast milk contains living white blood cells and active antibodies, both made in mom's body in response to infections mom has had in the past or even at the moment. If mom has a cold, for example, she is likely passing her baby antibodies or protection against that very cold virus every time she nurses. Our immune system, however, does not have to fight off disease alone. Our bodies host billions of "friendly" bacteria that make it harder for dangerous infections to get a foothold. Nursing inoculates a baby with these bacteria and provides nutrients that help these bacteria grow. In both of these cases, babies get protection not only from any infec-tion but specifically from the sorts of infections most common where they live. We know that breastfed infants and toddlers are less likely to contract ear infections, pneumonia, urinary tract infections, stomach bugs, and even some kinds of spinal meningitis.

Another benefit of nursing is that it protects children from developing allergies. Our immune system is designed to attack whatever it sees as "foreign." Human milk protein is therefore less likely to cause an immune reaction than cow's milk or soy proteins used in commercial infant formulas. Infants who are exclusively breastfed to age 4 months are less likely to develop food allergies, asthma, allergic rhinitis, and eczema than formula-fed infants. Studies also suggest breastfeeding protects children against sudden infant death syndrome, childhood leukemia, and obesity. Nursing even reduces a girl's risk of developing breast cancer as an adult.

Baby is not the only person who benefits from breastfeeding. The hormone that helps the breast release milk, prolactin (also called oxytocin), promotes feelings of love and attachment. Mothers often report sensations of relaxation, fulfillment, and joy when they're nursing. Prolactin has yet another job, which is to help the uterus contract, stopping the bleeding many mothers experience after childbirth. Breastfeeding helps the uterus shrink back to its regular size faster. Mothers who nurse also tend to lose weight faster, usually dropping around 1 to 2 pounds per month. The benefits of nursing can last for decades, protecting mothers against ovarian cancer, breast cancer, and possibly even osteoporosis later in life.

Yet another unique property of human milk is that it changes over time, in the short and long term. Over the course of a single feeding the components of breast milk change rather dramatically, starting with a more watery consistency and progressing to a thicker, creamier, high-fat milk toward the end. Human milk also changes as your baby grows, increasing in volume and evolving nutritionally to provide whatever nutrients your infant needs for that period in her development. Even the flavors of the milk change, carrying traces of spices and proteins from mom's diet. In this way your infant will learn to welcome flavors of whatever foods your family prefers. This may be the only scientific explanation for why I can eat pickled herring.

Many parents worry that nursing will make life more complicated, but nothing could be further from the truth. Breast milk is free, a big advantage over formula. You never have to run to the grocery store at 3:00 am when you look in the pantry and realize you're out of breast milk. If you don't enjoy doing dishes you'll appreciate the lack of bottles, nipples, and rings that can quickly overrun the top rack of your dishwasher. And while I have to admit that diaper bag manufacturers have made great strides in designing less embarrassing-looking luggage, there's a lot less stuff to haul around when you and your baby leave the house, so long as mom comes with you.

dad's role in breastfeeding

Let's say you and mom have talked about it and decided to go with breast-feeding. There are tons of things you can do to help, beginning even before the baby is born. While breastfeeding is instinctive, there can be a lot to learn to make sure it goes as well as possible. Many hospitals, obstetricians, pediatricians, and freestanding lactation centers offer breastfeeding classes, which they encourage expectant fathers to attend. The more you know about nursing, the more helpful you can be when the time comes.

Successful nursing depends on a host of factors, many of which you can help with. Positioning, for example, is key. Mom may need a pillow or help propping up to get baby lined up just right. At that moment she's probably not in the best position to jump up and grab a pillow for support from across the room—you're on it! In addition to all the other things prolactin does, it often causes mom to feel intensely thirsty just as her milk is really starting to flow. Does she have a glass of cold water? You know what to do. Nursing goes best when mom is relaxed and feeling happy about her baby. Can you adjust the lighting? Put on some music? Rub her back? These are all opportunities to be a hero.

If you really want to earn your cape, you'll remember the gastrocolic reflex. This is the medical term for the way the body makes room for in-coming food by eliminating waste. In other words, it's not your imagina-tion that your baby poops every time she nurses. Step in to handle this issue regularly and you can guarantee mom will be bragging about you to anyone who will listen. Seriously, this is the stuff women talk about—just run with it.

Listening, of course, is an especially important way you can help. Nurs-ing may be natural, but it can also be quite frustrating and uncomfortable, especially at first. Mom's nipples may crack and bleed; her breasts can become uncomfortably engorged or even infected. You can help here, too, bringing her ointment or preparing warm compresses. But at times it's even more important that you just listen and offer sympathy. Your support may literally make the difference in helping mom overcome the challenges of nursing.

how to know your baby is getting enough milk

One of the most common concerns parents have when their babies are nursing is how to tell if they are getting enough milk. Bottles are reassuring this way—you can see how much milk is in the bottle and how much your baby drank. The breast, however, isn't marked in ounces and milliliters, and parents naturally worry about babies becoming dehydrated or malnourished.

To begin with, it's important to know how nursing progresses from the time of birth. Making milk takes fluid, calories, and nutrients from mother's body. Humans didn't evolve to just start gushing milk the moment the baby is born. Instead, hormonal changes in mother's body ramp up milk production over a period that usually lasts 2 to 3 days. The first milk produced is a thick, yellowish, protein-rich substance called colostrum. Colostrum is full of protective antibodies and is great for newborns, but it is not high in volume or calories. Over the next few days mom's milk production normally increases dramatically in volume and calorie content, a process referred to as milk coming in.

Fortunately, human babies are born prepared. Babies born at full term have extra fat and fluid to carry them through the first few days of life as mom's milk production ramps up. Your baby should be weighed daily for the first 2 to 3 days after birth. In general, newborns can lose up to 7% of their initial birth weight in the first week of life without becoming dehydrated or malnourished. In some cases, even more weight loss is OK, but once weight loss exceeds 7%, most pediatricians like to monitor the baby closely until she starts to regain weight. Premature newborns are a different case. They may not have stored up adequate fat or fluid and often require special care to avoid excessive weight loss. As a rule, newborns should have regained their birth weight by 2 weeks of life.

Newborns may not feed all that often just after birth, remaining sleepy for a day or so. By day 2, however, expect your baby to nurse every 1 to 3 hours, on average. Newborns may cluster-feed, latching on almost continually for several hours, then napping for 3 to 4 hours. Your baby should be nursing 8 to 12 times in 24 hours. At the beginning she will often nurse for 30 minutes or more at a time, although as she gets more efficient she will drain the breast faster, often in 5 to 10 minutes. As mom's milk comes in, you'll hear your newborn swallowing and see milk pooled in her mouth when she releases the nipple.

when to call the doctor

If you notice that your baby is latching poorly, isn't feeding at least 8 times a day, or seems too sleepy to get a good feeding, alert her doctor.

Another way to gauge what is going in to your newborn is to see what's coming out. In the first 1 to 2 days of life, your baby will have 1 or 2 black, tarry-looking stools each day. By days 3 and 4, the stool should be turning greenish to yellow in color, and she should be having at least 2 bowel movements a day. By day 5 to 7, expect to see 3 or 4 yellow, loose, seedy stools a day; often newborns stool every time they feed. Your baby should pee at least once in the first 24 hours of life, with more every day until she's making at least 6 wet diapers a day around day 5 to 7. You may find it reassuring to keep a log of your newborn's feeds, wet diapers, and bowel movements for the first several days until you feel like she has a regular pattern. For you smartphone geeks, there's an app for that.

While human milk is a perfect food, it does lack one nutrient: vitamin D. Our bodies normally manufacture their own vitamin D using sunlight. If you think back through the history of human evolution, you'll realize only in modern times have we come to live almost completely indoors. At the same time the thinning ozone layer has made sunlight more dangerous, so we now counsel parents to keep their newborns out of direct sunlight and apply sunscreen to any exposed skin. As a result, humans, especially babies, are at grave risk for vitamin D deficiency. We therefore recommend every breastfed baby take a supplement containing 400 IU of vitamin D daily. These are available as drops over the counter at most pharmacies.

the formula behind formulas

While breastfeeding is growing increasingly popular, not every mother chooses to nurse her baby. She may take a medication that is not safe in lactation. Surgeries, such as breast reduction, can interfere with a mother's ability to nurse. Mothers who have had painful or traumatic experiences with nursing in the past are often reluctant to try again. Some rare metabolic conditions such as galactosemia make babies unable to tolerate human milk. Also, some mothers may breastfeed exclusively until they return to work, then find they are unable to pump enough milk at work to satisfy their growing baby's needs. For these reasons and others, commercially prepared formulas are available to provide babies the nutrients they need to grow.

A parent going to the store to buy formula today faces a dizzying array of choices. Bold letters on the canisters seem to shout, "For Fussiness and Colic"; "Now With Prebiotics and Probiotics"; "For Spitting and Reflux!" Looking at yards of brightly colored containers and competing claims, how are you supposed to pick one? ("Honey, I bought the one with the purple label. It was a little pricey, but I know that's your favorite color.") It helps to break down the basic nutrients and most common additives in formulas. When babies start having problems eating, this stuff matters.

The most basic way that formulas vary is by protein source. Human milk is composed of 2 proteins: casein and whey. Similar proteins are found in cow's milk, albeit in different ratios and with some structural changes. Around 80% of formula on the market today contains cow's milk proteins, separated out and remixed at ratios more akin to those in human milk. Other formulas derive their protein from soybeans, a plant whose protein is surprisingly similar in structure to that found in cow's milk.

When babies develop an allergy to formula it's usually a reaction to the protein component. For this reason, most manufacturers also sell partially hydrolyzed formulas, in which the casein or whey from cow's milk has been chemically broken down into smaller pieces. The idea is that the baby's immune system will not recognize these proteins and react to them. These formulas can be helpful for babies in whom regular cow's milk protein causes vomiting or diarrhea. Doctors often recommend partially hydrolyzed formulas for babies with other signs of allergies, such as rash (eczema), runny nose, or wheezing. If you or mom has a history of allergic disease, these formulas may help prevent your baby from developing similar symptoms, although breastfeeding exclusively for the first 4 to 6 months of life remains the best prevention.

Another class of formulas is called extensively hydrolyzed or elemental formula. In these formulas, cow's milk proteins have been chemically broken down into their most basic building blocks, amino acids. Elemental formulas are often quite expensive and they don't smell very good, but some babies with severe allergies can only tolerate this type of formula.

Another way formulas differ is by their carbohydrate, or sugar, content. Human milk contains lactose as its carbohydrate. Likewise, lactose is the main carbohydrate in most cow's milk formulas, except those whose labels read lactose-free. Soy formulas also contain glucose or sucrose in place of lactose. Many parents fear their newborns have problems with lactose, but while lactose intolerance is common in older children and adults, almost all human babies digest lactose perfectly. An illness that causes diarrhea, however, can temporarily interfere with lactose digestion. Your baby's doctor may advise using a lactose-free formula for a short time while she is recovering from a tummy bug, but in most cases the symptoms people attribute to lactose are actually caused by protein intolerance or stomach contents washing up into the esophagus (gastrointestinal reflux). In other words, don't waste your time or money on lactose-free formula without first asking your baby's doctor.

The third major nutrient in infant formulas is lipid, or fat. Cow's milk normally contains butterfat, but babies do not digest this lipid as well as vegetable oils and other fats. Among lipids, you'll see references to DHA, ARA, and linoleic acid, fatty acids found in human milk that contribute to brain and eye development. Although some controversy remains about whether they give any measurable advantage to full-term babies, there is enough concern that DHA and ARA are now almost universal formula additives. Some manufacturers contend that the lipids they use contribute to better calcium absorption and therefore help build stronger bones. While some literature supports this claim, the long-term implications for bone health are still in debate.

Infant formulas must be fortified with extra iron because the body absorbs iron better from human milk than formula. Some parents worry that iron in formula contributes to constipation or diarrhea, and in the past manufacturers sold low-iron formulas. Study after study has shown that iron in infant formulas does not cause any intestinal problems, and iron deficiency impairs growth and development. Iron-fortified formulas are the only acceptable substitute for human milk. Infant formula is also fortified with vitamin D; however, levels may vary depending on what formula your baby is taking. In many cases, unless your baby drinks more than 32 ounces of formula a day, she will still need to take a vitamin D supplement.

Some infant formulas are designed to meet very specific medical needs. Premature newborns, for example, need extra calories for growth as well as increased concentrations of minerals like calcium and phosphorous.

Where full-term infant formulas mimic the average caloric content of human milk (20 kcal/oz), preterm formulas may have 22, 24, even 30 kcal/oz. There are also special formulas for treating rare metabolic disorders like phenylketonuria, in which normal nutrients may actually pose a severe health risk to the baby. "Follow-up formulas" are marketed for older infants and toddlers, but a good, healthy diet with plenty of fruits, vegetables, protein, and iron is all a toddler really needs.

bottle-feeding basics

The most obvious difference between bottle-feeding and breastfeeding is that the bottle lets you see how much your baby is drinking. Depending on what kind of dad you are, this may make you feel better because you know what your baby is getting, or it may give you something new to obsess about. Whenever you read guidelines for bottle-feeding, remember that each baby is different. Bigger babies need more food. Your baby may go through a growth spurt and seem hungry all the time, and then she may have a period when she eats less for a while. In general babies know how much food they need to grow. If you attend to your baby's hunger cues, she'll tell you how much food she wants and when she's full.

Choosing a bottle can be as challenging as picking a formula. Manufacturers make all sorts of claims about their nipples working more like the human breast or their bottles preventing gas. I haven't seen good scientific literature that supports these claims, so I can't recommend one brand over another.

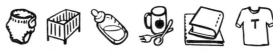

what you can do

More important than the type of bottle or nipple you use is how you position your baby when she eats. You'll want to support her in a semi-upright position, with her head cradled in the crook of your arm. Hold the bottle so that milk completely covers the nipple; that way your baby isn't swallowing air. Try not to bottle-feed your baby while she's on her back. Lying down increases the risk that she'll choke, and it allows milk to run into her eustachian tubes, possibly causing middle ear infections. In the first few weeks of life you may have to gently touch the nipple to her cheek to stimulate the rooting reflex.

Just like breastfed babies, bottle-fed newborns may start off slowly for 2 to 3 days, often taking only 1 to 2 ounces (30–60 mL) at a time. After the first 2 to 3 days of life she'll probably be taking 2 to 3 ounces (60–90 mL) every 3 to 4 hours. Sometimes your baby may sleep 4 to 5 hours between bottles, but she'll need a lot of food over the first month or so of life, so if she hasn't awakened to eat after 5 hours it's a good idea to go ahead and wake her up. You might even consider waking her up after 3 or 4 hours during the daytime, hoping she'll sleep a little longer at night.

After the first month of life your infant is likely to take around 4 ounces from the bottle every 4 hours or so, at least on average. That intake rises gradually so that by age 6 months, she'll take 6 to 8 ounces (180–240 mL) 4 or 5 times a day. Another way to think about normal intake is by weight; for every pound of body weight, your infant will consume around 2½ ounces (75 mL) per day. That said, every baby is different, and her doctor will weigh and measure her at each wellness examination to assess whether her growth is appropriate for her age.

Whether you're breastfeeding or bottle-feeding, your baby will give the same cues to let you know when she's hungry and when she's full. She will start rooting, scooting, sucking on her hand, and smacking her lips when she needs food. She will release the nipple, turn away, and often fall asleep when she's full. As she grows she may fall asleep less often and instead look up and grin at you. You can be pretty confident at this point that the feeding is over, especially if she's letting formula drip on your pants.

The 3 most common questions I answer about feeding, no matter the source, are, "Is she getting enough?" "Is she getting too much?" and "When will she stop waking up at night to feed?" The first question we've already answered. As for too much, it's rare for a baby to need more than about 7 or 8 ounces per feeding or more than 36 ounces in a day. She may be sucking for comfort rather than hunger. As for the last question, most babies will be able to make it through the night without feeding sometime between age 2 and 4 months or when they weigh more than about 12 pounds. That really unfamiliar, energetic feeling you'll have? It's called a full-night's sleep.

when to call the doctor
Overfeeding often results in spitting up and contributes to obesity. If your baby is taking more than 7 or 8 ounces per feeding or more than 36 ounces a day, address it with her doctor.

starting solid foods

Don't be surprised if you have relatives or friends who think your baby will win some sort of prize for eating solid foods, like if she'll just take a spoonful of rice cereal she'll get early admission to Harvard. They are, in fact, wrong. For Harvard she'll have to develop a new strain of pest-resistant rice that also cures river blindness and then eat a spoonful of that. In fact, pediatricians suggest she should be exclusively breastfed for about 6 months and begin eating solid food around 6 months of age.

It's important that your baby be developmentally prepared to start eating food. She should be able to support her head well. She should have lost the tongue-thrust reflex, an instinctive movement that is perfect for nursing at the breast but pushes food out of the mouth rather than toward the back of the throat. She should be at an age where she shows interest in eating solid foods and needs more calories than human milk or formula alone can provide. At around 4 months of age you'll notice your infant carefully observing you at mealtime. She may seem fascinated by the act of eating, carefully watching as the food travels from the plate to your mouth. It may be tempting to try feeding her at this point, but you probably want to wait until the moment she actually starts lunging for your food. If she grabs your fork in midair, it's a good sign she's developmentally ready to try some solids.

The baby food aisle in the grocery store is not exactly a relief from the chaos of the formula section. There are rows and rows of cereals, fruits, vegetables, meats, and combinations of these, and it continues in the refrigerated and frozen-food cabinets. Baby foods come in 3 stages, and many have more expensive organic versions. It's no wonder parents often find it overwhelming to decide what food to start with, what to try next, and how much to give.

Traditionally pediatricians have recommended starting with cereal, such as rice cereal. More recently some nutritionists have suggested that rice cereal, with its relatively simple carbohydrates, may contribute to obesity. They urge parents to start instead with meats, which supply more useable iron and zinc than cereal, at around age 6 months. When you do feed cereal, try a brown rice cereal, oatmeal, or other whole-grain option. Whichever you choose, go with the iron-fortified version.

At the beginning you can try one feeding a day from a spoon, not a bottle. Meals at this point can be as small as a couple of baby spoonfuls. If things go well, you can add another food every few days. The idea is to allow your baby time to grow accustomed to new flavors and textures as well as to identify reactions or allergies as they occur. That said, just because a food is new doesn't mean that it's the one that caused an allergic reaction. Children can develop allergies to foods they've had many times in the past.

Some pediatricians recommending starting vegetables before fruits, hoping the infant will not develop a strong preference for sweeter fruits. Preferences she does develop can often be overcome by repeated exposure. It may take 10 or more tries before your infant learns to enjoy a new flavor. One trick is to pair new foods with other foods she already likes. Studies remain inconclusive on the role of making airplane noises.

Over a few months, feeding amounts will grow to around an ounce or two, and your baby will eat around 3 times a day in addition to nursing or bottle-feeding. As solids become more important in her diet, you can add a little water in a bottle or sippy cup, but human milk or formula should still account for the vast majority of her fluid intake. Juice should be thought of as liquid dessert. It adds nothing useful to the diet, and it contains sugar babies don't need. If you do give juice, use 100% real fruit juice and limit the total volume to around 4 ounces a day.

The various stages of baby food refer mainly to the texture of what's in the container. The idea is to start with a smooth puree, sold as stage 1 food. You'll notice these containers are the smallest ones (2–2.5 ounces). Next, at stage 2, food will have a coarser texture and containers will be a little larger (3.5 ounces). At stage 3, foods will have actual small pieces in them, such as corn or peas, and containers will be larger still (6 ounces). There's no rush to progress through stages, so if you try a textured food and notice that your baby chokes or gags, wait a couple of weeks to give her time to develop a more coordinated swallowing motion.

By 8 to 9 months of age, your infant will develop motor skills necessary to pick up a small piece of food and put it in her own mouth. You may find yourself fighting her for control of the spoon at this point. She will enjoy finger-feeding, although you can expect a mess. It's important when selecting a finger food that you not expose her to the risk of choking. Some foods, like puffs or arrowroot cookies, are designed to turn to paste as soon as they contact saliva. This will look really gross, but just play like you think it's cute. You can also offer homemade vegetables or fruits, such as carrots or pears, so long as they've been cooked to the point of mushiness. When thinking about choking hazards, look at the tip of your baby's pinkie finger—her airway is roughly the diameter of her pinkie. Foods you give her should be soft or diced into pieces considerably smaller than her pinkie fingertip. Among the most common choking hazards at this age are peanuts and other whole nuts, popcorn, hot dogs, raisins, and raw carrots.

Increasingly, parents are interested in making their own baby foods. The market is rife with food grinders and mesh bags to make this process easier. It's tempting to season baby's food as you would your own, and a little flavor is great, but don't add salt. High salt intake in childhood is associated with high blood pressure later in life, and your infant does not yet share your taste for salt.

what you can do
If you're cooking food for everyone, put a portion aside for your baby before you pull out the salt shaker.

Parents often wonder about the advantages of using organic baby food. For many types of food, there is some evidence that pesticides used in their production can end up in the finished product; those chemicals can even be detected in babies' urine after they eat those foods. According to one study, fruits contained the highest levels of pesticides. What the effect is on an infant's ultimate health is still a matter of research, but there may be some value in paying the extra money for organic baby foods in certain cases. The Environmental Working Group provides guidance on which foods have the highest levels of contamination on its Web site (www.ewg.org/foodnews).

Babies are awfully smart about what they need to grow and develop. Whether looking for cues of hunger and feeling full, giving a spoonful of cereal to a 6-month-old who just grabbed your mashed potatoes, or letting your 9-month-old chase a green bean around her tray, you'll enjoy learning what your baby needs and providing it. The satisfied smile of a well-fed baby is one of the secret satisfactions of fatherhood, not to mention that it will impress mom.

4

the pit crew:
if you can change the oil…

is it just me, or are people fascinated with the stuff that comes out of babies? From your friends to grandparents to even the pediatrician, sometimes it seems like no one can stop talking about pee and poop. The fact is, a decent amount of early child care does involve diaper changes, from determining if one is warranted to worrying if there have been too many or too few. But really, if people are going to talk to you about it, maybe they should just come by and change a few diapers themselves?

By the time I was diapering my third child I was pretty proud of my technique. I wished there could be some kind of Daddy Olympics, where dads would complete for the fastest diaper change, and you'd get extra points for making the basket with the used diaper-ball. Of course you couldn't use real babies, or someone would get hurt. There's not a whole lot to know about changing diapers, but if you're smart you'll put the fresh diaper under your baby before you whisk the old one away. Also, if you have a girl, wipe front to back to keep nasty bacteria away from the bladder. Finally, there's no shame in simulating crowd-cheering noises if you score a 3-pointer in the trash can.

you're in urine

It's not obvious, but by the time your baby is born he has already been peeing for a long time. Amniotic fluid is actually made of urine, so he's literally been swimming in the stuff. Sometimes a low level of amniotic fluid is a sign of a problem with the baby's urinary system. Once he's born, your baby has 24 hours to pee (void) before doctors get concerned about his urinary tract. In most cases the first void occurs long before then. In the first few days of life he may only void 3 or 4 times a day, but once nursing is well-established, expect around 6 to 8 wet diapers a day. It's not uncommon for a newborn to pee every couple of hours, but in hot weather he may pee less, as few as 4 times a day.

when to call the doctor

Voiding fewer than 3 times a day is a worrisome sign of dehydration.

You may notice a pinkish, powdery-looking streak in your baby's diaper from time to time, the color of Pepto-Bismol. This is concentrated urine and not a cause for alarm, except in the unlikely event you've spilled Pepto-Bismol in his diaper. Parents of girls may also see a spot of blood in the diaper around 4 or 5 days after birth; girls may also have milky vaginal discharge. Both these findings result from mom's hormones affecting the baby's body. The blood is usually a small period, where the newborn sheds some uterine lining as a result of being removed from mom's hormones. The discharge may last longer, but it will usually slow down within a week or two after birth. Those same hormones also cause enlargement of breast tissue under the nipples in boys and girls. Sometimes this enlargement can be rather dramatic, and it can take months to completely resolve.

when to call the doctor

If your child seems uncomfortable every time he pees, tell his doctor. Urination should never be painful, and you should never see blood in urine. Parents often wonder about how their baby's pee smells. Urine that smells concentrated can just be a sign the baby needs to drink a little more. Pee that smells foul or stinky, on the other hand, may signal infection and warrants a visit to the doctor. Pee that smells like maple syrup means your baby has a rare and dangerous genetic condition.

making the cut...or not

Circumcising baby boys is an emotional and controversial topic in pediatrics. Some communities have seen efforts to outlaw circumcision, and anti-circumcision demonstrators are a reliable source of excitement at national pediatric meetings. In fact, the medical rationale for male circumcision is not very strong, and the procedure does expose male babies to complications including pain, excessive bleeding, and meatal stenosis, an abnormal narrowing of the hole where the pee comes out. While circumcision has declined in popularity in Europe, it remains a common procedure in the United States, where it is usually performed for religious, aesthetic, or cultural reasons, or because parents don't want their child to look different from other male family members. Those who favor circumcision point out that it can protect baby boys from contracting dangerous urinary tract infections. Opponents counter that these infections are quite rare in baby boys in the first place, so reducing their frequency doesn't make that big an impact in overall numbers. Circumcision supporters point to the power of circumcision to protect adult men and their sexual partners from certain sexually transmitted infections (STIs), including genital warts, cervical cancer, and HIV. Opponents note that condoms do a much better job of preventing STIs, and they ask if circumcision might give some men a false sense of security and actually reduce their condom use. Debate even rages about whether and how much circumcision decreases a man's enjoyment of sex.

If you are interested in having your son circumcised, there are some important questions to ask his doctor.

- Who will actually perform the procedure? In some hospitals only obstetricians perform circumcisions. In others it's always the pediatrician. Sometimes you'll have a choice.
- How often does that doctor perform circumcisions? In general, doctors are better at procedures they practice often.
- What does the doctor do for pain control? In the past, doctors thought newborns didn't really perceive pain, so they used no anesthesia. We now know that painful experiences in the newborn period can have long-term effects on pain perception, so pain control is critical. At a minimum the doctor should use a local nerve block, injecting anesthesia under the skin at the base of the penis to numb the nerves that carry pain signals from the tip. He may also use lidocaine gel to numb the surface of the skin. Taking acetaminophen and sugar water by mouth can also help control pain. Even with these measures, many babies are fussy or sleepy for 4 to 6 hours following the procedure. Ideally your baby would be healthy and feeding well at the time of circumcision.
- If there's a problem after circumcision, who will take care of it? Any doctor performing a procedure should have a plan in place for dealing with short- and long-term complications.

Post-circumcision care is relatively straightforward. If the doctor uses a clamp, you'll notice a raw, sometimes bloody appearance of the head of the penis immediately after the procedure. If you see a blood clot, leave it alone; it's doing the important work of preventing bleeding. Some doctors will leave a gauze dressing on the penis; the dressing will usually fall off within 1 or 2 diaper changes. You'll want to avoid soap and diaper wipes to the head of the penis for the first couple of days, and you should apply vitamin A&D ointment or petroleum jelly with each diaper change.

By day 2 you'll see patches of yellowish granulation tissue, which is where the skin is healing. These patches will shrink over the next 7 to 10 days until they are all healed. Continue applying vitamin A&D ointment until those patches are all gone; then you can stop. You may also see swelling around the head of the penis; this swelling can last 2 to 3 weeks. If your baby's doctor uses a type of instrument called a Plastibell, you may instead see a plastic ring around the head of the penis. (It's not really a bell.) It will fall off on its own in about a week.

Over time you may see that the remaining foreskin attaches itself to the head of the penis with scar tissue. This is a normal healing process called adhesions, and in most cases trying to pry them apart causes unnecessary pain and bleeding. They will usually disappear in the first couple of years of life. You may see some whitish collection, smegma, under the adhesions, which is normal.

when to call the doctor

Occasionally an adhesion is so dense it forms a skin bridge. If you see this happening, tell your son's doctor. These skin bridges sometimes need to be clipped under local anesthesia.

bowel movements

The very first stool your baby passes doesn't smell bad. That's because the black, tarry-looking stuff, called meconium, is sterile. Until the intestines are colonized with bacteria, there's nothing to make poop stinky. Don't go bragging about your baby's odorless poop, however; bacterial colonization begins with the first feeding. Some babies will actually pass meconium while still in the uterus, usually as a result of physiologic stress like an infection or a difficult delivery. When this occurs, the baby is at risk for lung disease, called meconium aspiration syndrome. Your newborn will most likely have his first bowel movement some time in the first 24 hours of life. When stooling takes longer than this, doctors look for problems such as intestinal blockages, an underdeveloped anus, or stool that is stuck, called a meconium plug.

Your newborn will continue to pass meconium over the first day or so, but if he is feeding well you'll notice that over a few days the stool goes from black to dark green to yellow in color. Breastfed babies usually pass poop that looks like Dijon mustard, watery with little whitish seedy-looking bits. Formula-fed babies may have less watery stool, usually pasty in consistency and yellow or tan in color. Many parents get concerned if they see the stool is green rather than yellow. In truth, all earth tones are fine, from yellow to green to brown.

when to call the doctor

There are 2 colors stool should *not* be. One is white. Stools the color of clay can be a sign of serious liver disease. The other is red. While blood in a baby's stool may simply have been swallowed at delivery or may result from mom's nipples bleeding, it's always wise to have a doctor check the baby out.

diarrhea

Parents often wonder if their baby is pooping too often. With newborns, "normal" varies widely. Many babies poop every time they feed, up to 12 times a day. This is a result of the gastrocolic reflex, where stretching of the stomach sends signals to the colon to make room for incoming food. Because normal bowel movements may occur frequently, it can be difficult to decide what to call diarrhea. Look for a sudden change in stool frequency, such as stools that are more liquid than usual, and signs of discomfort or illness in your baby.

when to call the doctor

If you see blood or mucous in the stool, you should alert your baby's doctor immediately. Fever in a baby younger than 90 days is always potentially alarming; call the doctor immediately if rectal temperature is above 100.4°F.

If your baby has mild diarrhea, he should keep taking human milk or formula. If he seems to be having excessive gas or discomfort with regular formula, you might switch to a soy or lactose-free formula for several days. Infants old enough to take solids can eat more starchy foods like potatoes, rice, cereal, or bananas. There are no medicines to give babies for diarrhea, but probiotics like *Lactobacillus* may help shorten the illness. If his diarrhea is more severe, or if he also has vomiting, you'll want to buy a commercially prepared electrolyte solution like Pedialyte to help keep your baby hydrated.

when to call the doctor

Be alert for signs of dehydration. Your baby should pee at least 3 times a day or every 8 hours. Knowing how much he has peed can sometimes be tricky when he is also having frequent stools. Other alarming signs of dehydration include dry mouth, crying without making tears, and decreased activity level. Poor skin tone, sunken eyes, and a sunken soft spot are signs of severe dehydration. If your baby seems dehydrated at all, contact his doctor immediately.

constipation

Parents also worry that their babies are not pooping enough, to which my answer is usually, "Seriously? That's awesome!" A baby eating formula usually has a bowel movement at least once most days. For breastfed infants it depends on age. During the first month of life, stooling less than once a day might mean your newborn isn't eating enough. After that, however, breastfed infants may go several days or even a week between bowel movements, using every drop they eat to make more baby, not poop. Infants normally work really hard to have a bowel movement, so straining at the stool isn't necessarily alarming, even when the infant cries or gets red in the face. For an infant to have a bowel movement is a major effort, and it shows. Just try to poop lying on your back and you'll get the picture. Actually, don't really do that. Imagining it should be enough.

For constipation concerns I always come back to the question of how the baby is doing. Is he excessively fussy? Is he spitting up more than usual? Is he having dramatically more or fewer bowel movements than before? Are his stools unusually hard, or do they contain blood? Does he strain for more than 10 minutes without success? These signs can all suggest actual constipation.

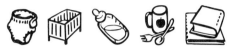

what you can do

After the first month of life, if you think your baby is constipated, you can try giving him a little apple or pear juice. The sugars in fruit juice aren't digested very well, so they draw fluid into the intestines and help loosen stool. As a rule of thumb, you can give 1 ounce a day for every month of life up to about 4 months (a 3-month-old baby would get 3 ounces). Some doctors recommend using corn syrup like Karo to get the same effect, usually around 1 to 2 tablespoons per day. Once your infant is taking solids you can try vegetables and fruits, especially that old standby, prunes. If these dietary changes don't help, it's time to call the doctor.

it's a gas, gas, gas!

One thing about babies—they don't care if they fart. People pass gas on average 14 to 23 times a day, but most of us use discretion or blame it on our kids. Babies, however, are always farting, and their thin abdominal walls allow you to hear every bubble as it works its way to the end. For this reason, gas sometimes seems like the scapegoat for everything that might make a baby fussy. Sometimes it may be the problem, but often it's just a distraction. Another thing about babies—even their farts are cute.

When we say "gas," we should really be saying "gasses." One form of gas is simply air your baby swallows while feeding, crying, or sucking on a pacifier. For a breastfeeding baby who seems to be swallowing too much air, mom might try adjusting latch or feeding position. If your baby seems to be gulping, unable to keep up with the amount of milk mom is producing, she might consider pumping a little first or nursing from only one breast each feeding. Bottle-fed infants may swallow air when the nipple is not completely covered with formula, the formula itself has been shaken until it's foamy, or the nipple is too short, too small, or too fast for the baby. Changing nipples or bottles may provide some relief.

A second source of gas comes from the chemistry of normal digestion. When acid from the stomach gets neutralized by bicarbonate from the pancreas, some gas arises, just like in the vinegar-and-baking-soda volcano you made in elementary school. Usually this gas volume is small, so if your baby has become a miniature Vesuvius, this probably is not the cause.

A major source of gas comes from bacteria acting on undigested food left in the colon. Foods high in fiber and sugars provide plenty of fuel for microorganisms to create methane. Infants whose formula has been thickened with rice cereal, for example, may have this kind of gas. Unless your baby's doctor has advised you to thicken formula to treat reflux, there is no reason to give your infant any solid foods until he's about 6 months of age. Starting solids too early can contribute to gas and stomach upset. For babies who have started solids, you might find that cutting back on fruits or juices helps with gas.

If you're worried about gas, feel your baby's tummy. Babies' bellies normally stick out, especially after a large feeding. Between feedings, however, they should feel quite soft.

when to call the doctor

If your child's abdomen feels swollen and hard, or if he has not had a bowel movement for more than 1 or 2 days or is vomiting, call your pediatrician. Most likely the problem is caused by gas or constipation, but it also could signal a more serious intestinal problem.

Store shelves are full of treatments for infant gas, from special formulas to gas drops (simethicone, eg, Mylicon). Some physicians recommend using simethicone, a medicine that breaks the walls of bubbles, turning little bubbles into bigger ones. Unfortunately, the best studies of simethicone find it works about as well as a placebo. That said, it is not absorbed by the body and is therefore at least harmless. Changing formula very rarely improves crying or gas, regardless of what it says on the side of the can.

burping

Go ahead and admit it—you love it when your baby burps, especially if it's loud enough that other people turn and look. It's OK; that's perfectly normal. Chances are you're not only looking forward to the day he'll win the burping contest at summer camp, you're also thinking he's averted a crying spell later on when that air would have found its way to his intestines. Burping a baby is more of an art than a science; your grandmother probably knows as much about burping as your pediatrician. I have had the advantage of listening to a lot of grandmothers!

Depending on how fast they're eating, babies can swallow air pretty quickly. Doctors (and grandmothers) often advise burping a baby between breasts if he's nursing or after every 2 to 3 ounces if he's bottle-feeding.

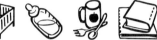

what you can do

The traditional approach to burping is to hold your baby to your chest in an upright position and gently pat his back, but sometimes a change in position helps. You can try holding him in front of you at about a 45° angle and swaying gently back and forth as well. Sometimes it takes a few minutes for the burp to find its way out, so patience is important. You can't rush a bubble! It is OK to give up if you've been trying for 5 to 10 minutes and your baby just won't burp. If you wait a day he'll probably make another attention-getting noise.

hiccups

Newborns have a lot of hiccups, but they often start a month or two prior to birth (mom may have even commented on them during her pregnancy). A hiccup is simply a spasm of the diaphragm. No one knows exactly why they're so common in babies except that newborns' nervous systems tend to be twitchy in general, as evidenced by all the sneezing and tremulous movements you'll notice in the first few weeks of life.

We tend to think, "If I were hiccuping like that, it would drive me crazy!" but hiccups don't usually bother babies. Sometimes a hiccup spell can make it hard to get through a feeding, so you might give your baby a break until it passes, stopping to burp him or change his position. If the hiccups don't go away, resuming feeding may actually help. You may also find feeding him before he gets terribly hungry will keep him from gulping and giving himself more hiccups.

umbilical cord

Depending on how involved you were in your baby's birth, how things went in the delivery room, and whether the obstetrician thought you looked pale, you may have gotten to cut your baby's umbilical cord. Some weeks before that you probably received information about saving umbilical cord blood in case your baby should one day need an infusion of the special blood cells (stem cells) it contains. Hopefully you did some reading at that time and learned that while free public cord blood banks save lives, private cord blood banking very rarely proves useful, in part because the baby's own stem cells are often affected by the same diseases that would require a stem cell transfusion to treat. While many communities are not equipped to accept cord blood donations, those that do have cord blood banks allow your family a no-cost, risk-free opportunity to save someone's life.

Usually once the umbilical cord has been clamped and cut, it is just in the way, waiting to dry up and fall off. The exception is for babies in the neonatal intensive care unit, where the 2 arteries and 1 vein in the umbilical cord can provide doctors with critical access to the baby's bloodstream. Assuming your baby does not require critical care, however, you're left working around the stump of the cord until it's gone.

The umbilical cord starts as a thick, squishy, translucent structure, usually with one or more plastic clamps applied to the end by the delivering doctor or midwife. The clamps are there to prevent bleeding shortly after delivery, when blood vessels in the cord may still be open. Those blood vessels close off in the first 24 hours of life, and the baby's nurse should cut off the clamps before hospital discharge. Over the first day or two of life the umbilical stump will dry into a hard mass of tissue. The stump will then separate from the navel, often in the first 1 to 2 weeks of life, but the process can take as long as 4 weeks.

Caring for the umbilical cord centers on preventing skin infections in the area around the navel. Because moisture and secretions collect around the cord, it sometimes serves as a source of infection (omphalitis). In the past, doctors used a variety of treatments to try to prevent these infections. Among these were a variety of antibacterial agents including a dark purple concoction called triple dye. More recent regimens have included applying alcohol to the umbilical stump with each diaper change. Now, however, most pediatricians advise doing nothing except to keep the umbilical stump clean and dry (dry care), as infection rates don't seem to be any higher in babies treated this way.

The key to dry care, as you might guess, is to actually keep the umbilical stump dry. This means the newborn's diaper should be tucked down so that it doesn't cover the stump, and you should sponge-bathe your baby rather than immersing him for baths until the stump falls off. Once the stump is gone, feel free to enjoy the little bathtub he got as a shower gift. You'll notice as the cord is separating from the body that there is a collection of somewhat stinky yellow goo in his umbilicus. Gross as it is, a small amount of this stuff is normal, along with the occasional drop or two of blood.

when to call the doctor
If you see larger volumes of pus or blood at the cord, or if you notice the skin around the navel getting red or warm, take him to the pediatrician immediately. While rare, omphalitis can be a serious, even life-threatening infection.

Once the cord falls off you may still see a little blood oozing from the area for a few more days. That's generally normal, but it shouldn't be more than a few drops. You may also notice a small mass of white or red tissue in the middle of the navel. This is called a granuloma and usually goes away on its own within a week or so. Sometimes granulomas persist and begin to ooze and bleed. In these cases your baby's doctor may want to cauterize the tissue with chemicals or heat.

when to call the doctor
If your baby still has his umbilical cord attached at 1 month of life, you should call his doctor. In rare cases, delayed cord separation can be a sign of an immune system disorder or a problem with the anatomy inside the abdominal cavity. Blood tests or an abdominal ultrasound may help determine whether there is really a problem.

innies and outies

Many babies start life as outies; that is, you can see a bulge in the area of the navel when they cry or strain. Sometimes this bulge persists even when the baby is not pushing with his belly, and sometimes the bulge can be rather dramatic. These babies actually have umbilical hernias, a condition in which space in the muscles of the abdominal wall for the structures of the umbilical cord has not completely closed. For some reason, this condition is a bit more common in children of African descent than in those of other ethnic groups. The good news is that umbilical hernias almost never cause any medical problems, and they almost always close on their own. Unless a hernia is very large or has not resolved by age 4 to 5 years, there's no need for surgery. Friends or relatives may tell you to strap a coin over the umbilicus, but just smile and nod, knowing this won't make the hernia go away any faster. You can, however, ask them to give you a coin.

let's not be rash

I've always found the name diaper rash misleading. After all, the diaper doesn't have a rash, the baby does! The other problem with diaper rash is that while it tells you where the rash is, there are several common causes of babies having a rash in that area, and different kinds of diaper rashes respond to different therapies.

The most common sort of diaper rash results from irritation from moisture or stool. You'll see some redness in the diaper area, usually most obviously where the baby's skin actually touches the diaper itself. Irritating rashes often result from not changing diapers quickly enough after your baby pees or poops. They become more common later in infancy, around

what you can do

A number of things will make common diaper rashes better. The most obvious, of course, is to increase how often you change your baby's diaper. You'll also want to give the area a chance to dry really well. If you can, allow your baby to nap without a diaper on a towel. You can also use a hair dryer on the "cool" setting to help dry his bottom before fastening the next diaper.

age 8 to 10 months, partly because of the changing composition of the infant's stool that is a natural consequence of eating more solids. These rashes can get especially bad when babies have diarrhea.

Wipes with alcohol or scent may be irritating; look for fragrance-free wipes or use a soft, damp paper towel or washcloth to clean him instead. You may use a little soap if he's soiled, but overusing soap can deprive his skin of protective oils. If your baby is very uncomfortable, you might find soaking his bottom in an oatmeal bath is soothing. Barrier creams such as Desitin, Triple Paste, Flanders, Balmex, and others all use zinc oxide, petrolatum, or a combination to keep stool and urine from contacting the baby's skin, and they can all help prevent or heal diaper rash. If your baby has actual sores on his skin, you should call his pediatrician and have him seen.

A second common type of diaper rash results from infection with a common yeast, *Candida albicans.* I find it sadly ironic that yeast, which gives us beer and pretzels, can also make our babies cry during diaper changes. *Candida* species love dark, damp places, and they tend to collect where skin touches skin. While an irritant diaper rash may create a friendly environment for yeast to get a foothold, the yeast rash differs in some ways from an irritant rash. Most obviously, *Candida* rashes are more prominent in the depths of the skin folds of the groin. The skin is often bright red and you may see a wet, cheesy, or bumpy appearance. Frequently, little red bumps called satellite lesions spread out from the affected area. Dryness and frequent diaper changes help treat yeast rashes as well, but doctors often advise using antifungal medications like prescription nystatin or over-the-counter clotrimazole.

A third cause of diaper rash is an allergy to a dye or scent included in the diaper itself. This type of rash might follow the elastic parts of the diaper or look like an irritant rash. Changing to another brand of diaper is often the cure. Cloth diapers may prevent this type of rash, but it depends on what sort of detergent they're laundered in. While some parents favor cloth diapers due to environmental concerns, the moisture-absorbing properties of disposable diapers seem to protect babies somewhat better against irritant rashes.

A fourth, increasingly common type of diaper rash is caused by skin infection with *Staphylococcus aureus* bacteria, usually methicillin-resistant *S aureus* (MRSA). This rash begins with one or more pustules that can then grow or coalesce into a nasty, deep skin infection. MRSA rashes only respond to antibiotics, drainage, or both.

when to call the doctor

If you see pustules or drainage in your baby's diaper area, call his doctor immediately. Methicillin-resistant *Staphylococcus aureus* infections are a leading cause of pediatric hospitalization, and early treatment is critical.

After reading this chapter, you can dare people to start talking to you about your baby's pee and poop. Just tell them everything you've learned, and chances are good next time they'll want to chat about something more appetizing.

5

crying foul: why is my baby crying and when will it stop?

quick, complete the following 2-word sentence: "Babies ____." What verb did you choose? Eat? Sleep? Poop? Even without reading the title of this chapter, chances are better than even you said, "Cry." Don't feel bad; it's everyone's first thought. Because babies do cry, sometimes a lot. Imagine for a moment you rely on other people to do absolutely everything for you, and on top of that you can't talk. You really only have 2 tools to get all your needs met: cry and look adorable. And looking adorable won't get your diaper changed.

a new language: "crynese"

Your newborn is probably not going to cry much for the first couple of days after delivery. You may be tempted to tell people she seems to be a really good baby, meaning one who seems content most of the time. While this period of calm is pleasant, it is also very likely to change as your baby becomes more alert and vocal in expressing herself. Crying more won't make her a bad baby, just a baby who is trying to tell you stuff.

72

5. Crying Foul: Why Is My Baby Crying and When Will It Stop?

The act of crying itself serves a number of purposes beyond simple communication. At the time of delivery crying helps push air into the air sacs (alveoli) of the lungs that had formerly been filled with fluid. Doctors no longer slap babies' bottoms to induce this response, but it often occurs naturally. While crying, your baby's eyes are closed, and she is making her own noise, shutting out visual and auditory stimuli she might find unpleasant. Crying also gives your baby a way to release pent-up tension or anxiety. Periods of crying or fussiness may give your baby a bridge between states of increased alertness and states of rest, ultimately allowing her to sleep better.

You've probably heard babies have a language of crying, and indeed after some practice, parents can usually make a good guess at what their babies need based on the sound of their crying. Just as with any language, different people have different accents or ways of expressing themselves. As with learning any language, the more you practice, the better you get. I tend to be skeptical of "crying dictionaries" that explain things like what type of cry means your baby's diaper is a little too tight on the left side. There are, however, some features of crying that are relatively universal. As your baby gets older, her cries will grow stronger and more distinctive. By the time she can say, "Excuse me, Father, but my nappy seems to be rather damp; would you please avail me of a new one?" she can just cry instead, and you'll get the message.

The most obvious type of cry signals pain or intense fear. This one starts suddenly, usually with one long wail that sounds like your baby is using up every bit of her breath. Often there's an uncomfortably long wait before she takes in a huge breath and starts again. Usually there's no missing this one. You'll be running to see what's going on long before you stop to pick up a book and read up on crying.

At the opposite end of the spectrum is the slight fussing that accompanies early hunger or fatigue. This cry may start more as a whine and ramp up gradually. You may also see your baby sucking on her hands or rooting around on whatever is touching her cheek. If you respond with a feeding it may never really get going, but the hunger cry has been described as a short, low-pitched cry that varies in pitch. Fatigue will sound much the same, but it may peter out with time. A tired baby will often cry with her eyes closed and mash her face into her crib or your chest.

Over time your baby will also start letting you know when she's just plain mad. This cry tends to sound like she's shouting at you, with a repetitive, rhythmic pitch. Sometimes when you hear it you'll be glad your baby has not yet learned to speak for fear of what she would be saying.

what you can do

The best way to learn how to respond to your baby's crying is to take a moment to feel your own instinct. This stuff is bred into us; if what you hear makes you want to check your baby's diaper, you're probably on to something! This observation is especially true when it comes to holding your newborn. There is a place for helping her learn to sleep on her own (see Chapter 8), and you won't hurt her by putting her down so you can cook dinner or use the restroom. But know that there is no such thing as holding a baby too much. No matter what well-meaning relatives and friends tell you, you cannot "spoil" a baby by holding her. If that's what she needs, do it! In general, if you teach your baby that her needs will be met reliably, she is less likely to be fussy. Of course, babies don't just have one need at a time. Yours may have a cry that means, "My diaper is wet; I'm cold; I'm tired, but I'm too hungry to sleep; and please pick me up." With this one you'll have to prioritize—diaper, hold, warm, feed, then nap.

Even parents who are completely fluent in crying get flummoxed sometimes. That's when the old troubleshooting checklist comes in handy. Checklists are particularly useful in the middle of the night when you're too tired to think constructively about the crying situation. If it helps, you can imagine yourself as a fighter pilot preparing for takeoff (not saying I've ever done that, but you know…). First, what's the diaper status? This one may take only a little sniff to determine. Second, does your baby need to be held? Third, is it feeding time again? Fourth, does she need to burp? Fifth, is there a source of physical discomfort such as bunched-up clothing, a too-cold room, or a hair wrapped around a finger or toe?

74

5. Crying Foul: Why Is My Baby Crying and When Will It Stop?

If you've run through your list and everything seems fine, it's OK to give your baby a little time to calm down and get to sleep, even if that means she's crying in her crib for a while. Many babies need a period of crying to help ease them into sleep. In most cases, 5 or 10 minutes of crying will do the trick. If the crying is lasting more than 15 to 20 minutes, you should probably check and see if her needs have changed.

Crying that is uncontrollable (inconsolable) suggests serious illness. Some babies habitually cry 2 to 3 hours a day (see "Surviving Colic" below) but in most cases, even colic responds somewhat when you pick your baby up or address her needs in some way.

when to call the doctor

A baby who seems to be in pain and just will not calm down no matter what you try may need emergent care. While fever does not always accompany serious disease in children, it can be a useful clue. If your baby has a rectal temperature of 100.4°F (38.0°C) or higher, call her doctor. If she is younger than 3 months, she should be seen immediately for any fever, even if it means a trip to the emergency department.

surviving colic

At least once a week someone will ask me, "What is colic?" This is an easy one—we really don't know. If we knew what caused it, doctors would have replaced the archaic word colic with something much harder to spell. But while current research points to some intriguing theories about bacterial colonization of the newborn's intestine, anyone who tells you they know what causes colic or how to cure it is selling snake oil. Snake oil, by the way, is great if you have a rusty serpent, but I wouldn't give it to my newborn.

We do know colic is quite common, affecting up to a quarter of all babies. While we don't know what causes colic, we can describe it quite well. Colic is crying that seems to serve no purpose—it does not indicate hunger, cold, discomfort, fatigue, or the need to be held. Babies often appear to be in pain. They may arch their backs, tense their abdominal muscles, or draw up their legs as though their tummies hurt. Whether actual pain is present no one knows, but the appearance of discomfort is one aspect of the crying that distresses parents. By the strictest definition, colic follows a rule of 3s: the crying lasts at least 3 hours a day, at least 3 days a week, for at least 3 weeks. That said, if your baby is screaming for 2½ hours a day, there's still a good chance it's colic.

The good news about colic is that, by definition, it will end. Colic almost never begins before about 42 weeks' post-gestational age. That means, for example, if your baby is born right on her due date, she won't develop colic for a couple of weeks. If, on the other hand, she was born 2 months' premature, she may develop colic around 10 weeks of life. Colic peaks at around age 6 weeks and should then peter off, stopping completely by around age 4 months, if not before. For this reason, some researchers theorize that colic represents a normal developmental stage, as the newborn's brain gets used to the world outside the womb.

Colic also tends to follow a daily schedule. Colicky babies usually cry more in the early evening and at night, just when you and any other children in the household would like to be sleeping. The crying spells are not related to feeds, and while they may improve when the baby is held or rocked, they often don't resolve completely no matter what you do.

Because of the way colicky babies behave, it's tempting to blame tummy pain from some source. Crying babies tend to swallow more air, which means they pass more gas. Many parents try gas drops (simethicone, eg, Mylicon) for colic symptoms, but they have not been shown to make any difference. Likewise, parents are often tempted to change what they're feeding the baby. A breastfeeding mom may want to try restricting common allergens such as dairy products or soy from her diet, but this strategy rarely works, so she shouldn't make herself miserable in the process. Also, if mom is breastfeeding, please don't change to feeding your baby formula unless the baby's doctor specifically instructs you to do so. Even then, mom may want to pump expressed milk until you see how the formula works. Lactose is the sugar in human milk, so lactose intolerance, while common in older children and adults, is rare in newborns. A small number of formula-fed babies seem to improve with a change to soy or hydrolyzed formula, but when there's no vomiting, blood in the stool, or allergic symptoms such as eczema or hives, the formula is probably not the problem.

Gastroesophageal reflux disease (GERD) is another cause of discomfort we are tempted to treat when babies get colic. Crying from GERD tends to happen after babies eat, and often babies have other symptoms, such as excessive spitting up, chronic nasal congestion, cough, or wheeze. Fewer

76

5. Crying Foul: Why Is My Baby Crying and When Will It Stop?

than 5% of babies with colic actually have GERD. Medications to treat GERD seem to carry little risk, so they may be worth a try, but when there are no convincing symptoms, don't be surprised if they don't seem to work.

Mothers with colicky babies are more likely to suffer postpartum depression. This type of depression is not just moodiness that often accompanies hormonal changes in the week or two following childbirth. Postpartum depression is a very real and potentially deadly psychiatric condition that requires appropriate treatment. Colic also contributes to marital conflict in affected families, as stress and sleep deprivation make parents less tolerant of the normal difficulties of family life. Babies who have colic are more likely to be abused, often by stressed, exhausted fathers who become frustrated and start shaking the baby violently. Finally, babies are emotional sponges; your own stress and frustration can agitate your baby and feed into a vicious cycle of crying and distress.

what you can do
The most important element of any colic strategy is to get a handle on how the crying is affecting you and mom.

Start by paying attention to your own feelings about the crying. Dealing with colic is among the most frustrating experiences known to humankind. As men we are eager to solve problems, and colic presents a problem for which there is often no good solution. Your baby was just born, you want to protect her, and already you feel helpless to do something about whatever is making her cry. Anger often accompanies frustration, so take a moment to feel if your heart is beating fast or your fists are clenching. If so, it's time to take a moment to calm down before you do anything else.

This may seem obvious, but I'll say it anyway: *never, ever shake a baby!* Shaken baby syndrome is a leading cause of severe trauma and death among babies. It's not usually bad people who shake babies, just people who get too tired and too frustrated and lose control for one tragic moment. If you're starting to feel that upset, make sure your baby is in a safe place and step away from her. She can cry in her crib or in another person's arms for a few minutes while you get a breath of fresh air, pour a cup of tea, or do whatever else helps you calm down.

If you're feeling calm, run through your checklist. Is there an issue you can fix? No? Then it's on to what developmental specialist Harvey Karp, MD, calls the 5 Ss. Dr Karp recommends a series of interventions to make your newborn feel more like she's back in the womb. Start by swaddling your baby, being sure to leave her legs enough room to move around (see drawings below). Next, rest her in your lap on her side or tummy. This is not a safe position for her to sleep, but if you're holding her and she's awake, it's fine. Third, give her something to suck on, such as your finger or a pacifier if she'll take it. The sucking reflex is one of the best ways a baby can calm herself. Fourth, jiggle her gently with your knees or hands. The idea here is to create the same sensation she would have if she were in her car seat on top of the washing machine while it's in spin cycle. Fifth, make a prolonged hushing or shushing noise in her ear, roughly the same volume as her crying. As the cry quiets down, so does your shushing. If all this works, you can try putting your baby back in her crib, face up of course.

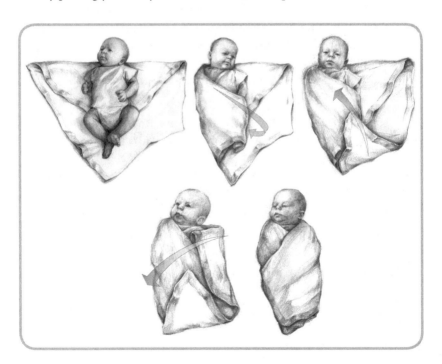

78

5. Crying Foul: Why Is My Baby Crying and When Will It Stop?

Of course these are not the only things you can try to address your baby's crying. Some parents find holding their baby while walking around helps. Others rely on a stroller ride, a bouncy chair, or the sound of a vacuum cleaner or washing machine to do the trick. Our own daughter calmed magically during Ricky Martin's performance of "Shake Your Bon-Bon" during the MTV Video Music Awards, inspiring us to buy 2 copies of his CD, one for home and another for child care.

Pharmacy shelves and Web sites are packed with products to treat colic, all with ringing endorsements from real parents! The thing to remember when looking at colic remedies is that colic gets better with time no matter what you do. That means whatever you were trying the day it went away appeared to work a miracle. Very few of these products have stood the test of scientific study, but there are a few that seem safe and possibly effective. Limited data suggest fennel extract, mixed herbal tea (with chamomile, licorice, fennel, and balm mint), and solutions of sugar water may decrease colicky crying somewhat. Other remedies, such as belladonna extract, are potentially dangerous, at least in theory. Remember that at this age your baby needs the calories contained in breast milk or formula. A regimen that includes more than an ounce or two of tea may interfere with her gaining weight appropriately. It's important to remember that plenty of things that are "natural" are not necessarily safe, especially for babies. We're still waiting to see if there are any long-term effects from exposure to "Shake Your Bon-Bon."

At 2:37 am, when your baby has been screaming for an hour and you hope you're awake because even your nightmares are better than this, you may feel like the crying is never, ever going to stop. The good news is that it will, and sooner than you think. The colicky period lasts even less time than Ricky Martin's musical career, ending when teething begins. Before long, when asked to complete the sentence, "Babies ___," you won't answer, "Cry." You'll say, "Drool."

6

that wasn't there yesterday: colors, spots, bumps, and rashes

there's no way I can prove this, but I suspect whoever coined the phrase, "As smooth as a baby's butt," had not really seen a lot of babies' butts. Our ideal of what skin should look like doesn't take into account the hard job it does for us: to protect all the squishy stuff inside us from the harsh assaults of the outside world. On top of that, skin plays a major role in regulating our temperature and, through its colors and smells, signaling others about our internal states. Because skin is the part of us everyone else can see, even minor skin issues can draw a lot of attention. It's worth our time to think a little about childhood skin issues, including those that affect baby's butts.

blue-blooded babies

The first thing you might notice about your baby's skin at birth is that he looks kind of blue. Don't worry, you have not fathered a Smurf. The blue color you're seeing (cyanosis) is not the color of the skin but of the underlying blood. Understanding why it looks blue takes knowing a little about fetal circulation, but this part is important because it will also help explain why some babies turn yellow in the days after birth.

Red blood cells have a basic job: take oxygen from where there's a lot of it and give that oxygen to tissues that need it. The amazing molecule that makes this possible is called *hemoglobin,* a protein in red cells that serves as a sort of cage for an iron molecule. It's this iron in the middle of the hemoglobin that actually holds onto the oxygen, releasing it when the time comes. When iron is oxygenated, hemoglobin is bright red in color. When the iron has given away its oxygen molecule, hemoglobin looks more blue.

In the womb the fetus relies completely on mom's bloodstream for oxygen. This means the fetus's red blood cells have to actually "steal" oxygen from mom's bloodstream as the blood cells pass near each other in the placenta. There are 2 differences between the fetus's blood and mom's that make this process more efficient.

The first difference is that fetuses have more blood cells in their blood than moms do. One way we measure blood's thickness is to see how much blood volume is made up of red cells. This percentage is called the *hematocrit.* A fetus's hematocrit is almost double the mother's, around 60% compared with her 30%.

Fetuses also make a slightly different kind of hemoglobin than their mothers. This fetal hemoglobin (hemoglobin F) is "stickier" for oxygen than mom's adult hemoglobin (hemoglobin A). This means that in the placenta oxygen molecules jump from mom's blood to the fetus's. Fetal hemoglobin, however, also breaks down faster than the adult kind, one cause of newborn jaundice (see "You Yellow-bellied…Baby?" on the next page).

What does all this have to do with blue-looking babies? The more red cells you have, the more blue your blood looks in the veins. Because newborns have thicker blood, their skin looks more blue than an adult's even when they have plenty of oxygen. While most healthy babies will pink up within a few minutes of delivery, you may still see a purple appearance to the hands and feet for a week or two after birth, a phenomenon called *acrocyanosis.* When your newborn is cold or agitated, his extremities look more purple, a result of blood flow slowing down in the hands and feet as blood vessels there tighten up. Acrocyanosis improves by the end of the first month of life, by which time your infant's hematocrit will have fallen by nearly half, to around 30%.

It's important to distinguish between acrocyanosis, a blue or purplish appearance to the hands and feet, and *central cyanosis,* a blue color of the face or chest. Central cyanosis is never normal; it may arise from serious heart disease, breathing problems, or seizures.

when to call the doctor

If your newborn has central cyanosis, check his airway, breathing, and pulse, and call emergency medical services (EMS) (911).

you yellow-bellied...baby?

Some babies take on a yellowish hue in the first few days of life. This condition, called jaundice, is often normal, but in severe cases it can cause life-threatening and irreversible brain injury. Monitoring and treating jaundice early can almost always ensure a good outcome.

To understand jaundice, we have to go back to the whole thing with fetal hemoglobin. Remember, babies are born with a relatively high hematocrit, and their red blood cells contain the less-stable hemoglobin F. Once newborns start breathing air, they no longer need all this extra hemoglobin, and having it there makes more work for the heart and lungs. The fetal hemoglobin starts to break down rapidly after birth, and during the first month of life the baby's hematocrit falls to nearly half of what it was in the womb. As all these red cells break down, the body has to recycle the hemoglobin that is released.

One by-product of this process is an orange-yellow chemical called *bilirubin*. (My father is a pediatrician, and I grew up thinking he had a troublesome colleague I'd never met, Dr Billy Ruben.) At low levels, bilirubin is perfectly harmless, but at higher concentrations bilirubin can cross from the newborn's bloodstream into the brain tissue, where it can cause permanent brain damage and, rarely, death. Babies who are weak from an infection, were born prematurely, or have a severe illness are at higher risk for this type of brain damage, called kernicterus.

Sometimes babies' blood cells break down faster than normal. This occurs most commonly when mother and fetus have different blood types, especially when the Rh factor is different. The Rh factor accounts for the "positive" or "negative" you hear when people talk about blood types. If the fetus has Rh-positive blood and mom does not, mom's immune system may make antibodies that attack the newborn's blood cells. The same thing can happen if the fetus has a different blood type, but the reactions are not usually as severe.

Jaundice first appears in the whites of the eyes. As bilirubin levels rise, a yellow tinge becomes noticeable in the face, then chest, then abdomen, and finally the legs. As bilirubin levels fall again, the yellow color appears to creep back up the body, disappearing last from the eyes. In the past doctors would guess the severity of jaundice by looking at how far down the body they could see yellow. This measure alone, however, is far from adequate to judge jaundice because anything from the baby's own skin pigment, to the light in the room, to the observer's inherent ability to perceive colors can affect the results.

Instead we use 2 methods to measure jaundice. Most newborn nurseries now have handheld bilirubin testing devices that measure jaundice levels by shining a special light through the newborn's skin. These devices are handy, but they don't measure bilirubin with enough precision to guide therapy. When the handheld meter suggests a concerning level of jaundice, we still have to prick the baby's heel and send a few drops of blood to the laboratory for testing.

Every hour the newborn is alive his brain gets better at protecting itself from jaundice. That means a "normal" bilirubin level is a moving target, with the number going up by the hour until the baby is around 5 days old, when numbers level off. A bilirubin value that is quite alarming at 24 hours of life may be no big deal just 1 day later. Since 2004, pediatricians have had a reliable chart to show us exactly how worried to be about a given bilirubin value based on the newborn's age and other risk factors for kernicterus.

To understand how we treat jaundice, you have to know a little more about bilirubin. In its initial form bilirubin dissolves better in oil than in water. (If you put it in vinaigrette it would rise to the top, but don't.) To get most toxins out of our bloodstream, our bodies have to convert them to a form that dissolves in water. For bilirubin this process involves a chemical reaction, called *conjugation,* performed by the liver. Bilirubin arrives at the liver in its unconjugated form; the liver conjugates it and sends it to the gallbladder, where it becomes part of bile and does the job of lending a greenish tint to poop. Some conjugated bilirubin is also cleared by the kidneys, which send it out with urine.

Anything that slows down the baby's peeing and pooping also slows down the release of bilirubin, so babies who are feeding poorly or becoming dehydrated are at higher risk of serious jaundice. This is one reason we advise parents to bring their newborns in for an examination a day or two after hospital discharge, so we can check the babies' weight and make sure they are not getting too yellow. Sometimes just eating more frequently is enough to improve jaundice.

There is, however, another way to alter the bilirubin molecule so it will fall to the bottom of the salad dressing, and that involves light. Light in the blue wavelength breaks down bilirubin into a different, water-soluble molecule called *lumirubin*. We use this process, called *phototherapy*, to treat most cases of jaundice. For mild cases, a blanket of fiber-optic threads can supply enough light directly to the newborn's skin. In more severe cases, we use 2 or even 3 different light sources to maximize the dose. Before phototherapy was widely available, doctors told parents to put their babies in sunshine. That was also before central air conditioning and the hole in the ozone layer. Today we prefer to use medically approved phototherapy devices rather than putting babies at very real risk for low body temperatures, skin cancer, or sunburn.

In rare cases, jaundice progresses so rapidly that even phototherapy is not adequate treatment. In those cases doctors perform an exchange transfusion, literally taking out a portion of the newborn's own blood and replacing it with donor blood. Fortunately, this once-common practice has grown quite rare as we've gotten better at preventing jaundice and treating it in its early stages.

One harmless cause of jaundice can be breastfeeding itself. Human milk contains enzymes that actually cause unconjugated bilirubin, leading it to be absorbed back into the bloodstream. Breastfeeding jaundice, however, is not dangerous and does not usually require treatment. Sometimes the baby's doctor will have mom stop nursing for a day or two just to prove that it is the cause of jaundice, but once the cause is known it's safe to resume breastfeeding.

One tip, however, will save you a needless trip to the doctor—if you have a jaundiced looking infant who has started eating solids, look first to see if the whites of his eyes are yellow. Beta-carotene in carrots, sweet potatoes, and other yellow-orange vegetables can lend the skin an orange color, but this color does not affect the eyes.

when to call the doctor

When jaundice appears anytime after the first several days of life, it can be a concerning sign of disease. The bottom line is that if you think your baby looks yellow, make sure the doctor checks him out.

birthmarks of distinction

There are a variety of common skin discolorations you might notice as soon as you hold your newborn. One of the most common is the stork bite, salmon patch, or nevus flammeus. All 3 terms refer to a reddish-pink discoloration of the skin that is not at all raised. Stork bites got their name because they occur most commonly on the back of the neck in the hairline, where you might imagine the proverbial stork was carrying the baby. They are caused by mildly dilated blood vessels under the skin. Stork bites on the back of the neck rarely go completely away, but over time they often get covered by hair.

Another creatively named birthmark is the mongolian spot. These are broad, non-raised areas of darker pigmentation, often on the back or buttocks. I'm guessing they got their name because that's where you might imagine the proverbial Genghis Khan was carrying the baby, but check me, I might be wrong on that one. Mongolian spots occur more commonly in more darkly pigmented children. They almost always disappear by age 5 years.

Another skin condition that tends to affect more darkly pigmented babies is called *pustular melanosis.* It got its name because these babies develop small pustules on the skin that pop and leave dark marks with increased

when to call the doctor

If you notice any pustules on your baby's skin, be sure to alert his doctor. While pustular melanosis is completely harmless and goes away on its own, other causes of pustules include skin infections with *Staphylococcus aureus* and herpes simplex virus, both of which can be life-threatening.

skin pigment (melanin). Sometimes the condition occurs in the womb and all you see when the baby is born are the spots.

Many babies are born with little, white, raised pearly lesions, especially on the nose, chin, and cheeks. These lesions, called *milia* after the Latin word for seed, come from retained glandular secretions in the skin. They go away on their own within a few weeks and do not require any special scrubbing. The confusingly named miliaria (same root) is better known as prickly heat or heat rash and results from blocked sweat glands. These lesions are red and tend to occur in skin folds. They occur when newborns get overheated from warm weather or being bundled.

On the subject of little white bumps, my least favorite rash name is erythema toxicum, or E tox if you're lazy. These lesions look like ant bites, with tiny white bumps surrounded by small, flat red areas. They come and go over a period of hours, and usually they only occur in the first couple of weeks of life. There is nothing at all toxic about them, and they affect up to 70% of newborns. Historians attribute the name to the ancient Mesopotamians, who first described the condition and thought it was "nature's method of cleansing the child of impure blood of the mother" (I'm not making this one up).

Two more common types of birthmarks are named after food and drink. One is the strawberry hemangioma, known to doctors as capillary hemangioma. These birthmarks are caused by a tangle of enlarged blood vessels. They may begin as pale patches, but they turn red in the first week or two of life. Lesions often grow larger over the first year, but they usually shrink and fade or even disappear completely by school age. Another birthmark, the port-wine stain, is also caused by enlarged blood vessels, but these purple-red lesions are not at all raised. They often cover broad areas of the face or neck. Port-wine stains do not go away on their own, but dermatologists and plastic surgeons have a variety of therapies to treat them.

acne for babies

The same maternal hormones that cause breast development, vaginal discharge, and even small periods in newborns can also cause acne, at least for the first 3 to 4 months of life. The lesions are the same as you see in adolescents, with blackheads and whiteheads *(comedones)* and sometimes red pustules in the "T-zone" (for those of you who don't watch MTV, that's the forehead, nose, and chin). Because the acne will eventually go away without scarring, pediatricians rarely recommend treatment beyond washing the baby's face with mild soap and water. For severe cases, some doctors use benzoyl peroxide, mild steroids, or an antifungal cream called ketoconazole.

cradle cap

Another version of an adult disease that affects newborns is *seborrheic dermatitis* (dandruff), except that when we see it on a baby, we call it cradle cap, at least when it involves the scalp. Seborrheic dermatitis can spread to the oily areas of the skin behind the ears, beside the nose, and at the neck. In addition to the scale you may see areas of redness or even cracking of the skin.

The easiest way to remove scales from your baby's scalp is to apply baby oil to the affected area and brush gently. Seborrheic dermatitis also responds to the same treatments we use for adult dandruff: selenium-containing shampoos like Selsun Blue and Head & Shoulders and mild topical steroids like hydrocortisone. You'll just want to be careful to keep the shampoo out of your newborn's eyes because it's not necessarily pH balanced.

yeastie beasties

We talked in Chapter 4 about yeast *(Candida)* rashes in the diaper area. Another place yeast can strike is in the folds of the neck, especially around 4 to 9 months of age when infants are drooling a lot and their necks are comparatively short. Like in the diaper area, the neck folds become the sort of warm, moist, dark environment yeast just loves. As with diaper rash, the drier you can keep this area, the better. The same antifungal medicines, nystatin and clotrimazole, can treat infections in both locations.

eczema

Eczema is one of the most common skin conditions affecting babies and children. You'll see signs of skin inflammation including rough scaly patches, clusters of tiny bumps, or red, cracked skin. The location of these lesions depends somewhat on the age of the child. Infants often get eczema on the face, neck, and chest, while toddlers and children tend to get flares in the folds of the elbow, behind the knees, and at the wrists and ankles. The abdomen, back, and buttocks are common locations for eczema at any age.

Eczema is really a version of allergic disease, just like allergic rhinitis and asthma, and some of our treatments for eczema include allergy medicines like hydroxyzine (eg, Atarax), cetirizine (eg, Zyrtec), and loratadine (eg, Claritin). The inflammation, however, tends to get much worse when the skin loses its natural oily barrier against allergens, so much of eczema therapy focuses on keeping or replacing these oils. Bathing, for example, removes oil from the skin. To prevent or treat eczema, you should only bathe your baby when he clearly needs it, usually every 2 or 3 days. Keep baths short and use lukewarm rather than hot water because hot water removes more oil. Go light on the soap, which is really just a chemical designed to wash away oil from the skin's surface. In severe cases you can even add a few drops of mineral oil to the bathwater.

what you can do

Because scents and colors in skin products may worsen eczema, it's better to restrict yourself to using only creams or lotions that don't look or smell pretty, even if they are marketed for babies. Likewise, scented diaper wipes, shampoos, laundry detergents, or dryer sheets may worsen eczema. When looking for a moisturizer to treat eczema, remember, thicker is better. Oils like baby oil don't have a lot of sticking power. Lotions are a little thicker, but they still have high water content and don't tend to add a lot of oil back to the skin. Creams are better, especially if they're thick enough that you have to scoop them out of a pot with your fingers. The most effective moisturizers are ointments, usually petrolatum-based. Because ointments can lend a certain sheen to the skin, many parents save them for use at bedtime or in areas normally covered by clothes.

Corticosteroids applied to the skin address the allergic part of eczema and the need for moisture. These drugs are not like the steroids some athletes or body builders use to pump up; instead, corticosteroids suppress the overactive immune system that causes allergic reactions. Corticosteroids come in different degrees of strength; only the weakest forms of hydrocortisone are sold over the counter. Stronger steroids can cause permanent changes in the skin that look like stretch marks (striae), especially when people use them for prolonged periods. We rarely use them on the face for this reason. If your child's doctor has prescribed a steroid for eczema, be sure you read the directions carefully and only put it where directed and for no longer than specified.

In some cases, food allergies can make eczema worse. Doctors will sometimes advise parents to change formulas or avoid feeding certain foods to make it better. This strategy can be worth a try, but most cases of eczema don't get better with dietary changes. Unless your child has been diagnosed with a known food allergy, it's often a wild goose chase trying to figure out what food to eliminate.

when to call the doctor

Because inflammation from eczema damages the skin's protective layers, children with eczema are targets for skin infections like impetigo or cellulitis. If you see that your child has a yellowish crust or weeping sores, make sure a doctor sees him immediately. In most cases these infections require antibiotic therapy.

ringworm: it's not a worm

You can stop reading now if you want. For many people, just knowing ringworm is not caused by a worm is all they really need. You, however, may want to know that this common childhood rash is actually caused by a fungus. Ringworm (tinea corporis) usually starts as a little red bump but then spreads outward in a circular or oval shape, creating a slightly raised, reddened border and a flat, scaly inner area. There may be more than one ring, but if you see lots of them chances are it's another kind of rash, like eczema. Ringworm may itch, but often the itching is mild.

what you can do

Treating ringworm is straightforward as long as it does not involve the scalp. Tinea on the body or face responds very nicely to any number of over-the-counter antifungal medications, including clotrimazole, miconazole, terbinafine, and tolnaftate. You can find these medications in the athlete's foot section of your drug store; athlete's foot (tinea pedis) is just a variation on the same infection. So, for that matter, is jock itch (tinea cruris).

The fungi that cause ringworm come from so many sources it's hard to say where any given child picks it up. Direct contact with an infected person's skin is one way to contract ringworm, but cats, dogs, and even soil harbor the same fungi. Ringworm in the scalp may be carried on a comb, hairbrush, or hat, so an infected child shouldn't share these items with others.

There are 2 important things to remember when treating ringworm. First, the fungi are actually growing beyond the visible ring, so you need to apply the cream about an inch past the border of the lesion. Second, you should treat the area for about a week after the visible lesion is gone to make sure it doesn't come back. This is hard to do because you no longer have the spot there to remind you. Count on treating anywhere from 2 to 4 weeks to get the best results.

when to call the doctor

When ringworm gets into the scalp (tinea capitis), treatment gets more complicated. Because the fungi are growing down in the hair follicles, medicated creams and shampoos can't reach them. Instead, your child's doctor will prescribe an oral medication, usually griseofulvin. It usually takes 6 weeks of daily therapy to ensure a cure. You may also want to use an antifungal shampoo (terbinafine or ketoconazole) to control itching and prevent your child from infecting others.

don't touch that! poison ivy/oak/sumac

An ardent nature explorer, I spent my childhood in an intense personal study of the effects of poison ivy, which, as far as I could tell, was the only plant widespread in my neighborhood. Regardless of the offending plant, these rashes are all forms of contact dermatitis, a skin allergy against the oils produced by these weeds. Contact dermatitis develops slowly, often 1 to 3 days after a child actually contacts the plant that caused it. Remember that even if your child hasn't played outside, pets can bring the oils inside on their fur and transfer them to your child's skin.

The rash often spreads over the next few days, with red bumps or water blisters starting in the areas that got the heaviest exposure and working toward more lightly exposed skin. This pattern gives the illusion that scratching is spreading the rash, but unless the child hasn't had a bath or shower since the exposure, this is not really the case. Most cases of contact dermatitis are terribly itchy, and controlling the itch is the best way to prevent secondary skin infections like impetigo.

Because contact dermatitis is an allergy, corticosteroids and antihistamines work best to control it. You can buy low-strength hydrocortisone cream over the counter, but for more severe cases your child's doctor may want to prescribe something stronger. In cases involving the face or large areas of the body surface, we sometimes use oral corticosteroids like prednisone. For itching control, oral antihistamines like diphenhydramine (eg, Benadryl), cetirizine (eg, Zyrtec), or loratadine (eg, Claritin) can be very helpful. Benadryl lotion applied to the skin doesn't really seem to do much, and old remedies like calamine lotion are not as effective as steroids. Cool compresses might help control the itching and cut down on scratching. The rash usually takes 2 to 3 weeks to go away.

bugging out

Among the most common skin lesions of childhood are simple insect bites and stings. The most common offender is the mosquito, but fleas, bedbugs, and no-see-ums (biting flies) also find kids tasty. It is important to distinguish between insects that bite and insects that sting; while insect bites may cause really big, itchy bumps, they don't cause life-threatening allergic reactions.

Especially in toddlers, insect bites can leave surprisingly large, itchy bumps. Mosquito bites will be scattered on exposed areas, whereas flea bites tend to cluster on the ankles and legs or where clothing is tight, such as at the waistband. Bedbugs may bite in a row of 2 or 3 lesions, and they like to work the night shift. Bites respond to the same hydrocortisone cream and oral antihistamines used for contact dermatitis, and cool compresses can help control the itching.

Parents often have questions about the safety of insect repellents. Most insect repellents sold in the United States contain DEET (N, N-diethyl-meta-toluamide), in concentrations between 6% and 30%. Higher concentrations of DEET last longer but don't repel insects any better, so use the lowest concentration needed for the time your child will spend outdoors. DEET is not approved for infants younger than 2 months. Regardless of the child's age, one application a day is all that is safe. Putting DEET on repeatedly increases the risk of toxicity. A newer alternative to DEET is picaridin, for which the same safety rules apply.

Insects that sting actually inject venom into the skin, causing a painful, burning, itching local reaction. Stinging insects include bees, wasps, hornets, and fire ants. Fire ants bite with one end while stinging with the other, making them the only insect that does both. Bees often leave their stingers in the skin, where they continue to inject venom. Remove the stinger cleanly with a credit card or your fingernail as soon as possible, taking care not to squeeze the attached venom sac.

when to call the doctor

If your child has any wheezing, light-headedness, or swelling beyond the immediate area of a sting, call EMS immediately. Also call EMS if the child develops hives all over instead of one bump at the site of the sting.

Ticks represent a special kind of insect bite, as ticks can carry diseases including lyme disease, Rocky Mountain spotted fever, and ehrlichiosis. The good news is that of the millions of tick bites children suffer every year, very few of them actually result in any disease. As many as 80% of tick bites occur without the victim even knowing, as the ticks attach, feed, and fall off painlessly. If you do see a tick on your child, however, there is a right and a wrong way to react.

Let's knock out the wrong stuff first, just in case you're already holding a match. Put the match down before you hurt someone. Do not then pick up petroleum jelly, nail polish, alcohol, or any sharp, hot, or cold objects. These also will not work. Instead get a pair of fine-tipped tweezers or one of those special tick-removal tools you can buy at your local wilderness outfitters.

You're aiming for the tick's head, taking care not to squeeze the abdomen and the tick's gastric contents into your child's bloodstream. If you can, grasp the head, flip the body straight up, and pull steadily upward, trying to dislodge the tick's mouth parts from your child's skin. If the tick is still moving, you know you've done it perfectly. With the smaller deer tick it may be impossible to isolate the head, in which case you'll have to use a credit card or similar object to scrape the tick from the child's skin. When you're done, wash the area with soap and water and apply a little antibiotic ointment. If you can't get all the mouth parts or head out of the skin, you might have to have a doctor examine your child. In some cases the skin will shed the parts without help, but they can sometimes cause skin infections.

when to call the doctor

Few tick bites require a doctor's care, but there are some things to be on the lookout for. If your child develops a fever, severe headache, joint pain, or red, non-raised spots within 2 weeks following a tick bite, the doctor should see him. Lyme disease usually starts with a target lesion, a bull's-eye–shaped ring around the site of the original bite. While lyme disease is potentially dangerous, it usually responds well to antibiotic therapy when caught early. Any sign of skin infection, such as pus, warmth, a lump, or a red area, deserves a doctor's examination.

mastering MRSA

In the past a chapter on common skin conditions would not have needed a section on methicillin-resistant *Staphylococcus aureus* (MRSA). Thanks to overuse of antibiotics in humans and livestock, however, MRSA lesions now account for a shockingly large number of pediatric office visits and hospitalizations. Two properties make MRSA special. First, the bacteria are resistant to many commonly used antibiotics. As if this were not scary enough, they also have a mutation that makes them better able to invade body tissue and cause large, deep lesions compared with garden-variety staph infections. Around one-third of children are thought to harbor MRSA, although it does not usually make these kids sick.

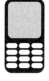

when to call the doctor

As a rule, lesions that drain pus are never normal and always require a doctor's attention. If you see a growing tender, red lesion on your child's skin, he needs to see a doctor as soon as possible. Sometimes these lesions respond to oral antibiotics or simple drainage, but they can easily progress to a stage that requires intravenous antibiotics and surgical drainage.

Staph lesions start as red areas or small pustules, but they often grow quickly to become large, red, warm, pus-filled abscesses. In younger children they commonly affect the diaper area, where chronic skin irritation and poor hygiene create an inviting environment for infection. In older children the lesions can appear anywhere.

what you can do

Preventing methicillin-resistant *S aureus* is a matter of good skin care practices. Keep kids' fingernails short so they don't scratch themselves. Keep their hands clean and wash cuts and scrapes with soap and water, then protect them with a clean bandage and change the bandage daily. Discourage your child from sharing towels, washcloths, or clothing with other kids, even if those kids look clean and lesion-free.

this is zit

No discussion of common skin lesions would be complete without a nod to acne, the near-universal condition that seems to say, "So you thought adolescence wasn't already hard enough?" At its root, acne is a case of too much of a good thing. During puberty, oil glands that protect the skin from conditions like eczema go into overdrive, producing an excess of the oil, sebum, that keeps skin moist. These glands also shed dead skin cells, which can collect and block pores, causing whiteheads and blackheads (together called comedones). As these lesions become inflamed and infected, they can produce pustules, nodules, or cysts. Cysts only affect about 5% of patients, but these deep-seated lesions sometimes cause permanent scars.

Acne seems tailor-made to frustrate teens. Just at the moment they care the most about their appearance, lesions crop up on their faces, backs, and chests. At a time of life marked by haste and urgency, treating acne requires patience, and the goal is to reduce severity of lesions rather than make them disappear completely. You'll have to remind your teens that most of the kids they see on television and in magazines have clear faces only thanks to the magic of makeup and digital correction.

Acne will tempt your teen to do things that make it worse. Face-washing, for example, is a good idea done twice daily with a mild soap or a product like salicylic acid that dissolves dead skin cells. Washing more often or rubbing too hard with a washcloth, however, is likely to make things worse. Likewise, the compulsion to squeeze acne lesions is nearly universal, but it's also a good way to turn a mild zit into a really severe one by driving the inflammation into deeper layers of the skin.

The best over-the-counter acne treatments share one ingredient: benzoyl peroxide. Benzoyl peroxide comes in a variety of forms, including washes, lotions, and gels. Concentrations range from 2.5% to 10%. This is a drug that requires patience to use. Starting with too high a concentration will just inflame the skin and cause redness and peeling. Your teen should start just once a day with a wash or lotion; if the skin isn't red or peeling, he may first increase applications to twice a day, then increase concentration, making no more than one change a week. The 10% gel is the strongest form available over the counter.

Retinoids are another class of acne medications that can be applied to the skin, but they require a doctor's prescription. Products, including Retin A, Differin, and other brands, come as creams or gels. Kids using retinoids are at greater risk of sunburn, so it's important they avoid strong sun exposure and, of course, tanning salons. Just as with benzoyl peroxide, it's a good idea to start with a low-potency form and move up slowly if needed.

Pustules and cysts in acne usually contain a bacteria called *Propionibacterium acnes,* a bacteria that thrives on the excess sebum teen oil glands secrete. Antibiotics applied to the skin or taken in pill form can help control these lesions by fighting the bacteria. Some prescription acne preparations actually combine antibiotics and benzoyl peroxide.

The strongest acne medication is also the riskiest to use. Isotretinoin, sold as Accutane, Amnesteem, Claravis, and Sotret, is a pill for severe cases of cystic acne. Isotretinoin can cause liver disease and severe birth defects, so doctors often require blood and pregnancy tests prior to prescribing it. It may also worsen depression, so close monitoring is important for patients who have a history of psychiatric problems. Because isotretinoin requires so much specialized care, it's best prescribed by a physician who has extensive experience using it.

Skin is an organ that's easy to take for granted, but it has a big job to do, and it's always visible. Working with your child's doctor, you should be able to address most skin issues with simple interventions. With proper care even your baby's butt may be as smooth as…as, uh…OK, I got nothing.

7

a good shot: vaccines and common sense

let me clarify right now: my 3 children are all vaccinated, fully and on time. All of the people I work with can say the same thing, as can the overwhelming majority of pediatricians in the United States today. Every week a parent tells me some scary vaccine story passed on by an uncle, a friend, or a well-meaning coworker (the same one who asks why you wore that tie with that shirt), and I talk to parents every day about why the benefits of immunizations far outweigh the risks, using my own kids as examples. I hope the parents I speak with feel the same way I do whenever I board an airplane and look at the pilot—if he didn't believe this thing were safe to fly, he wouldn't be in it with me!

Vaccines save lives. In the course of my own career I've seen hospitalizations from rotavirus and invasive *Pneumococcus* infections fall off dramatically. My father, also a pediatrician, has witnessed the near-disappearance of *Haemophilus influenzae* type b, a bacterial infection that was once a common cause of deadly meningitis, intellectual disability, and deafness. Deaths and severe disability from measles have nearly vanished from this country, and polio, once a common cause of childhood paralysis and death, is now essentially unknown. Chances are you've never heard of anyone dying of lockjaw (tetanus), whooping cough (pertussis), or diphtheria, even though in 1921 diphtheria killed 12,230 Americans. Pediatricians who practiced before the modern vaccine era feel we're living in an age of miracles.

The problem with successful preventive practices is they create the illusion that they are not necessary. What happens if you change your car's oil? Your engine doesn't lock up. If you change your home's central air filters? Your heat pump doesn't conk out in January. And if you vaccinate your child? She doesn't end up hospitalized or dying of a vaccine-preventable disease. In other words, dramatic success looks like…nothing. Naturally, some people ask, "If nothing ever happens, then why should I do it?"

The answer is that while vaccine-preventable diseases have grown rarer, they are still out there, and in some cases they remain shockingly common. We have enjoyed the luxury of retiring one vaccine, for smallpox, once the disease it protected against was eliminated all over the world in 1977. Whooping cough, on the other hand, remains a common illness in American teens and adults, who can transmit it easily to unvaccinated children. Measles have seen recent dramatic resurgence in unvaccinated American populations. Tetanus remains one rusty nail away from every child. As much as we would love to eradicate these diseases, their threat is far from gone. In some cases, it's as close as the person next to you.

nuts, bolts, and antibodies: how do vaccines work?

Like a modern jetliner, the immune system is an incredibly complex mechanism that does what would seem to be a simple job. The immune system is supposed to identify whether a given thing in your body is supposed to be there and attack whatever doesn't belong. It does this by recognizing parts of proteins or carbohydrates, called antigens. Each antigen has a specific shape, like a key. The cells of the immune system generate proteins, called antibodies, that fit these keys like a lock. When these antibodies come into contact with a familiar antigen, they stimulate the immune system to attack it in a variety of ways. Once your body makes antibodies against a particular invader, those antibodies hang out for years, sometimes for the rest of your life. When the invader reappears, they can mount a rapid attack and defeat it before you get too sick.

If the immune system has never before seen a given antigen, it can take a while to build up a strong enough response to fight off the disease. The response occurs much faster when antibodies that recognize the invader already exist. With many illnesses, such as colds, the body is able to generate a response before the infection overwhelms its defenses. Other diseases move too fast, causing serious illness and death before the immune system has time to fight off the first infection. Vaccines give us a way to teach the immune system to battle a given disease without exposing the child to the risks of actually getting the illness. In some cases we use a weakened form of a live virus, like measles or varicella (chickenpox), to introduce antigens without risking harm to the child. In many cases, vaccines only include a handful of proteins from the infectious agent.

No vaccine is 100% effective. Effectiveness rates actually vary from 85% to 98% depending on the vaccine. Some children have defects in their immune systems that limit how well they can fight off certain diseases. In other cases, natural genetic variations in the child's immune function keep her from mounting a vigorous response. Some children, like those on immunosuppressive medications for cancer or organ transplant, cannot safely receive vaccines against some diseases. Finally, because many vaccines require multiple doses to become fully effective, infants and young children may only be partially protected against a disease, even when they've had all their vaccines on time. For this reason, we rely on what's called herd immunity. If most children are successfully protected against a given disease, the chances of a vulnerable child getting it are very low. This herd immunity has a tipping point. With measles, for example, when less than 90% of the population is protected, the whole group becomes a powder keg, awaiting the spark of just one infected child to blow up in an epidemic.

but i heard...

Rumors and suspicions about vaccines would seem to be a modern phenomenon, born of the Internet and the 24-hour news cycle. In reality, however, myths about vaccines have circulated ever since 1796 when English physician Edward Jenner discovered he could protect people against smallpox by giving them the benign infection cowpox instead. As Jenner was attacked in pamphlets and editorial cartoons, you know he had to be like, "Uh, guys, I'm saving you from a scourge that has wiped out entire civilizations. A little thank-you, maybe?" Thus was set the tone of the vaccine debate for the next 2 centuries and beyond. But think about this—thanks to Jenner and those who followed him, smallpox no longer exists as a human disease.

At times people have had good reasons to be concerned. Live polio vaccine, for example, used to cause polio in a handful of Americans every year. Compared with the number of cases the vaccine prevented, benefits far outweighed the risks, but as the threat of polio shrank we stopped using the live form of the vaccine, and today we only use the inactivated polio vaccine, which contains a handful of antigens instead of a weakened live virus.

Likewise, the whole-cell pertussis vaccine used to cause very high fevers in a substantial number of children. While these fevers were not dangerous, they were unpleasant. We now use an acellular pertussis vaccine with a much lower rate of adverse effects. The Food and Drug Administration (FDA) recalled the older version of rotavirus vaccine as soon as it became clear the vaccine could cause rare cases of intestinal obstructions. When newer versions of the rotavirus vaccine came out, the Centers for Disease Control and Prevention (CDC) followed millions of patients in Mexico and Brazil and 800,000 patients in the United States, finding that so far any increased risk is minute for both vaccines. In the meantime the vaccines have prevented tens of thousands of infant hospitalizations.

The system we use to ensure vaccine safety is aggressive and proactive, and it errs on the side of caution. In addition to extensive pre-approval testing and post-approval monitoring, we have the Vaccine Adverse Event Reporting System (VAERS). Through VAERS, doctors and family members can report any medical incident that seems related to a vaccine. The CDC and FDA investigate the incident to determine whether the vaccine played a role. VAERS receives around 30,000 reports a year, most of them for mild symptoms like fever or irritability.

Figuring out cause and effect in medicine is not as easy as just saying, "This happened, then that happened, so this caused that." By that logic you could decide that geese flying south cause leaves to change color in the fall. Instead we have to know how often a given outcome happens, then see if it happens any more often after the suspected cause. One example of this process involves a rare nerve disease called Guillain-Barré syndrome. In Guillain-Barré, the immune system attacks cells that insulate nerve fibers, causing muscle weakness. Normally, about 1 child in a million develops

Guillain-Barré syndrome each year, usually following a viral infection like a cold or influenza. Through extensive monitoring we've learned that the nasal influenza vaccine (using a weakened virus) increases that number to about 2 children in a million. The vaccine saves many more lives than that, and most children who contract Guillain-Barré recover, but we no longer offer the live influenza vaccine to children who have had the condition before. To discover a side effect that is literally a one-in-a-million event requires studying millions and millions of children, but that's exactly what VAERS does.

It's the same sort of monitoring that tells us that vaccines do not cause autism. Children get vaccines in the second year of life, and autism symptoms often become obvious in the second year of life. It's not at all unusual for a child to be diagnosed with autism within days or weeks of getting her vaccines. To know whether the vaccine caused autism, however, you need to know how often kids are diagnosed with autism when they have never been vaccinated. As it turns out, we have that answer, and not just in one study or in a small study but in a number of truly vast studies. In fact, unvaccinated children are diagnosed with autism just as often as vaccinated children.

Many of the vaccine rumors have to do with mercury, specifically a mercury-based preservative called thimerosal. Again, multiple studies of huge numbers of patients have proven that thimerosal in vaccines never harmed anyone, but even if those studies were never done it still wouldn't matter—vaccine manufacturers voluntarily removed thimerosal from childhood vaccines in 2001 (it remains in a single type of influenza vaccine that we usually only administer to children older than 3 years, and it remains in barely measurable amounts in others). If thimerosal had been the cause of autism, rates of autism diagnosis should have plummeted since then, but of course they have not.

Once mercury became a nonissue in vaccines, rumors turned to aluminum, which is used in small amounts to boost the body's immune response to some vaccines. We don't realize it, but aluminum exposure is a routine part of life on Earth. The amount of aluminum in vaccines compares with that contained in just 33 ounces of infant formula. Other rumors involve vaccines containing antifreeze, which is ethylene glycol, a poison to humans. Vaccines don't contain ethylene glycol; in some cases they contain small quantities of polyethylene glycol, a different chemical that is safe.

Yet another common misunderstanding involves vaccines "overwhelming" the immune system. Understandably, parents look at their vulnerable-appearing babies and worry that they should limit how much work their immune systems have to do. Some parents fret that vaccines will "weaken" their baby's immune system somehow. These beliefs stem from a misunderstanding of how the immune system works. First, the number of antigens in the currently required vaccine regimen from birth to age 5 is a bit more than 200. Compare this with the thousands of antigens a single cold virus introduces to the body, and then consider that most babies get multiple such infections in the first year of life. The antigens in vaccines are a tiny drop in a very large bucket as far as the baby's immune system is concerned. What vaccines do is strengthen the immune system by helping it fight diseases that, without vaccines, are likely to overwhelm the baby's defenses.

None of the above will satisfy your coworker who read that vaccines are the product of a vast conspiracy of pharmaceutical companies, doctors, and government agencies. As a doctor the medical literature is what enables me to do my job; I trust it. I also have never heard of any conspiracy theory that could be disproved by mere evidence.

tear-free vaccination, even for your baby

Many children and parents associate a trip to the pediatrician with shots. Not infrequently, new moms tell me they plan to make dad hold the baby for vaccines while they leave the room. There are actually a couple of vaccines that we don't give as an injection, specifically the oral rotavirus vaccine and nasal influenza vaccine. It would be great if we could give them all by mouth, but vaccines contain proteins and complex sugars that are digested quickly in the stomach, so the only way to get most of them into contact with the immune system is to inject them into the skin or muscle.

The good news is that pediatricians have gotten better at minimizing or even eliminating the pain of vaccination. For one thing, we can often administer multiple vaccines in a single injection. The current record is 5 (diphtheria, tetanus, acellular pertussis, inactivated poliovirus, and *H influenzae* type b). Thanks to combination vaccines, the most separate injections many children receive at any given wellness examination is 3. We usually give these vaccines in the thighs during the first few years of life and in the shoulder muscles after that. When staff are available, they can use both legs at the same time to minimize the duration of discomfort.

Because what pain there is tends to be experienced as a single event, I discourage parents from spreading vaccines out over multiple visits. There is no medical reason to do so, and it tends to prolong the discomfort for everyone.

We now also have a variety of effective pain-control techniques. Cooling spray can numb the skin just before shots are given so there is no poking sensation. Another method uses a plastic plate covered with small points to block pain sensation. Topical anesthetic creams can work in as little as 15 minutes to achieve the same effect. For babies who are nursing, breastfeeding during a vaccination can provide significant pain relief as well. Even without using any of these techniques, most babies calm down very quickly after their shots with being held. The calm in your voice and the firm reassurance of your embrace tell your baby that everything is fine. Remember, the shots may hurt for a moment, but the protection they're giving your baby is good for a lifetime.

By far the most common adverse reactions following vaccination are fever and fussiness, and sometimes there may be a little redness or swelling at the injection site. Many parents ask if they should give acetaminophen (eg, Tylenol, PediaCare Fever Reducer) or ibuprofen (eg, Motrin, Advil) prior to the vaccine visit. In the past we have encouraged using these medications to reduce any discomfort or potential fever from vaccines. Some newer studies have questioned whether giving acetaminophen might make the vaccines slightly less effective, so some pediatricians are no longer recommending it.

when to call the doctor

No symptoms after receiving vaccines should be dramatic. If your child has a temperature above 102°F or a fever that lasts more than a few days, or if she is unusually fussy, you should still consult her doctor and not just assume her symptoms are from vaccines.

Any medication or vaccine has the potential to cause an allergic reaction, sometimes a severe one. Rates of severe allergic reactions with vaccines run in the 1 per million range, making them quite rare.

when to call the doctor

If you notice your child getting hives, wheezing, or seeming unusually ill shortly after she gets vaccines, alert office staff if you're still there or call emergency medical services (911) if you're not.

One last note on improving the wellness examination and discipline in general: please, please never tell your child, "If you don't behave, that doctor's going to give you a shot." First of all, she will think injections are punishment, not a way to make or keep her healthy. Second, if you make threats you can't keep, your child will quickly learn to ignore you. You can't make the doctor give her a shot, so if she calls your bluff, you got nothing. I swear the next time I hear a parent say that I'm going to turn around and give the parent a shot. Except that in my practice the doctors don't actually give the shots.

hepatitis B: more livers are living

The first vaccine your baby will be offered is against hepatitis B. Hepatitis B is a virus that infects the liver, leading in some cases to liver failure and death. This vaccine is unique in that we can start protecting babies as soon as they are born. It has been a massively successful vaccine, reducing childhood and adolescent deaths from hepatitis B by more than 95% since its introduction in 1991. The vaccine is given as 3 or 4 doses in the first year of life.

Hepatitis B is transmitted through infected blood and sexual fluids. For this reason, many parents ask why we would vaccinate babies, as they are unlikely to share needles or have sex. The answer is that hepatitis B is so contagious that a simple scratch, bite, or paper cut is enough to transmit it. Even using an infected person's toothbrush can spread the disease. Mothers who carry hepatitis B can give it to their babies at birth, and there are special precautions to take when we know a mom is infected. Before the vaccine, thousands of children contracted hepatitis B infections every year.

rotavirus: when "tummy bug" is an understatement

There are tons of viruses that cause vomiting and diarrhea, but rotavirus is especially nasty, infecting infants and young children and causing life-threatening fluid losses. Rotavirus is highly contagious, able to live for days on contaminated surfaces and toys. There is no medicine to treat rotavirus once a child contracts it; therapy focuses on replacing fluid lost through vomiting and diarrhea.

Prior to the approval of the rotavirus vaccine in 2006, these infections caused more than 200,000 emergency department visits, 55,000 to 70,000 hospitalizations, and 20 to 60 deaths a year in the United States. The vaccine has cut hospitalizations by 98% since its introduction. Rotavirus vaccine is given by mouth, not as a shot. Infants get the vaccine in 2 or 3 doses depending on the timing and brand of vaccine, at age 2 months, 4 months, and in some cases, 6 months.

diphtheria, tetanus, and pertussis: the trifecta

Vaccines against diphtheria, tetanus, and pertussis have been available in some combination for decades. Formulations vary by age, with the DTaP vaccine recommended for 5 doses between birth and age 5 years, then a booster of Tdap at age 11 to 12 years. Additionally, adults younger than 65 and older teens who have never gotten Tdap should get at least one Tdap injection to protect against pertussis. The Td vaccine protects against tetanus and diphtheria only, and adults require a booster every 10 years. Td also protects patients who have suffered burns or severe cuts and are vulnerable to tetanus.

Tetanus, or lockjaw, may be the disease most familiar to most people. Tetanus infections occur when the bacteria *Clostridium tetani* enters the body from contaminated cuts, burns, or bites. The bacteria excretes a toxin that causes muscles to lock up, starting around the mouth. The disease progresses quickly to total paralysis, killing around 1 in 4 people who get it. Prior to the vaccine, there were around 1,300 cases of tetanus a year in the United States. Since the vaccine became available, tetanus cases have fallen by more than 96%, with most victims being unvaccinated.

Diphtheria, thankfully, is almost unknown now, although at one time it infected 175,000 Americans each year. Thanks to the vaccine, diphtheria now infects around 5 people a year in the United States. Diphtheria is a bacterial infection that creates a membranous covering over the back of the throat. The bacteria, *Corynebacterium diphtheriae,* also secretes a toxin that can cause paralysis, breathing difficulty, heart failure, and death. The death rate from diphtheria is around 10%. Diphtheria is spread by infected people, including carriers without symptoms. Victims can also contract it through contaminated objects or foods.

Pertussis, or whooping cough, is not rare at all, although widespread vaccination has held down the contagion among children. The immunity from childhood pertussis vaccine wears off by late adolescence, so many teens and adults harbor pertussis and can pass it to vulnerable children. The disease, caused by the *Bordetella pertussis* bacteria, results mainly in a cough. That doesn't sound too bad until you understand that this is not just any cough. The cough of pertussis comes in prolonged spells that often lead to vomiting and may cause victims to turn blue or pass out from lack of oxygen. As the victim tries to breathe in through an inflamed airway, she makes the whooping sound that gives the disease its name. The cough may also cause bleeding in the retina, broken ribs, hernias, and even strokes. Pertussis may lead to pneumonia, ear infections, seizures, brain damage, and of course, death. In general, the younger the patient, the worse the disease. Newborns who contract pertussis face a 1 in 100 risk of death; that risk falls to 1 in 200 over the first year of life.

Haemophilus influenzae type b: the b stands for bad

Because no one wants to pronounce the full name of this bacterial infection, just about everyone calls it Hib. Despite having a similar name, Hib does not cause influenza. (That's another vaccine-preventable disease, caused by one of the influenza viruses.) What Hib does cause is meningitis, throat infections (epiglottitis), skin infections, bone infections, heart muscle infections, and death. Meningitis is an infection of the tissues and fluid around the brain that can lead to permanent brain damage and hearing loss in survivors. Until the vaccine became available, Hib was the leading cause of meningitis in the United States. Epiglottitis causes swelling of the flap (epiglottis) that closes your airway so you can swallow without choking. Inflammation of the epiglottis can completely block the airway leading very quickly to death.

Prior to the introduction of Hib vaccine in 1985, Hib caused severe disease in around 20,000 American children a year, killing around 1,000.

Vaccines decreased Hib infections by more than 95%. Children receive the vaccine 4 times between the ages of 2 and 15 months.

Streptococcus pneumoniae: no, not that strep

This is not the strep that causes strep throat (that's called *Streptococcus pyogenes*). *Streptococcus pneumoniae*, also called pneumococcus, is a bacteria responsible for nasty infections in the brain and spinal cord (meningitis), lungs (pneumonia), bloodstream (bacteremia), joints (arthritis), ears (otitis media), sinuses (sinusitis), and eyes (conjunctivitis). These infections are often aggressive and can cause death, especially from meningitis and pneumonia. There are more than 90 subtypes of pneumococcus, some more dangerous than others. The vaccine we give children currently protects against 13 types that cause most of the worst disease.

Before the vaccine became available in 2000, pneumococcus was the most common cause of invasive bacterial infection in children. While pneumococcus is still the most common cause of bacterial meningitis, infections have fallen by 77% since the vaccine was introduced. Healthy children should receive 4 doses of pneumococcal vaccine (PCV13) between the ages of 2 and 15 months.

measles, mumps, rubella, and varicella: a grand slam

Measles, also called rubeola, was once common, infecting 3 to 4 million Americans a year and killing 500 a year prior to the vaccine's creation in 1963. Measles still killed 164,000 children worldwide in 2008. Starting with cold symptoms, red eyes, and a fine, red, bumpy rash, measles may lead to deadly pneumonia or brain infection (encephalitis). Of all the vaccine-preventable diseases, measles may be the most contagious—more than 90% of unvaccinated people exposed to measles will contract the disease. People infected with measles can spread the illness for 4 days before the rash appears and 4 days after it disappears. Measles virus can remain in the air and cause infection for up to 2 hours after an infected patient leaves the room!

The good news is that the measles vaccine is highly effective in preventing the disease, around 98% in healthy patients. Children receive 1 vaccine at age 12 months and another at age 4 to 5 years, providing lifetime immunity. The measles vaccine is combined in most cases with vaccines against mumps and rubella.

Mumps is almost unknown in the United States today thanks to vaccination, but as recently as 2006 an epidemic caused by an unvaccinated child entering the United States from the United Kingdom reminded us how unpleasant this vaccine-preventable disease is. A viral infection, mumps usually causes painful swelling of the salivary glands around the mouth, especially the big ones in your cheeks that squeeze when you taste lemon juice. That's not to say mumps cannot kill; encephalitis and meningitis from mumps can and do occur, causing brain swelling and in some cases, death. Mumps can also lead to permanent hearing loss and, in males, sterility from infection of the testes. Vaccination at age 12 months and again at age 4 to 5 years provides lifelong immunity.

Rubella, also called German measles, is unique among vaccine-preventable diseases in that children who contract the disease don't tend to get terribly ill. Symptoms include a rash that starts on the face, spreads to the trunk, and then fades, usually over about 3 days. Mild fever, swollen lymph nodes, fatigue, headache, eye redness, and joint pain are common as well. The problem with rubella is that infected children pass it on to pregnant women, who may go on to have miscarriages or severely disabled babies as a result of the disease. Vaccination of children at age 12 months and again at age 4 to 5 years has essentially eliminated stillbirths and severe disability from the infection in the United States.

Varicella is better known as chickenpox in its childhood form and shingles when it affects adults. Prior to the vaccine becoming available in 1995, varicella infections killed about 100 people and hospitalized 10,000 each year in the United States, mostly adults. In 2004, by comparison, 8 Americans died of varicella infection.

Chickenpox begins like a cold, with runny nose, cough, and fever. About a week later the classic rash appears, first on the body and scalp, and then spreading to the face, arms, and legs. Chickenpox lesions start as little red areas with water blisters, but the blisters grow and pop, leaving open sores which scab over and heal. The rash tends to be very itchy, and the hallmark of chickenpox is that the lesions come on at different times, meaning you'll see some new lesions while others are healing. In general the disease lasts about 2 weeks.

While chickenpox is very rarely fatal, it can cause pneumonia, severe skin infections, or rarely, brain damage. Children who have been vaccinated may get the disease anyway, but usually their symptoms are quite mild and not dangerous. Varicella vaccine is usually given at age 12 months and again at age 4 to 5 years.

hepatitis A: yeah, there's another hepatitis

The only thing hepatitis A and hepatitis B have in common is that they are viruses that infect the liver. Hepatitis A is transmitted by eating food or drinking water contaminated by the virus, but children can also pick it up from close, personal contact with infected individuals. While childhood disease tends to be milder than adult disease, about 1 victim in 5 requires hospitalization, and 3 to 5 out of 1,000 die of the infection. Hepatitis A starts as a flu-like illness with fever, nausea, vomiting, and fatigue. Inflammation of the liver can cause tenderness in the upper right abdomen and a yellow discoloration of the skin. The disease tends to last weeks to months, and treatment is purely supportive.

Children get hepatitis A vaccine in 2 doses 6 months apart starting as early as the 12-month wellness examination. The vaccine is 97% to 99% effective in preventing hepatitis A, and immunity lasts about 20 years.

meningococcal infections: if freddy krueger were a bacteria

Among the nastiest organisms that infect the human species, *Neisseria meningitidis,* known more commonly as meningococcus, holds a special position. This bacterial infection passes among victims through sneezing, coughing, sharing a drinking glass, or other forms of close physical contact. Up to 15% of adults carry the bacteria without displaying any symptoms. In some cases, most commonly in young children and teenagers, meningococci invade tissues around the brain, causing severe inflammation. In other cases meningococci infect the bloodstream, causing bleeding in the skin and internal organs. Both types of infections progress rapidly, with mortality rates ranging from 10% to 50%. Survivors may suffer hearing loss, brain damage, limb amputation, and severe skin scarring.

The vaccines we have for meningococcal disease work best for children aged 11 years and older. Certain high-risk children should also be vaccinated starting at age 2 years. A single dose of the vaccine given at age 11 is 85% to 100% effective in preventing disease from the more common strains of meningococcus. It's not clear how long immunity lasts, but we know it lasts at least 3 years.

human papillomavirus: your child is not sexually active—that's the point

Human papillomavirus is another one of those medical names that's so long even medical people won't say it, calling it HPV instead. HPV is the virus that causes genital warts, which in turn cause cervical and, rarely, penile cancer. Every year about 10,000 American women are diagnosed with cervical cancer, and 3,700 women a year die of it. Cervical cancer is the second most common cause of cancer death in women worldwide, and with vaccines most of these deaths are now preventable. Newer studies have implicated HPV as a cause of oral and esophageal cancer in men and women.

Genital warts can be transmitted to babies from the birth canal, but usually they are sexually transmitted. HPV is actually the most common sexually transmitted infection (STI) in the United States, affecting more than half of the sexually active population at some point in their lives. HPV is highly contagious, and people often transmit it without showing any symptoms of the disease. There are 2 vaccines against HPV. Gardasil protects against the types that cause the vast majority of genital warts and cervical cancer; Cervarix protects against the cancer-causing types only.

Girls should get Gardasil or Cervarix in 3 doses over 6 months, starting at age 11 or 12 years. Boys can also get Gardasil starting as early as age 9. It's hard as a parent to look at your 11-year-old and consider giving her a vaccine to prevent an STI, but the idea is to give the vaccine before the child gets exposed to the disease.

We know that to protect every girl from cervical cancer, we have to give the vaccines before adolescence. She may be 11 now, but in another 11 years she'll be 22, and these vaccines could be her ticket to seeing age 44 and beyond.

influenza vaccine: one lifesaver, 2 flavors

Because it's so common, it's easy to forget what a formidable killer influenza virus is. In an average year the flu hospitalizes 200,000 Americans and kills 30,000. That is, by anyone's count, a lot of people. Children succumb to influenza more often than adults, so it's especially important to protect kids against the flu.

Influenza passes from person to person easily through coughing, sneezing, and touch. Influenza begins like a really bad cold, with fever, runny nose, sore throat, cough, and headache. Unlike a cold, influenza also causes vomiting, diarrhea, and muscle aches. Influenza virus is especially nasty in the lungs, where it damages the usual immune defenses. Potential results include viral pneumonia from influenza itself, bacterial pneumonia, or a noninfectious lung disease called *respiratory distress syndrome.* Any of the 3 can lead to hospitalization and death.

The tricky thing about vaccinating against influenza is that there are really scores of different types of influenza virus, and the viral antigens are constantly changing. To begin with, we group influenza into 2 major types, influenza A and influenza B (virologists are not all that creative). You can fight off an influenza A virus early in the season only to be infected with influenza B later. On top of that, influenza A viruses carry 2 antigen groups, called H and N. Different strains of flu have different types of H and N antigens, which means that just because your immune system fought off the flu last year doesn't mean it will recognize this year's strain. For this reason, vaccine manufacturers sample infected patients and animals around the world and reformulate the vaccine each year to protect against the types of influenza that seem likely to cause the most disease. In any given influenza season, the vaccine can be between 50% and 90% effective, but even partly effective vaccine may prevent hospitalization and death.

Manufacturers offer an inactivated (killed) vaccine and a live, weakened vaccine that may cause some mild flu symptoms but may also work a little better. Children as young as 6 months can take the inactivated vaccine, which is given as an injection. Starting at 2 years of age, children can receive the live vaccine, which is sprayed into the nose. Some children younger than 9 years will need 2 doses of vaccine if it's their first year to be vaccinated. Children with asthma or other lung or heart disease may not qualify for the nasal spray vaccine; your child's doctor should have a short list of screening questions to see which version would be best.

The flu vaccine myth I hear most often is that the vaccine causes people to get the flu. There are a couple of reasons this rumor just won't die. One is that for the live vaccine it's kind of true—the vaccine causes some very mild flu symptoms but does a great job preventing hospitalization and death from the wild influenza virus. The other is that we give flu vaccine during the fall and winter, when people tend to get colds and influenza anyway. It takes about 2 weeks for the vaccine to work. So a certain number of people are going to get the vaccine and then contract influenza 2 days later, before the vaccine has taken effect. Many more people will go on to contract a garden variety cold, which they will suspect is the flu. The truth is this—influenza hospitalizes and kills a lot of people every year, and vaccine is by far the most effective tool we have for preventing senseless tragedy.

Hopefully this chapter has provided some reliable information to consult next time a well-meaning coworker, friend, or relative assaults you with sincere but inaccurate advice about vaccines. As soon as someone starts that conversation, you can always do what I do—change the subject to stock tips, sports opinions, or even better, fashion advice.

great sources for reliable vaccine advice

www.HealthyChildren.org

www.chop.edu/service/vaccine-education-center

www.vaccinesafety.edu

www.cdc.gov/vaccines

8

the big sleep:
helping your child learn to
sleep, over and over

If you're reading this chapter, there's a good chance you're tired.
You may even be severely sleep-deprived, exhausted to the point that you
start reading something and soon you're not sure if you're still awake
or dreaming. The unicorn beat his golden wings and mounted into the
lime-colored sky bearing the goddess on his back, swerving to dodge the
dragons' fiery breath. For example, do you think you just read a sentence
about a flying unicorn? Dude, you need some rest!

If you are cooperating with another human being in raising your child,
now is a good time for the 2 of you to stop and talk. Sleep challenges can
serve as a microcosm of your whole relationship. Do you step up and help
each other out? Do you map out a problem-solving strategy? Or do you
yell, point fingers, and see that the other one is doing everything wrong?
Before you end up in relationship counseling, make sure you and your
partner in child-rearing are, if not on the same page, at least in the same
universe. If you're not, this may be a good time to sit down with a third
party and work through some issues. You know how cranky you both
get when you're tired.

what to expect when you're expecting sleep

Sleep is an essential function of pretty much every organism with a brain. Sleep seems to help with growth, immune function, and memory, among other things. Our sleep cycles are regulated by hormones, which in turn respond to light cues and elapsed time to help keep us on schedule. Even before birth, the fetus is spending time sleeping, alternating between rapid eye movement (REM) sleep and the other 4 phases of sleep, collectively called non-REM sleep (have I mentioned that doctors are not that creative in naming things?). REM sleep is when dreams occur, and you may see your newborn twitching, startling, or looking around behind his eyelids. No one knows what babies dream about, but I suspect it has something to do with showing up to school wearing only a diaper.

Your newborn will sleep a lot, around 16 hours a day on average. Don't panic if your baby sleeps 14 or 18 hours; people vary. Those hours, however, won't all be in a row. Your baby also needs to eat frequently to grow, so expect him to wake up every 2 to 4 hours at first. Depending on how well your newborn is gaining weight, his doctor might even recommend waking him up after 4 or 5 hours to feed, especially in the first few weeks of life.

Many parents of newborns say their babies have their days and nights mixed up. It's not so much that they're mixed up as that they just don't know the difference. The whole day/night thing is a fresh concept, and it takes the newborn's brain a while to adapt to the cycle. There are some steps you can take to move this process along. Light is a very strong cue to help our brains regulate sleep. Don't be afraid to keep your baby's environment bright during the daytime, even at nap time. By contrast, make his nighttime sleeping space as dark as you can without risking injury on your way to the crib. Sound and activity will also serve as sleep cues. It's probably a good thing if there's a little noise around the house in the daytime, but try to keep the night quiet. Even your voice can serve as a signal that it's time to relax. Try singing a lullaby while channeling Barry White. (If you don't know who Barry White is, stop right now and download some of his songs; it will be good for your relationship.)

The good news is that this phase will come to an end. Even by the end of the first month you'll find your newborn sleeping some longer stretches at night. By 3 months of age many infants are able to sleep 8 or more hours a night. At 1 year of life your baby will sleep somewhat less in each 24-hour period, just under 14 hours on average.

Now is a time some friends and relatives might feel like jumping in with advice, and not always because you asked. Some might tell you that rigidly controlling your baby's sleeping and eating schedules will lead him to live a more disciplined life in the future; there are even books that make this assertion. If you hear this theory, just smile and nod politely, knowing that it has absolutely no basis in science and may even pose risks to your baby's weight gain and emotional attachment.

Another popular but misleading bit of advice you're likely to hear involves cereal. The idea is that if you give your baby a bottle containing some cereal before bedtime, he'll stay full longer and wake up less. It's a compelling theory; it just doesn't happen to be true. Multiple studies have shown that eating cereal does nothing to prolong periods of sleep. While doctors do sometimes use thickened cereal for babies with gastroesophageal reflux disease, we worry cereal may cause excessive weight gain in healthy babies.

You may want to map out a coping strategy for dealing with this period of sleep interruptions. If your baby is nursing, you might agree to be the one to get the baby out of his crib and change the inevitable post-feeding diaper while mom stays in bed to nurse. If your baby is taking formula, you might alternate who gets up so each parent can grab 6 to 8 hours of uninterrupted sleep. Work schedules can play a role, too, making some times better or worse for one parent to deal with lost sleep. There is no one-size-fits-all solution except to work together.

yes, even sleep can be dangerous

We tend to associate sleeping with safety, unless of course we do it while also driving. Babies, however, are at risk of sudden infant death syndrome (SIDS). This mysterious condition is exactly what it sounds like—babies die in their sleep for no obvious reason. While SIDS rates have dropped dramatically since 1992 when doctors began advising parents to put babies to sleep on their backs, SIDS still remains the leading cause of death in the first year of life. SIDS rates peak between 2 and 4 months of age, and about 90% of cases occur by age 6 months.

Theories abound on what causes SIDS. Most likely there are multiple underlying causes. Much research points to problems with sleep arousal or with the brain's ability to respond to increasing levels of carbon dioxide in the bloodstream. The good news is that doctors are learning more effective ways of preventing SIDS.

SIDS prevention actually begins before birth with smoking cessation. Babies of mothers who smoke during pregnancy are more likely to die of SIDS. Even exposure to secondhand smoke may make a difference. Likewise, babies who live in houses where people smoke are at higher risk for SIDS. Make sure smokers always take it outside.

The single most important thing you can do to prevent SIDS is to always put your baby to sleep on his back. Before 1992 we had a theory that went something like this: if your baby is sleeping on his back and spits up, he may choke on his gastric contents and die. The theory was just plain wrong. It turns out that healthy babies don't do that. As doctors began to study SIDS, it became clear that babies were twice as likely to survive if they slept faceup rather than facedown. Some babies seem to prefer sleeping on their tummies, which can be frustrating, but remember, this really is a matter of life and death. Many parents find swaddling helps their babies sleep better on their backs. We used to say back or side, but some babies will roll from their sides to their fronts, so we now recommend babies only sleep face up. If someone gives you a foam device or pillow to prop your baby on his side, write a nice thank-you note and then repurpose it as a doggy toy.

Other soft stuff does not belong in a safe sleeping environment, starting with the mattress itself. Look for a firm mattress and sheet set that has been certified safe by the Juvenile Products Manufacturers Association. Adult beds, couches, chairs, and air mattresses are not safe places for babies to sleep. Babies who sleep in bed with their parents are more likely to die of SIDS, even more so if the parent has been drinking. Fluffy blankets, crib bumpers, comforters, soft toys, and stuffed animals can all be adorable, but none of them should be in the crib or bassinet while the baby is sleeping there. Any of these objects might cover the baby's face and block his breathing.

Overheating can also contribute to SIDS. While you want your baby to be cozy and warm, he does not need to be much warmer than you do. If you see him sweating, flushing, or breathing too fast, unbundle him or adjust the room temperature. Ideally, his sleep area will be at a temperature you would find comfortable if you were wearing a t-shirt.

It's critical if your baby spends time in the care of other people that they understand the rules for safe sleep. About one-fifth of SIDS deaths occur in child care settings. When you're touring these centers, be sure to peek

what you can do

If there's room, the best place for your baby to sleep is in a crib or bassinet close to your bed. This makes it easy to check on him, feed him, and change his diaper when needed. It also makes it easy to put him back in his bed to sleep. He'll learn to sleep better if you lay him down while he's still a little bit awake but getting sleepy. Whatever way he learns to get to sleep is the method he is likely to depend on. If you rock him to sleep or feed him until he is completely asleep, he will learn that those are the ways to settle down.

in on the babies' room and see if all the younger babies are sleeping on their backs. Don't be shy about educating friends and family members about safe sleep practices as well. Things have changed some since your parents raised children, and some people simply have not gotten the memo.

Just because your baby should sleep on his back doesn't mean he has to look at the ceiling all the time. Doctors have noticed 2 unintended consequences of the US government's Back to Sleep campaign. One is a condition called positional plagiocephaly, in which the baby's head becomes flattened in the back from prolonged time spent lying down. The other is that many babies have a slight delay in developing some motor skills, such as the ability to roll from front to back. When your baby is awake and playful, spend some tummy time building muscles to help him raise his head and arch his back. Not all babies enjoy this time. You might find having him on your chest makes it more fun, but even if your baby is crying, he's still getting needed exercise. Don't leave him unattended in this position, in case he does fall asleep.

Once your infant can roll from back to front (usually around age 6 months), you really can't keep him from sleeping facedown. The good news is that by this point, the risk of SIDS is much lower than just a couple of months ago. That does not mean, however, that it's time to fill his crib with toys, pillows, and puffy blankets or haul him in bed with you. SIDS remains a risk for the whole first year of life.

shouldn't you be asleep?

By age 6 months infants will usually sleep 8 to 10 hours at night without interruption. Most infants can keep enough food in their tummies to make it through the night at this point. Some will continue to require a nighttime feeding up to age 12 months. Most infants nap some during the day to fill in however many hours of sleep they need to get their full 14. Some will take 2 naps, while others take just 1 long nap. If your baby is sleeping poorly at night but then napping for 5 hours during the daytime, you might think about shortening the daytime nap a bit, hoping to move that sleep to the evening.

Sleep, whether for babies or adults, depends very much on routine. Bedtimes go best when they're at the same time every night. Maintaining a consistent bedtime can pose a challenge on weekends or when traveling, but to the extent you can do it, you'll be glad you did. Rituals also help your baby transition from a wakeful state into restfulness. A bath, a special song, or a period spent rocking can all reinforce the idea, "It's nighty-night time now." You may find that feeding your baby just before bedtime actually keeps him awake more than feeding a half hour or an hour before bed. After your baby is 1 year old you can use a special blanket, stuffed animal, or item of your own clothing as a transition object to help him calm down and sleep.

Dealing with crying can challenge parents, especially when the parents are so tired they may want to cry, too. Some degree of crying often helps babies release stress and get themselves to sleep. Babies also may cry from fatigue itself. A baby's cry carries tremendous emotional power. It tells parents there's something wrong that they need to fix. But responding to a cry inappropriately may reinforce bad sleep habits that can then become very hard to reverse.

By the time your infant is 6 months old, you probably can tell when he's crying from sleepiness, fear, or discomfort. If you hear an alarming cry, by all means, go find out what's happening. But if your infant has just awakened and seems sleepy or cranky, try giving him a few minutes to calm down before rushing to check on him. If he's still crying, you might check his diaper, feel for a fever, and make sure nothing is hurting him, but then it's OK to reassure him, pat him on the back, and encourage him to go back to sleep. If you need to pick him up and hold him for a minute that's fine, but he'll learn to get back to sleep better if he's still a little awake when you lay him down.

Some babies don't take this sort of practice lying down, so to speak. They may scream for a half hour or more, wanting to eat, play, be held, or even sleep in bed with the parents. If you suspect this is what's happening, the first step is to talk to your parenting partner, in most cases mom. Start by asking questions. How does she perceive the crying? Does she feel it's a problem? Do you both agree it's something you'd like to change? If you find the 2 of you disagree about the issue, you might want to meet together with the baby's pediatrician and talk about what seems appropriate. The pediatrician may also be able to reassure you that your baby isn't crying because of an ear infection, hunger, or an undiagnosed illness.

what you can do

If you agree that your baby's sleep routine needs to change, pick a date to start. Weekends and holidays are probably better times than, say, the Sunday night before that big Monday job interview. Responding consistently to the crying will be critical, so both partners will need to commit to the process.

Starting on the appointed night, respond to awakenings by waiting a few minutes, then checking on and reassuring your baby, then leaving the room. If he's still crying in 5 minutes, you can come back and check on him again. At some point he will fall asleep, but you may repeat this cycle quite a few times before he does. After a night or two of this pattern add another 5 minutes between checks, so if you were checking on him every 5 minutes, it's now every 10 minutes. Chances are excellent using this system that you will not get to the 30-minute mark, although every baby is different, so yours may be the exception. Another approach to the same problem is to check on him every 5 minutes, but stand a little farther away each time you do.

that was fun—let's do it again!

Establishing good sleep habits in the first year of life creates a strong foundation for healthy sleep later, but these habits will likely require reinforcement from time to time. As your baby's development progresses, his sense of the world around him evolves in profound ways. By 6 months, for example, he recognizes that you have not disappeared just because you left the room; by crying he might summon you back. At 9 months he will be able to pull himself to a standing position on the crib railing and jump up and down to get your attention. At 15 months he will be able to call out some words. Each developmental stage brings with it new reasons for your child to wake up at night and new tools for expressing his desires. While your child is confined to a crib, you always have the option of putting him back in it. But what do you do when he moves to a bed?

The first step is to remember that whatever ritual or routine your child has grown accustomed to is what he'll rely on. If you've gotten in the habit of letting him fall asleep in your bed, while watching television, or with a bottle of milk, you're in for a much rougher transition. Even a child who has a more traditional bedtime routine now has the tools to prolong that routine almost indefinitely. Your child can now request another book, another hug, another sip of water, or an explanation of the meaning of life. Setting boundaries about what bedtime entails will be important to prevent it from stretching into the wee hours. Enforcing these boundaries may lead to temper tantrums at the time, but come morning you'll be glad you stood your ground.

The rules for addressing sleep behavior with a toddler are the same as for addressing any other behavior. First, state your expectations clearly. "This is your bed; this is where you sleep. If you leave it, you'll come back here to sleep. You can get up to use the potty, and you can come get me if you need me, but only if it is an emergency. Then you'll go back to bed." At the end of the bedtime ritual ask, "Do you need anything else?" and respond to any reasonable request. This step will set the stage for later in the night when he makes more demands you'll have to ignore. You can also stack the odds in your favor by starting with a later bedtime and then clocking it back 15 minutes a week until your child is going to bed at a more reasonable time.

You can explain your reasoning ("I want you to feel good when you wake up in the morning"), but don't expect a preschooler to follow this rationale and agree with you; that's not how they see things. Offer a reward for each good night's sleep, such as a sticker or a special breakfast. You may also take away a privilege after a bad night's sleep, such as eliminating television time or removing a toy for a day (but not the transition object!).

Some children are frightened to sleep in their own beds. Be proactive with these children, promising you'll come check on them rather than having them come to you. If you peek in for a few seconds every 15 minutes, you'll eventually find your child asleep. If you find him awake but in bed, take a moment to let him know how proud you are of him for staying there. If he does wake up frightened, take time to reassure him, but lead him back to his bed and tuck him in again, letting him know that he's safe and you're nearby if he needs you. There's nothing wrong with having a dim night-light in the room.

Other interruptions may also require your attention at night. A trip to the potty, a blanket issue, or an earache are all really good reasons to attend to your child. You should have met all his other needs during the bedtime ritual, so you may just have to turn away and close the door when he's demanding that sixth hug.

Toddlers and preschoolers often throw fits when they don't get what they want, so you'll have to be prepared for some crying, screaming, and door-kicking. In this case you can use the bedroom door as a reward. Tell your child that when he stops crying you'll leave the door open, but while he's crying it will need to stay closed. Open the door every 15 minutes to check and see if your child is in bed yet, and let him know that as soon as he's back in bed you'll leave the door open.

If your child leaves his room at night, return him to his bed quietly and calmly and let him know you'll have to close his door if he keeps coming out. In extreme cases you may have to bring your superior hardware skills to bear, installing a gate, putting in a privacy lock that works from the outside, or using a chain latch. This step is especially important for children who may wander around the house at night and endanger themselves.

If you're consistent with these principals you can expect a few nights of crying, but within 2 weeks most children will adapt to their new routine. If your child seems unusually fearful or if you've tried these measures for

2 weeks without success, it's time to talk with your child's doctor. Even if you are successful, don't be surprised if you have to repeat the process a few months later.

Development never stops, and as your child grows he will face new challenges to good sleep. Television and video games are stimulating experiences that can leave your child way too cranked up to sleep. Never put a television or video game in your child's bedroom; not only do they interfere with sleep, but you'll know less about what your children are watching or playing. Children metabolize caffeine more slowly than adults, so a caffeinated beverage or chocolate dessert can interfere with a child's sleep hours later. As kids acquire mobile phones at younger ages, it's important to establish guidelines about when they can be used. Have a rule that phones go in their chargers outside the bedroom at night.

mares and terrors:
it's just a dream, unless it's not

Everyone knows what a dream is. Dreams occur during REM sleep and involve simulated experience. While we dream our muscles are usually in a state of relative paralysis, so we don't go running around and hurting ourselves. When dreams are frightening, we call them nightmares.

While babies spend a lot of time in REM sleep, children don't seem to begin having nightmares until the second year of life. Nightmares are more common during the second half of the night, when REM is more intense. Children often awaken from nightmares frightened, and they need reassurance that whatever was scaring them was not real. They may be able to tell you a little about their dreams, and they may remain frightened for a while afterward. Nightmares don't necessarily reflect any increased stress in the child's life, but if they persist on a nightly basis you might want to talk with your child's doctor. Remember that toddlers don't distinguish between the imaginary and the real, so frightening television shows or video games may manifest themselves in nightmares.

Night terrors seem like nightmares in that they occur during sleep and the child appears scared, but the key difference is that night terrors tend to scare the daylights out of parents and leave children unscathed. Children don't usually experience night terrors before age 4 to 5. They tend to occur during non-REM sleep, often in the first couple of hours after bedtime. Children awaken suddenly and appear terrified. They may scream, kick, hit, or cower from some unseen threat. Children who have awakened from nightmares usually acknowledge your presence and cling to you for reassurance. Children with night terrors don't seem to be awake at all, staring right through you or ignoring your presence altogether. They are often impossible to console; you just have to keep them safe until they fall back to sleep.

Night terrors usually last from 5 to 15 minutes. In the morning the child will have no recollection of the event, but you will probably remember it vividly. Kids tend to grow out of their night terrors within a few years, whereas nightmares persist into adulthood, or I really do take tests unprepared and naked on a regular basis.

Sleep issues remain one of the most common and contentious challenges parents face. With perseverance, cooperation, and good coffee, you, your relationship, and your child can all survive and even awaken well-rested. It does take some work, but with persistence you can have your baby sleeping like a…a…someone help me out here…yeah, again I got nothing.

9

the air force: congestion, coughing, and wheezing in babies

If you're like most dads, you'll find yourself compelled to watch your newborn breathe. For several days it's more fascinating than Monday Night Football. At some point you're guaranteed to wake up in the middle of the night and stand over her crib to make sure your baby is still breathing. She is, just like she was before you woke up and just like she will continue to do after you go back to bed. Monday Night Football, on the other hand, will eventually end, although it may go into overtime.

If you watch your baby breathe for too long, however, you'll freak yourself out. That's because newborns breathe in a pattern first described by 2 Irish doctors in the early 19th century. John Cheyne and William Stokes wrote a book on breathing in which they noted that new babies and some severely ill adults alternate between periods of breathing fast and breathing slowly. This pattern, called Cheyne-Stokes respiration or periodic breathing, is normal for newborns, whose brains are learning to respond to varying levels of oxygen and carbon dioxide in the bloodstream. Over a period of a minute or two you'll see your baby almost panting at times; at other times she may pause for a period that feels uncomfortably long but is usually only 2 or 3 seconds. Now you can go back to bed or, if it's Monday, return to the game.

sleep apnea: in support of breathing

As much as you are likely to worry about your baby's breathing, healthy term newborns generally breathe well whether you watch them or not. There is such a thing as sudden infant death syndrome (SIDS), which we discussed in Chapter 8, but thanks to the Back to Sleep campaign SIDS now occurs only once in every 2,000 births, way down from once in every 650 births in 1980.

Sleep apnea occurs when a sleeping person stops breathing long enough for her blood oxygen level to fall to below normal levels. While sleep apnea is a problem for some children and adults, among newborns it's pretty much confined to babies born prematurely or with other severe medical conditions. Babies admitted to the neonatal intensive care unit following delivery usually have their breathing monitored for a bit. If that monitoring shows they have sleep apnea, they may be discharged home with an electronic monitor to keep track of their breathing and heart rate. Sleep apnea is not related to SIDS, and home apnea monitors do nothing to reduce SIDS rates. If your baby is discharged from the hospital with an apnea monitor, her doctor should have talked to you about how to respond to alarms. You should also have some idea of how long you must use the monitor and when you'll know it's OK to stop.

nosy babies

Newborns use their airways differently from older children and adults. If you watch a baby nurse, you'll notice she may go for 20 or 30 minutes, even longer, without stopping to take a breath. That's because she breathes through her nose the entire time. In fact, newborns are generally unable to breathe through their mouths except when they're crying. In rare cases a baby may be born with an underdeveloped nasal airway (choanal atresia), which is a life-threatening emergency, especially if it affects both sides of the nose. These babies will cry some to breathe, but when they're not crying they may turn blue and suffer respiratory failure. They are also unable to breathe and feed at the same time. Later in infancy your baby will learn to breathe through her mouth, but even then she will find nasal congestion annoying.

For the first few months of life babies rely on mom's antibodies to protect them from cold viruses. This does not mean they cannot catch a cold; they can and they do. The worst kind of viral upper respiratory infection in newborns is respiratory syncytial virus (RSV), which causes potentially life-threatening wheezing (see "Wheezer" on page 128). Any cold can cause a runny nose and swollen nasal passages, which provide your newborn an extra challenge when trying to feed or sleep.

The best tools at our disposal for dealing with newborn nose issues are saline solution and suction bulbs. Chances are good your baby left the hospital with one or more rubber suction bulbs, usually blue or red in color with a tapered tip. If you cannot find them among all the baby stuff, you should be able to pick up a replacement in the baby section of the nearest pharmacy. This alien-looking instrument is designed to suck snot. As obvious as this is, there are right and wrong ways to slurp boogers out of a baby's nose.

If secretions are dry or sticky, you'll want to loosen them up first with a little saline solution. Saline will also help shrink tissues inside the nose to aid in breathing. One or 2 drops to each nostril should do the trick. You can buy inexpensive commercially prepared saline solution at the pharmacy, but in a pinch you can also make your own at home, using a half teaspoon of table salt and 1 cup of water. The salt will dissolve better in warm or hot water, but be sure to let it cool to body temperature or below before you use it. Using the suction bulb, medicine dropper, or cotton ball, dribble a drop or two in each nostril and then wait around 30 to 60 seconds. Be aware—few babies enjoy having water dribbled in their nostrils; expect some fighting, coughing, and sputtering.

Next, bring the tip of the suction bulb just to the opening of the nostrils. There is no advantage to jamming it way up in the nose, where trauma could actually worsen the swelling. You should also know that the airway starts at the nostrils and goes straight back into the head, not upward. Angle the tip of your suction bulb at 90° to the face for best effect. A couple of suctions on each side should do the job. Your baby will probably need a few minutes to calm down before eating or sleeping. As your baby grows, she'll get better at fighting you off. By age 4 to 6 months you'll probably want a partner to help you with the process. Finally, while you may be tempted to perform suction every 5 minutes, try to limit your interventions to just before she eats and nap times. Overdoing it may cause more swelling.

Another weapon in your battle against nasal congestion is the cool mist humidifier. The idea here is to help moisten the baby's airway and loosen secretions. Steam vaporizers also add humidity to the room, but the risk of burns from contacting hot, invisible steam makes them a poor choice for settings where children play. While many pharmacies sell medicine to put in the humidifier, what you're really after is just the moisture; water alone will do. Humidifiers, like everything else, can pose a risk if not properly maintained. Put in fresh water every day, ideally distilled water to prevent buildup of mineral scale. Scrub out the basin of the humidifier regularly so that scum and fine particles don't collect. If you use bleach or harsh chemicals in cleaning, be sure to rinse them out thoroughly before using the machine again. Finally, know that dust mites love humid air; if you think your child has an allergy to dust mites, the humidifier may be part of the problem, not part of the solution.

wheezer

Many parents I talk to aren't quite sure what wheezing is. That's probably because wheezing is often so quiet it cannot be heard without a stethoscope. Parents sometimes say a child is wheezing when they mean the coarse, rattling sounds that come from a congested airway. The best way to understand the difference is to take an imaginary trip down the windpipe.

You can imagine the human airway as an upside-down tree. The trunk of the tree is the trachea. A little way into the chest, the trachea divides into 2 mainstem bronchi, one for each lung. These bronchi then branch many more times, getting smaller with each division, until they reach their smallest twigs, the bronchioles. At the end of each bronchiole is a cluster of air sacs called alveoli. It's in these alveoli that oxygen actually passes from air into the bloodstream.

All cold viruses cause increased mucous secretions in the lungs. This mucous can clog up the larger branches of the pulmonary tree, causing cough and the rattling sounds we call rhonchi. These are usually the longest-lasting symptoms of a cold, continuing for up to 3 weeks.

Wheezing, however, doesn't happen in the larger branches of the tree. Wheezing comes from mucous or inflammation in the bronchioles, which traps air in the alveoli. Wheezing only occurs when a baby is breathing out, not when she's breathing in. Because wheezing involves smaller airways, doctors often find it alarming when a sick baby is wheezing.

when to call the doctor

If you think you hear a wheeze, make sure your baby sees a doctor quickly. Her doctor can give her breathing treatments and sometimes steroids to try and help her breathing. Younger babies often require hospitalization until their breathing improves.

A handful of other signs can alert you that your baby is having serious breathing problems. First, watch her nostrils. If they flare with every breath, it's a sign she's working too hard to get air. Second, look at the skin between her ribs and under her rib cage. You should not see the skin pulling inward in those areas when she inhales. Third, listen for a grunting sound every time she breathes out. If she pauses and makes a noise with each breath, she's trying to expel air trapped in her lungs. Fourth, try to count how fast she's breathing. Because her breathing will vary, check a full minute's worth of breaths. If she is breathing more than 60 times a minute, a doctor should see her. At respiratory rates that high many babies can no longer breathe well enough to get an adequate feeding.

In older children wheezing is often a sign of asthma, but with babies the cause of a wheeze is not always so clear. Babies have smaller airways, which means viral illnesses that might not cause an older child to wheeze may cause wheezing in a baby. As mentioned previously, RSV is often associated with dangerous wheezing in young babies, but other viruses can do the same thing. While wheezing from asthma often responds to medicines like albuterol (bronchodilators), babies whose wheeze comes from a viral infection may not get any better with breathing treatments.

cough analysis

Most surveys put cough at the top of the list of reasons parents bring their children to see the doctor. Cough gets your attention. It seems to advertise that something is wrong with your child. In most cases, however, cough results from a common viral infection; it's one of the body's most effective defenses against illness.

Our airways are lined with a layer of mucous designed to entrap any invaders before they can penetrate into our lungs. This mucous doesn't just sit there; it rides on a carpet of tiny, waving, hairlike structures called cilia that propel it upward and out of the lungs into the throat, where we swallow it all day long without usually being aware of the process. Acid in our stomachs kills whatever organisms were trapped in the mucous, and we stay healthy.

When we get sick, however, our lungs respond by making more mucous. To get this mucous out of the airway we first close our throats, then build up pressure in our lungs, and finally release this air pressure forcefully by suddenly opening our throats. This reflex is so natural and protective it's not clear if any of the medications sold to reduce the symptom of cough even really work. As annoying as it can be, the cough reflex is a good thing.

when to call the doctor

Some types of cough are not normal. Whooping cough is especially dangerous for babies and causes prolonged coughing spells that may cause the child to turn blue. Cough that also comes with wheezing or signs of respiratory distress is always concerning and deserves a doctor's attention. A cough from a cold should go away within 3 weeks. Any time you feel like your baby is unusually sick, seek medical attention for her.

what you can do

Babies younger than 3 months rarely get coughs, but when they do a humidifier is the only intervention that is safe. Older than 3 months, you can try a tablespoon of corn syrup like Karo or you can try giving her a few teaspoons of warm fluid such as apple juice. There are no cough medicines that have been proven safe and effective for babies or, for that matter, children younger than 4 years.

strident about stridor

If wheeze is a sound babies only make when they're breathing out, you can think of stridor as its opposite. Stridor, the rough sound of air passing through swollen vocal chords, tends to occur more when the baby is breathing in. The most common cause of stridor is croup, a viral infection that targets vocal chords and the trachea. Croup can be life-threatening, especially in babies; if yours seems like she can't get enough air, you might even have to call emergency medical services (EMS) (911).

what you can do

If your baby's croup symptoms are milder, there are some things you can try. Humid air seems to help croup symptoms; many doctors recommend bringing your baby into a steamed-up bathroom or shower stall. Cool air may also help, so a trip outside is worth a try, at least when the weather is right. A vaporizer can simulate the same environment indoors.

when to call the doctor

Regardless of what you try, if your baby still has stridor after 15 minutes or if you hear the noise when she breathes in and out, get her to a doctor's office or hospital. Croup often responds to steroid treatment, but when some children get sick enough it's safer to watch them overnight in the hospital.

Croup is not the only cause of stridor. As your infant develops the ability to move around the floor and put things in her mouth, she may get a foreign body lodged in her airway. The same thing can happen if she gets a piece of food that's not safe for her. If you suspect either of these events, call EMS immediately.

Once you know all the stuff you don't have to worry about, watching your baby breathe can be a great way to relax after a hard day. Sometimes, at night, when the weight of fatherhood wakes you up, it's just the thing to do. Of course, on Monday night, during football season, there's also the game, but I haven't met many men who would describe watching that as peaceful.

10

eye, captain:
eye boogers, the red eye,
and when to worry

among the deepest joys of fatherhood is the experience of
gazing into your baby's eyes. If he's awake, take a moment to do it now.
Amazing, isn't it? Don't you just marvel at the personality there, the yearn-
ing to comprehend the universe around him? It feels like you can see right
into his soul. Except, what's that booger doing there in the corner? Can
you maybe get a washcloth or something and get that out? Yuck. OK,
that's better. Now, where was that soul again?

whose eyes does he have?

New parents often ask what color I think the baby's eyes are going to be.
I never answer this question until the child is at least 1 year old; I mean,
what if the parents believe me and use my answer to make major life
decisions? When we talk about eye color, we're really talking about the
appearance of the *iris,* the muscular ring around the pupil that controls
how much light enters the eye. After all, the pupil will always be black,
except in flash photos, and the whites *(sclera)* should stay pretty much

white, although jaundice may turn them yellow and inflammation may make them look pink or red.

Iris color, just like hair and skin color, depends on a protein called *melanin*. We have specialized cells in our bodies called *melanocytes* whose job it is to go around secreting melanin where it's needed, including in the iris. When your baby is born his eyes will be gray or blue, as melanocytes respond to light, and he has spent his whole life in the dark.

Over time, if melanocytes only secrete a little melanin, your baby will have blue eyes. If they secrete a bit more, his eyes will look green or hazel. When melanocytes get really busy, eyes look brown (the most common eye color), and in some cases they may appear very dark indeed. Because it takes about a year for melanocytes to finish their work it can be a dicey business calling eye color before the baby's first birthday. The color change does slow down some after the first 6 months of life, but there can be plenty of change left at that point.

Eye color is a genetic property, but it's not quite as cut-and-dried as you might have learned in biology class. Two blue-eyed parents are very likely to have a blue-eyed child, but it won't happen every single time. Two brown-eyed parents are likely (but not guaranteed) to have a child with brown eyes. If you notice one of the grandparents has blue eyes, the chances of having a blue-eyed baby go up a bit. If one parent has brown eyes and the other has blue eyes, odds are about even on eye color. If your child has one brown eye and one blue eye, bring it to your doctor's attention; he probably has a rare genetic condition called Waardenburg syndrome.

Parents also often note that their newborns' eyes appear to cross from time to time. For the first 6 months of life this can be normal. To begin with, to look at something the brain has to know where to point the eyes. For the first 2 to 4 weeks of life vision is not accurate enough for the baby's eyes to find a target a lot of the time. Parents often feel like their newborns are looking past them rather than at them, because they are. By the fourth week of life, however, your baby will focus on your face if you're cradling him.

Most visual development occurs in the brain, not in the eyes themselves. One of the greatest challenges for the developing brain is to coordinate visual signals from one side to the other. Nerve signals from the eyes travel through optic nerves and split off to both sides of the brain. To make sense of those signals, the 2 sides of the brain have to cooperate, comparing information and coordinating eye movement in the desired direction. Until age 2 months you may notice your infant will follow your face or a toy a little way, then lose it as it crosses from one side to the other. By 2 months, however, he should be able to track from right to left and back again.

The next big visual milestone occurs at 6 months of age. By this time the 2 sides of the brain are on good terms with each other. Until this point the eyes track together as long as they both have something to look at, but if one is deprived of input (from being covered by a hat, for example), it might drift off in its own direction. By 6 months of age the eyes should continue looking the same direction even if one of them is covered temporarily. We test this in the clinic by covering 1 eye for 3 seconds, then suddenly uncovering it and looking to see if it's still tracking with the opposite eye. We call this test (with our usual creativity) the *cover-uncover* test.

Sometimes the shape of a child's face makes it look as though the eyes are crossed even when they are not. A child with a broad nasal bridge may appear to have an inward-looking eye, when in fact he's just looking off to the side. You can check this by watching the light reflection in your child's eyes from a window or lamp; if it falls in the same place on each eye, the eyes are working together.

Even with office screening, however, we don't always catch an eye that tends to deviate. Deviations occur more often when the child is tired. If you ever notice that your 6-month-old or older child has an eye that doesn't always look the same way as its partner, alert his doctor. It's critical that an eye specialist (ophthalmologist) examine the child. What some people call a lazy eye *(amblyopia)* may be a sign that one eye doesn't see as clearly as the other. When the brain is forced to make 1 picture from 2 very different inputs, it starts to ignore the signals from the worse eye. Over time this process becomes irreversible, leading to partial blindness in the weaker eye. In most cases, you should address the problem before the child turns 3 to ensure he'll grow up with normal depth perception. Treatments for amblyopia vary based on the cause and severity of the condition. Some children require glasses or patches that force the brain to pay attention to signals from the weaker eye. Other kids need surgery to shorten or lengthen certain muscles that control eye movement.

should i let them put that goo in my newborn's eyes?

In short, yes. That goo, in most hospitals, is erythromycin ointment, and it serves as a simple, harmless, cost-effective means of preventing blindness. The blindness in question results from infection with 1 of 2 sexually transmitted infections, chlamydia and gonorrhea (often people get both at the same time). Both infections can progress rapidly in newborns' eyes, damaging the clear part over the pupils (corneas) and causing irreversible harm. Men and women can harbor chlamydia and gonorrhea infections without any symptoms. Obstetricians test most women for these infections during their pregnancies and treat them if their tests come back positive, but mothers can still pick up those diseases after their tests come back, so to be safe we treat everyone.

Erythromycin ointment is close to 100% effective in preventing gonorrhea eye infections, but chlamydia infections can still pop up as long as 2 weeks after delivery. When this happens, only oral antibiotics provide effective treatment. Because of the danger from chlamydia, most pediatricians test newborns' eyes for the disease before prescribing antibiotics. Other eye infections may also threaten a baby's vision, including herpes simplex virus and *Staphylococcus aureus*. There are several other reasons a baby might develop eye discharge in the first few weeks of life, including a rare allergic reaction to erythromycin.

when to call the doctor

If your newborn develops thick, yellow discharge from one or both eyes, make sure a doctor sees him quickly.

the tracts of my tears

The good news is that the vast majority of newborns with eye drainage will just have blocked tear ducts. Also called nasolacrimal ducts, these are the tiny tubes that start at the inner corners of our eyes and drain tears into our nasal cavities. These tiny passages are blocked in up to 10% of newborns, although you may not be able to tell until the baby is 2 or 3 months old and his tear production increases. Babies with blocked tear ducts may have one eye that waters all the time, although nearly one-third of affected babies have blockages on both sides. Matter or mucous often collects in the corner of the affected eye and may require cleaning several times a day.

when to call the doctor

Pus is never normal; if you see thick, yellow discharge in your baby's eye or if you find the eye stuck shut after he's been sleeping, it's time for a doctor to get a look at him. He has almost certainly developed an infection in the eye.

Antibiotic drops or ointment will clear an infection up within a few days, but in the meantime you'll want to clean the eye with warm water and a soft washcloth or cotton ball, soaking dried secretions to loosen them up, then gently wiping them away. Be sure to clean the eye out prior to using the medicine because drainage may keep antibiotics from getting to the infection site.

Traditionally, pediatricians have told parents to gently massage the area of the blocked tear duct, just under the inner corner of the eye. Whether doing this actually clears up the blockage no one knows, but it at least makes you feel like you're fixing something. As babies grow their tear ducts also enlarge, and about 90% of these blockages resolve by 12 months of age. Ophthalmologists treat the ones that don't improve by probing the duct, usually once the child is approaching his first birthday.

when to call the doctor

Any time you see a red, swollen eyelid you should call the doctor and have your baby seen immediately. These types of infections can be very dangerous if untreated.

not so pretty in pink

Pinkeye is a word that says everything and nothing at the same time. It does tell you exactly what you're looking at—the part of the eye where it ought to be white is pink. But there are many reasons for that color change, and pinkeye doesn't really tell you the cause or what to do about it.

What all cases of pinkeye have in common is the pink part. It's conjunctiva, a thin, clear membrane that covers the sclera and also lines the eyelids. Normally, blood vessels in the conjunctiva are so tiny you can't see them, but when something inflames the tissue the blood vessels swell, giving it a pink appearance.

Swollen blood vessels are not the only symptom of conjunctivitis. The conjunctiva is full of disease-fighting cells; it also secretes mucous to lubricate the eyes and trap germs and dust. When something inflames the conjunctiva it works overtime, secreting mucous and even pus onto the eye, which you'll see as discharge. The conjunctiva itself can even swell, giving a rough appearance to the eye surface. A child with conjunctivitis will also produce excess tears, and he may complain of itching, burning, or the feeling that something is in his eye.

when to call the doctor

Two eye symptoms are always alarming and should never be ignored. Pain with light (photophobia) suggests the eye is inflamed at a deeper level than just the surface. If your child closes his eye in the light or won't go into a bright setting because of discomfort, alert his doctor immediately. Causes range from serious infections to corneal injury to glaucoma, all of which deserve quick attention. The second alarming sign is change in vision. A child with conjunctivitis may have some mucous on his eye, but once you wipe it away he should see fine. If he reports blurred vision, someone should evaluate him that day.

The most common cause of pinkeye is bacterial infection, often with the same bacteria that infect sinuses or the middle ear. These infections tend to cause panic in schools and child care because they look gross and your child may indeed pass them to other children by hand-to-hand contact (more accurately, hand-to-eye-to-friend's-hand-to-friend's-eye contact). Pediatricians, however, don't panic, knowing most of these infections tend to resolve on their own eventually. Antibiotic drops or ointment do clear them up faster and decrease transmission.

The idea of putting drops or ointment in a child's eye gives many parents the willies. The key is to remember that you don't actually have to touch the eye. In fact, it's a really bad idea; don't do that. Instead, put your finger on the lower lid of the affected eye. Try to pull it down to form a cup for eyedrops or ointment, and then pretend you're a bomber, aiming for that lid. Eye medicine is very forgiving. As long as some runs into the eye, it should work.

It's tempting to grab an old bottle of eyedrops and try to treat conjunctivitis yourself, but this is a bad idea for a few reasons. The most important is that without a good history and physical examination, you don't know you're treating the right thing. One case of pinkeye may look a lot like the next, even when they result from very different causes. Second, pinkeye in young children is often a red flag that alerts us to a middle ear infection. *Haemophilus influenzae* bacterial infections are notorious for attacking the eye and ear simultaneously. Not all children run fevers or grab their ears with infections, so the only way to make sure we're not missing an ear infection is to look in there and see. Third, the best way to create antibiotic-resistant bacteria is to treat an infection with old antibiotics or treat it partially then stop because you ran out. You've heard the expression, "What doesn't kill you makes you stronger"? It's especially true for bacteria. Nail them properly or leave them alone, but treating them halfway just makes them mad. Fourth, in the worst case scenario you might grab a vial of antibiotics combined with steroids, in which case you run the risk of doing very real and permanent damage to the eye. Instead, call the doctor and have your child seen.

The next most common cause of pinkeye is viral infection. In some cases viral conjunctivitis causes a more watery discharge with less pus, but it's not always obvious which one you're dealing with. Adenovirus is a common cold virus famous for causing dramatic eye symptoms, but there are dozens of others as well. The vast majority of viral eye infections resolve without treatment, causing only mild symptoms.

Two viral infections of the eye, however, are dangerous. One is herpes simplex virus. With herpes you might notice a cold sore on the lip or an erosion elsewhere on the face in addition to pinkeye. This type of infection deserves immediate attention from an ophthalmologist. Shingles (varicella zoster) is a type of infection with the virus that causes chickenpox. Again you'd probably see bumps on the face in the area of the eye along with the eye irritation itself. Either of these infections requires treatment in the hospital with intravenous medication and close follow-up by an ophthalmologist.

Allergies cause conjunctivitis symptoms as well, although with some hints as to what's going on. Allergic eyes tend to itch, often dramatically. They drain tears and sometimes mucous but never pus. Itching often starts within seconds or minutes of contact with the offending allergen. Several over-the-counter and prescription medicines treat allergic conjunctivitis, but don't forget you can also use oral antihistamines like diphenhydramine (eg, Benadryl), cetirizine (eg, Zyrtec), and loratadine (eg, Claritin). Cool compresses and artificial tears also help with symptoms, especially when you can't get to a pharmacy. Allergic conjunctivitis that doesn't respond to these measures probably deserves an ophthalmologist's attention.

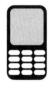

when to call the doctor

Contact lens wearers have special concerns when they get pinkeye. Contact lenses can harbor infections or cause allergies. The most important first step if your child or teen wears contacts and has pinkeye is to take out the contacts. The second step is to call the eye doctor who prescribed them and ask what the third step should be.

in the eye of the beholder

Childhood can be tough on eyes. Kids spend a lot of time down where all the dust, sand, sticks, and bugs are, and they don't always begin an activity with the question, "I wonder what risk this might pose to my eyes?" It's not unusual for children to get stuff in their eyes or be struck in the eye with a foreign object, such as a sibling's finger. These are good times for dad to play hero, as long as you know what you're doing.

A child with a foreign body in the eye might know exactly what it is and how it got there, or it may be a mystery. Stray eyelashes are the most common foreign bodies, along with dried bits of mucous, but anything that fits can end up in a child's eye. He is likely to keep his eye closed, but he may also rub at it. The first step is to calm him down and stop the rubbing so he doesn't end up injuring his cornea.

Be aware that whatever is in there, it cannot end up behind the eye. The conjunctiva follows the front of the eye up and down about a quarter inch to where the lids are, then folds back on itself to line the eyelids, forming a pocket above and below the eye. The foreign body will stay in that pouch or travel back onto the eye's surface.

when to call the doctor

There are some foreign bodies you should leave to the professionals. Anything sharp, such as a shard of glass or metal, should be removed by an ophthalmologist or trained emergency physician. Chemicals, such as powdered fertilizer or laundry detergent, should be flushed immediately with large volumes of water, and the child should be examined as soon as possible. Foreign bodies propelled at high speed (for example, from an explosion or a lawnmower) deserve professional evaluation. A foreign body that appears to be stuck on the eyeball and won't float around needs urgent medical evaluation as well.

Assuming it's just a garden-variety particle, you now face the problem of how to get the thing out of there. If you're dealing with multiple particles, such as a face full of sand or dirt, you'll first want to dab or rinse off the other particles before they, too, end up in your child's eye. Next, if he's cooperative, you can have your child submerge his face in a pan or a sink full of water and blink. A younger child probably won't buy into this plan, so you'll need to gently pour warm water onto his eye while holding the lid open (no one said being a hero would be easy). To make the experience as pleasant as possible, you might even dissolve half a teaspoon of table salt in a cup of water to make normal saline if you have time.

If you can see the particle in the corner of the eye, you can try taking a moistened washcloth or a cotton swab and gently wiping it out of the eye. You can approach particles lodged in the lower lid the same way, pulling the lid out and swiping gently with a moist cloth or swab. Alternately, you can pull the lid down and pour a little warm water over it. The most common place for a foreign body to get trapped is under the upper lid, which poses a greater challenge.

when to call the doctor

If blinking underwater and irrigating the eye don't work, you can try pulling the upper lid out and over the lower lid, hoping the lower lid will capture the invader for easier removal. If none of these measures work, you're heading to the doctor's office, urgent care center, or emergency department.

Tearing and discomfort should improve over the next hour or two after you've successfully removed a foreign body from the eye. If symptoms fail to go away or worsen, chances are good there is more stuff in there or the child has suffered a scratch to the cornea. Other concerning signs include a cloudy spot on the cornea or any change in vision. Any of these symptoms should prompt an immediate trip to the doctor.

What about that cornea, anyway? The clear part of the eye over the pupil and iris is a very delicate organ, full of nerves to sense any injury. If a fingernail or grain of sand injures the surface of the cornea, it will register as discomfort and the child may feel like there's something in his eye, even if there's not anything there anymore. Corneal abrasions may hurt more with exposure to light or cause blurred vision. Your only clue to a corneal abrasion might be that your child is constantly squinting with one eye.

A corneal abrasion may get infected or it may scar, causing loss of vision. The good news is that most corneal abrasions are mild and resolve without causing any problems. Corneal abrasions can be invisible to the naked eye. If she suspects an abrasion, your child's doctor may use a little strip of paper to dye tears with fluorescein, a chemical that collects wherever the cornea is injured and glows bright yellow in ultraviolet light. Doctors may use antibiotics or eyedrops to relieve symptoms and prevent infection. Special contact lenses can also function as bandages to protect the cornea while it heals.

a bump in the lid

A variety of things cause eyelid swelling in children. Some of them are very likely to go away on their own or with minimal intervention on your part. Others threaten vision, even the child's life. It helps to have an idea which is which.

One common cause of eyelid swelling is getting hit in the eye with something. Trauma like this usually causes bruising, and as the dad you're also likely to hear what happened. Bruising around the eye (a black eye) may take weeks to resolve, but the swelling should go away within a day or two.

when to call the doctor

If your child has been struck in the eye, it's a good idea to have him examined urgently to make sure all the structures of the eye are intact. If the child reports any vision problems, it's especially important to have him seen.

Allergies can cause some generalized swelling of the eyelids. As we discussed earlier, allergies often cause dramatic itching and eye watering but do not cause pain.

The eyelids contain hundreds of tiny glands that secrete oil and sweat (yes, your eyelids can sweat). When these glands become blocked they can swell and grow tender, causing a sty, which doctors call a hordeolum because sty doesn't sound fancy enough. When the blocked gland is located along the outside of the eyelid where the eyelashes are, it tends to form a little pimple, which then resolves on its own in a matter of weeks. Applying warm compresses to the eyelid may help speed this process some. Sometimes the blockage occurs deeper inside the eyelid, and you see a bump that looks more like a mass than a pimple. Sties in both locations often harbor staph or strep infections, and doctors usually prescribe antibiotic ointment or drops to treat them.

A chalazion looks very much like a deep sty, appearing as a bump in the body of the eyelid. Chalazia, however, are not infected and don't tend to hurt or form pustules. If a chalazion doesn't go away after several weeks, an eye doctor may have to remove it.

when to call the doctor

Other structures in and around the eyelids may also harbor infections. The tear glands themselves may become infected, a condition called dacryoadenitis. Those glands lie above and outside the upper lid. When tear ducts become infected, swelling occurs just below the inner corner of the eye. You might even see pus come out of the little opening where the tear duct starts. Both of these infections require treatment with antibiotics, sometimes in the hospital.

One of the most dangerous infections in childhood involves the eyelids and surrounding tissues. When the infection is limited to the lids and tissue in front of the eye, we call it periorbital cellulitis. When it gets behind those structures it's orbital cellulitis. With these infections you'll notice the entire eyelid is swollen and red, sometimes above and below the eye. Orbital cellulitis may cause the eye to bulge forward. These infections often strike children who have had cold symptoms for a while and have developed sinus infections. Bacteria find the tissue around the eye especially easy to penetrate, and it's a short trip from eyelids to the vulnerable nerve and artery that supply the eye from behind. Infections in this area may also extend to the brain and surrounding fluid.

when to call the doctor

If you notice your child has a red or swollen lid not just in one spot but all over, you need to get him medical attention immediately.

do you see what i see?

To work well the eyes have to be pretty much round. Unfortunately, the same way some people are taller than others, some eyes are rounder than others. A child whose eyeball is a little long may have trouble seeing objects at a distance, a condition we call nearsightedness or myopia. If his eyes are a little shorter, he may find it difficult to see things up close, which we call farsightedness or hyperopia. If the cornea isn't perfectly even, he may have distortion of his visual field, like looking through wavy glass. Together we call these conditions refractive errors because they involve problems with how light bends as it travels from the front of the eye to the retina. All of these conditions may be inherited, but they rarely become evident before the school years.

If you notice your child has to sit close to the television or can't read signs at a distance, it's kind of a no-brainer to get his vision checked. The same thing would be true if he has to hold books far away like his grandparents. Visual problems, however, can affect learning and school performance before they become that obvious. Starting at age 3 your child should have his vision screened at his annual wellness examination. Any problems that arise from the screen deserve follow-up by an optometrist or ophthalmologist.

Many parents ask to have their children's vision checked because of headaches. While children with headaches may also have vision problems, those problems very rarely cause headaches. Migraine headaches, which are common in children, may cause bizarre visual complaints, such as wavy lines or flashes in the visual field or objects appearing distorted in size. We will discuss headaches in detail in Chapter 22, but for now let's just say I'd start at the pediatrician's office, not the eye doctor, for this problem.

If your child is diagnosed with a refractive error, your first thought as a dad might be, "How is my child going to play sports if he wears glasses?" Hopefully you've watched enough sports by now that you already know the answer—plastic or polycarbonate lenses, a secure head strap, and confidence.

You might also wonder whether your child will get bullied because of his glasses. The short answer is if he gets bullied, it probably isn't the eyewear. There are tons of resources available for parents to help deal with bullying, but the key is for you to help your child feel confident so he is less likely to attract the attention of bullies. Let him pick out a pair of glasses he feels makes him look good, and let him know you think he looks great wearing them. Remind him of all the things he'll be able to do better now that he can see clearly.

Contact lenses are an option for many teens with refractive errors, but ophthalmologists and optometrists are very reluctant to prescribe them to kids before the teen years because without proper care and attention, they put children at risk of eye infection and injury. Surgery for refractive errors should wait until your child has finished growing completely because his eyes are still growing, too. For that reason, you'll also want to make sure he keeps his scheduled appointments with the eye doctor. Just because those glasses were perfect last year does not mean they're still doing the job.

One final word on vision issues and learning. Claims that eye exercises or vision training therapy can help children overcome learning disorders have failed to survive the test of science. There are a variety of effective therapies for dyslexia and other learning disabilities, but they don't really focus on the eyes.

Your child's eyes are truly amazing. He's using them to watch you, and you're using yours to watch his watch you, and looking at his to see what he thinks about you watching him while he's looking at yours to see what you're seeing in his. In short, there's lots of looking going on. But the bottom line is this: when it comes to the health of your child's visual organs, just keep an eye on him.

11

keep it down:
infant spitting up and vomiting

each time we announced we were having a baby all sorts of people congratulated us, but no one seemed quite as excited as our dry cleaners, except perhaps my mother. No, scratch that. The lady at Carolina Cleaners just about leapt over the counter to hug us, knowing that each baby we had would boost her business by 50% for at least a year. I had shirts that looked like Rorschach tests, pants like Jackson Pollock's famous drip paintings if Pollock had worked in curdled milk. If I'd had any sense I would have donned a poncho before holding any of our babies, but I was too sleep-deprived for that kind of forethought, and besides, I sort of enjoyed my trips to the cleaners.

gastroesophageal reflux: déjà eww

To some extent spitting up is a normal part of human infancy. You'd think as precious a substance as human milk is we would have evolved not to waste any of it, but recent studies suggest that spitting up may actually serve a purpose. Mom's milk contains important protective bacteria, and when that milk washes up into the baby's upper airway it spreads those bacteria around, helping protect the baby from invaders. An alternate theory holds that the purpose of spitting up is to enrich the dry cleaning industry.

To understand spitting up, it helps to know how the plumbing works. Milk gets to the stomach by way of a muscular tube called the *esophagus.* At the point where the esophagus meets the stomach, a ring of muscle called the *lower esophageal sphincter* opens up to let food in, then tightens to keep gastric contents where it belongs. At the other end of the stomach is another muscular ring, the *pyloric valve,* which opens intermittently to allow food into the first part of the intestines, the *duodenum.* When all these parts are working properly, food progresses in an orderly fashion in one direction, from mouth to intestines.

Babies, however, tend to have weaker lower esophageal sphincters than older children and adults, allowing gastric contents to wash up into the esophagus and often into the mouth and nose. (Many parents are alarmed to see spit-up coming from their babies' noses, but rest assured this phenomenon is normal and may one day prove a big hit in the school cafeteria.) This sort of passive backwash is called gastroesophageal reflux (GER), and it is a nearly universal phenomenon in babies.

Vomiting, on the other hand, is a more active process, involving contractions of the stomach muscle, diaphragm, and abdominal muscles. These contractions expel gastric contents forcefully up the esophagus and out of the mouth. Vomiting is a protective reflex, designed to rid the stomach of ingested toxins. At the extremes anyone can tell the difference between vomiting and reflux, but there is a gray zone of large-volume reflux where it may not be so easy to tell.

Once gastric contents are on your shirt it's easy to overestimate their volume. Your baby may appear to spit up his entire feeding, but even with forceful vomiting a child really can't fully empty his stomach. (This is one reason we no longer induce vomiting when a child swallows a poison; it doesn't work well enough to make a difference.) For fun, pour a tablespoon of half-and-half onto an old shirt to see how much it spreads out. Two of those tablespoons make an ounce, and most babies eat at least 2 ounces per feeding, often more.

Many parents are alarmed to see that their babies' spit-up appears curdled, like cottage cheese. This reflects normal chemical changes that occur in milk proteins when they contact stomach acid; it's just that we don't usually have to look at it. Mucous is also a normal part of gastric contents, although you may see more of it if your baby has a cold.

Newborns often spit up some in the first 24 hours after birth as they clear the airway, esophagus, and stomach of amniotic fluid and maternal blood. After that spitting up tends to calm down for several weeks, in part because feeding volumes start relatively small and feeding tends to take a long time. Reflux becomes more common and dramatic as infants approach 4 months of age, when symptoms peak. From that point they gradually resolve, and by 12 months of age most children spit up rarely, if at all.

Some practices predictably worsen reflux. The most common problem is overfeeding, which we see more frequently in bottle-fed babies. A newborn's stomach is roughly the size of a walnut, and in most cases it doesn't hold more than about 2 to 3 ounces comfortably. By 4 months of age many infants tolerate 4 to 6 ounces, but think of the stomach like a water balloon—overfill it and you'll be getting some of that stuff back.

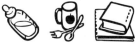

what you can do

It may seem obvious, but anything that compresses a baby's abdomen will increase pressure inside the stomach and drive out gastric contents. For 30 to 60 minutes after a feeding you'll probably want to avoid jostling your baby, putting him in a swing, or strapping him to your chest and doing wind sprints. Also, respect the force of gravity—feed your baby at least 30 minutes before laying him down for a nap to minimize the chance he'll spit up all over his crib.

If your baby has spit up, don't try to feed him again immediately in an attempt to make up for the lost meal. Wait for his next feeding and trust him to know how much he needs. Frequent burping may reduce spitting; burp him after the first few minutes (if he's nursing) or first ounce (if he's taking a bottle). Some babies seem to gobble milk so fast that they don't know they're full. If your baby seems to be one of these, you might give him a little break partway through his feeding to assess his appetite. You may also find that shrinking his feedings by an ounce and feeding more often helps. Cigarette smoke not only causes GER in adults, it contributes to GER in babies. Add reflux to the long list of reasons no one should smoke in a house where infants or children live.

how much is too much: gastroesophageal reflux disease

While spitting up is a normal part of infancy, there are times when it poses a health hazard. Some babies with more severe reflux cough, wheeze, or suffer chronic nasal congestion. They may also develop esophageal irritation that makes them reluctant to eat, leading to poor growth and malnutrition. When we see these symptoms we call the condition gastroesophageal reflux disease (GERD).

You might think diagnosing GERD is pretty straightforward, and sometimes it is—your baby is growing poorly, coughing, crying after feedings, and spitting up like a fountain. But not all cases are so obvious. For one thing, because spitting up is so common, doctors can't always tell when it's the cause of the problem or just coincidental. For another, not all babies with GERD spit up. Gastric contents sometimes reflux into the esophagus and even the lungs without coming out the mouth or nose. Some people call this silent reflux.

In many cases it's simpler to perform a trial of therapy than test for GERD, but there are some tests available to help sort out challenging cases. The simplest and most common of these involves feeding the baby formula or expressed breast milk laced with a dye that shows up on x-ray films, then performing x-rays to see if it comes back up. This test, called an upper gastrointestinal (GI), can identify when reflux is occurring, although it cannot tell doctors if GERD is the cause of a baby's symptoms. Sometimes, too, a baby with GERD just doesn't reflux during his upper GI. In another type of test doctors insert a probe down the baby's esophagus to monitor changes in acidity or electrical activity that indicate gastric acid may be causing irritation. Very few babies require testing this extensive, and many of these babies suffer other chronic illnesses as well.

Treating GERD is not always as simple as it might seem. The single most effective measure we have is not to give a medication but to thicken feedings with infant cereal. Traditionally pediatricians have recommended rice cereal for this purpose, but some doctors now worry that introducing refined carbohydrates early contributes to obesity; they prefer whole-grain cereals. In most cases we advise adding 1 level teaspoon of cereal for each ounce of formula or human milk. Be sure to use a measuring spoon and not just whatever you happen to have around for stirring coffee.

Thickening feedings serves 2 purposes. One is to add substance to the gastric contents so they don't flow into the esophagus. The other is to add calories so you can cut the volume of each feeding by about an ounce, stretching the stomach less. Infant nutrition companies now market thickened formulas for treating GERD, but these formulas don't have increased calories, so you cannot plan on cutting back on feeding volumes if you're using them.

If a baby is formula-fed, his doctor may recommend changing to a less allergenic formula to improve GERD. Some children develop allergies to cow's milk or soy proteins in many infant formulas, and these babies may spit up or vomit depending on the severity of their allergies. Even nursing babies can react to traces of these proteins in mother's milk, so some moms try eliminating these foods from their diets for a couple of weeks to see if reflux improves. Unfortunately, food allergies only account for about 2% to 5% of cases of GERD, so this approach rarely works.

Medical therapies for GERD have spotty success. Most medications we use for reflux reduce the quantity of acid the stomach produces. Many doctors start with a class of acid reducers that interfere with type 2 histamine receptors in the stomach. Ranitidine (eg, Zantac) is the best known of these H_2 blockers, but the class also includes nizatidine (eg, Axid), cimetidine (eg, Tagamet), and famotidine (eg, Pepcid). These medications have a long history of newborn safety, but their effect tends to wear off with time.

A newer class of antacids blocks the proton channels in stomach cells that actually secrete hydrochloric acid. The chemical abbreviation for hydrogen is the letter H, so we call these medicines H_1 blockers or proton-pump inhibitors. Omeprazole (eg, Prilosec) and lansoprazole (eg, Prevacid) are the best-known members of this class. While these medications appear safe when used in place of or alongside H_2 blockers, recent studies have questioned how well they work for infants and children.

A third class of medications, called *promotility agents,* signal the intestines to move food along more rapidly. These medications include metoclopramide (eg, Reglan) and the antibiotic erythromycin. As you might imagine, these medications can cause diarrhea as a side effect. Doctors usually save them to use as backup therapy when nothing else is working for severe GERD.

Surgery remains an option for babies with severe GERD. Often these babies are born prematurely or have other chronic health issues like cerebral palsy. The surgery, called a Nissen fundoplication after the surgeon who pioneered it, involves wrapping the upper part of the stomach around the lower part of the esophagus to form a cuff. Children who have had this surgery often cannot vomit.

beyond spitting up

While GER and GERD account for much of baby vomiting, they are not the only causes. The most dramatic vomiting occurs with a condition called *pyloric stenosis*. Under normal circumstances the pyloric valve, or pylorus, lets food out of the stomach and into the first part of the intestines (duodenum) at regular intervals. The pylorus works kind of like a bouncer at a hot night club, making sure entry occurs in an orderly fashion.

Some babies, however, develop an overly muscular pyloric valve. Because the pylorus is ring-shaped, overgrowth of the muscle closes off the passageway into the duodenum, so milk or formula can only leave the stomach the same way it came in, often with a shocking amount of force. We call this phenomenon projectile vomiting. Projectile vomiting doesn't mean you were holding your baby in your lap and he threw up on your shoes. It means you were holding your baby in your lap and he threw up on the shoes of the guy sitting across from you on the subway. Vomiting with pyloric stenosis usually occurs within 30 minutes of each feeding.

Pyloric stenosis affects boys more than girls. Vomiting usually starts by the third week of the baby's life, but symptoms may not appear until as late as 5 months. After 6 months pyloric stenosis is almost certainly not the cause of an infant's vomiting. Affected children require urgent hospitalization and surgery to correct the condition.

You might think the small intestines are stuffed into the abdominal cavity randomly, like spaghetti in a bowl. In fact, however, they're tucked in more like a parachute, in a specific way that keeps them all from getting tangled. During the fetal period the intestines develop outside the body and are then drawn into the abdominal cavity. If something goes wrong with that process, it results in malrotation. The easiest way for doctors to diagnose malrotation is to feed a baby formula or breast milk laced with a dye that shows up on x-ray images. The process is the same as the upper GI we discussed earlier, but this time radiologists follow the dye as it pro-

when to call the doctor

Vomit that contains bright green or yellow fluid is always concerning because it suggests a blockage in the intestines. If your baby has this type of vomiting, his doctor may want to hospitalize him and perform studies to determine what is wrong. Causes of such intestinal blockages include a condition called volvulus, in which a baby's intestines become twisted on themselves. Volvulus is a medical emergency that requires surgery. Usually babies with volvulus also have a condition called intestinal malrotation, another potential cause of severe vomiting.

gresses into the small intestine. Malrotation usually requires surgery, although the surgery may not be urgent if the child is not also suffering volvulus (see above).

Intussusception may also cause babies to vomit bile. Intussusception occurs when one segment of intestine slides inside another, like a telescope closing. Swelling and blockage result, causing vomiting, abdominal swelling, and often bloody stools. Intussusception is another medical emergency; if not treated quickly, bowel can die and cause overwhelming infection. Most often doctors diagnose intussusception by filling the colon with dye that shows up on x-ray films. In some cases the radiologist can actually fix the condition by filling the large intestine with enough dye to push the telescoped segment back out. When this method fails, urgent surgery is the only option.

when to call the doctor

An incarcerated inguinal hernia may cause bilious vomiting as a symptom. The giveaway here is that your baby is likely to have a bulging, painful scrotum. Girls can also get hernias, but they are much more common in boys; girls will have a painful bulge in the groin instead of in the scrotum. An incarcerated hernia is also a surgical emergency, so don't delay getting care if you think you see one.

when to call the doctor

A baby who suddenly starts vomiting may have a disease far from the gastrointestinal tract. Ear infections, pneumonia, meningitis, kidney infections, and brain tumors may all present with unexplained vomiting. If your baby vomits hourly for more than 8 hours in a row or for more than 24 hours, it's timeto get him to the doctor.

why just vomit?

For the first few months of life, mother's antibodies protect babies from many common intestinal infections. That said, even young babies may contract rotavirus, *Shigella*, *Salmonella*, influenza, *Clostridium difficile*, and other infections that can be quite dangerous in some cases. In most cases, these infections will produce diarrhea and fever along with vomiting. **Remember that any fever in an infant younger than 3 months is alarming and deserves immediate medical attention.** An older infant may have fever with an intestinal infection, but the infant's temperature should not be above 104°F and it should not last more than 3 days.

Even if he has an infection, your baby shouldn't vomit for more than 1 day. He may have tummy pain when he vomits or a bowel movement, but his tummy shouldn't hurt in between these episodes. Most parents are appropriately alarmed if they see their baby vomiting blood, but stomach acid can give blood the appearance of coffee grounds, so vomiting that looks like that is also grounds to call the doctor. (Get it? Grounds? Yeah, I know. Good one, right?)

when to call the doctor

Any time you see blood or lots of mucous in the stool, it suggests a more serious infection, and you should call your baby's doctor immediately.

waterworks

Babies dehydrate pretty easily, so any time a baby suffers vomiting and diarrhea you want to be on the lookout for signs his tank is getting low. Decreased urine output is among the most reliable. We like to see a minimum of 3 pee diapers a day or 1 every 8 hours, but when a baby is having frequent watery stools, it can be tough to judge what sort of liquid is filling the tenth diaper of the afternoon. Look also at where fluid should be—if your baby's mouth looks dry or he cries without making tears, he may be seriously dehydrated.

when to call the doctor

If your baby's skin seems loose or he's difficult to arouse, his dehydration is probably severe, and he needs quick medical attention. Also, if your baby vomits more than 8 times in 8 hours, he should probably see a doctor, especially if he's also having diarrhea.

In many cases you have the power to keep your baby from becoming dehydrated. Remember that even with vigorous vomiting, the stomach does not completely empty. That means you may be able to keep enough fluid going in to catch up with what's coming out. If your baby is breast-feeding, he should continue to do so, with one 10-minute feeding every hour or two for mild vomiting or a 5-minute feed every 30 to 90 minutes for more severe symptoms. Additionally, you can use a commercial electrolyte solution like Pedialyte for hydration. Unlike plain water, juice, or sports drinks, these fluids contain a balance of salt and sugar that helps the body absorb as much water as possible. To avoid causing more vomiting, you want to give just a little at a time, about a teaspoonful, but offer it frequently, around every 5 minutes or so. If you imagine a leaky faucet, you'll get a picture of how much fluid that can end up being over time.

Once vomiting has subsided, continue to give your baby breast milk or electrolyte solution for around 8 hours before trying food. He may seem hungry, but you don't want to lose ground. Once the 8 hours have passed, try something bland, like bananas or single-grain cereal, before getting adventurous.

Once your adventure with a vomiting baby is over, you'll have war stories to tell, and people will be impressed. You will have earned your stripes as a dad. Some of those stripes may not come out, either, even with repeated dry cleaning.

12

heating and cooling: fevers and what to do about them

. . . .

dad tip

Instead of alternating ibuprofen and acetaminophen

for fever, just pick the one that seems to work best.

You can always use the other if the first one

doesn't seem to be helping.

. . . .

of all the symptoms known to pediatrics, none seems to frighten parents quite as much as fever. Here's a typical complaint in my office: "Doc, I'm worried because my daughter had a temperature last night of a hundred and two! She also levitated off the bed, her head spun around, and she cursed me with the voice of a beast while green flames shot from her eyes. What can I do for the fever?"

As a dad, you might take pride in calming everyone down. In that case, you'll be happy to know that while fever can be a sign of serious illness, it's almost never a problem itself. A sick child cannot generate a fever high enough to damage her brain, for example. Getting a child's temperature down is a matter of comfort, not of life and death. As for the green eye flames, I recommend 2 drops of holy water every 6 to 8 hours, and call me if a bottomless chasm suddenly appears in the backyard.

catch the fever

You know what a fever is, don't you? Sure you do! It's whenever someone's body temperature is higher than normal. And normal body temperature is…were you going to say 98.6°F (37.0°C)? Of course you were! Every schoolboy knows that, ever since the German physician Carl Wunderlich stuck his foot-long thermometer in the armpits of 25,000 adults in 1868 (they didn't have a lot to do for entertainment in 1868). The number he came up with was the average of all those temperatures. More recent research actually moved the peg down a little to 98.2°F (36.8°C).

The problem with that number is that it's an average and does not take into account that normal human temperatures vary by time of day and other factors, including a person's age, sex, physical activity, and even the surrounding air temperature. What we really want to know is what body temperature indicates a child may be sick. That answer depends on how and where you take the temperature.

Just like a thermostat controls the temperature in your house by making adjustments when the air gets too hot or too cold, the brain controls body temperature. Our brains do an amazing job of keeping our body temperatures within the very small range at which our systems all function well. When you think about humans living everywhere from the Arctic Circle to the Kalahari Desert to New Jersey, you have to marvel at the mechanism that makes it possible (especially New Jersey). When our bodies get too cold, our muscles create heat by shivering; our cells generate heat by burning chemical fuel called adenosine triphosphate (ATP); our blood vessels direct blood away from the skin and deeper into the body; we bundle or curl up in the fetal position. When we get overheated those processes work in reverse. Our skin flushes, we unbundle, we move slowly, and we sweat.

Viral and bacterial infections cause the vast majority of fevers in children. Research in animals and test tubes suggests fever helps us defeat infections. When the brain detects signs of inflammation from an infection, it bumps the body's thermostat up. Your child may be in a comfortable room, but she will feel cold; she will shiver, bundle up, and look pale as her body tries to conserve heat. Then, when the fever breaks, she will sweat and throw off her blankets, and her skin will look flushed.

you want to put that where?

Prior to modern times there was only one way to check a child's temperature: you'd feel her forehead with your hand and go, "Yep, you've got a fever!" This method remains the most commonly used for obvious reasons, but it's not very accurate. For one thing, different people are more or less sensitive to cold or heat. Women are more sensitive to cold than men, so don't be surprised if you and mom disagree about the child's temperature. Mom's own temperature will also vary depending on her hormone levels, so what feels normal to her one week may feel warm the next. Likewise, if you just came back from a workout, you've elevated your own core temperature and may think everyone else feels cool. Overall, parents using the hand-to-forehead method miss about 20% of fevers. If your child feels warm and she also seems sick, chances are around 50% to 80% she really does have a fever. If you can, however, go ahead and actually check your child's temperature; it will make her doctor happy.

The brain regulates temperature, so the temperature we'd really like to know is the temperature in the brain. There's no easy way to get that number, so instead we try to get as close as possible to measuring the temperature inside the body, called the core body temperature. First you have to have a thermometer. There are several types to choose from, and they're not all appropriate for every age.

If you have an old glass mercury thermometer lying around, check with your local waste disposal provider about its hazardous waste collection plan. What you have there is an incredibly potent nerve poison encased in a thin, fragile tube of glass, and now you have a child. If that thermometer breaks, vaporized mercury can cause permanent brain or nerve damage in anyone who inhales it; children are especially vulnerable. This is not the sort of thing you just throw in the trash either, unless you plan to poison your whole community. Instead, find a disposable plastic container, fill it with absorbent kitty litter, insert the thermometer in the kitty litter, write "Mercury—Do Not Open" on the container, then put the container in a cardboard box and deliver it to the collection site in the trunk of your car. Really. It's that dangerous.

Once you remove your hazmat suit, it's time to run by the pharmacy or grocery store and pick up an inexpensive digital thermometer. If you're just itching to spend more money, you can opt for a tympanic thermometer that reads the temperature of the eardrum, but know that these thermometers are very difficult to use in infants younger than 6 months and that earwax, crooked ear canals, and squirming children can all interfere with their accuracy. Another pricey option is a temporal artery thermometer that reads the temperature of blood flowing through a vessel on the side of the forehead. These devices are baby-friendly but relatively new, and most of the studies on their accuracy come from the manufacturers. Likewise, it's not clear how well pacifier thermometers work. The least helpful thermometer is a strip of plastic containing liquid crystal, like a rectangular mood ring you place on the child's forehead. These devices are probably OK to monitor the temperature in your fish tank, but they're not adequate for medical use.

Assuming you went with the digital thermometer, your next big decision is where to stick it. If your child is 4 or 5 years old, she should be able to hold the thermometer under her tongue long enough to get a reading. This site gives a good approximation of core temperature unless she's just finished a popsicle or a cup of hot soup. For babies and younger children, many parents start with the armpit (axilla). Axillary temperatures are not very accurate because the armpit serves as the body's heat pump—as a child is mounting a fever, her body will keep blood away from the skin, so the armpit temperature will lag behind core temperature. As her fever breaks, blood will rush to the skin and the thermometer may read a little warm. A lot of parents have heard they should add a degree when reporting an axillary temperature, but that's not quite right. Just tell the doctor what the temperature was and how you took it, and the doctor will take it from there.

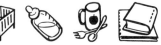

what you can do

To get a good rectal temperature safely, turn on the thermometer (don't forget that step); next, coat it with petroleum jelly, K-Y, or another lubricant. Some thermometers come with thin, plastic, disposable wrappers you can apply first. Have the child on your lap, in her crib, or on another firm surface where you can help keep her still. She can be face up with her legs up (the diaper-change position) or facedown with her knees under her. Gently insert the tip of the thermometer about ½ to 1 inch into her bottom and wait for the beep. That's it, you're done, and her doctor will be so proud of you! *Note:* If you don't use the little wrappers, you want to have one thermometer for rectal use and another for the mouth. Either way, clean the thermometer with alcohol or soap and water when you're done.

Rectal measurements provide the most accurate temperatures, and newer digital thermometers make taking a rectal temperature a quick and easy process. Some parents are squeamish about putting a thermometer down there, but you're a dad now, which means you've had ample opportunity to get over that. Parents also fear they might damage a child's rectum with the thermometer. Unless you use a ball-peen hammer to insert it, this complication is seriously unlikely.

So now you know your child's temperature, but is it a fever? That depends on how you took it. Here are the cutoffs.

- Rectal, tympanic (ear), or temporal artery temperature: 100.4°F (38.0°C) or higher
- Oral or pacifier temperature: 100°F (37.8°C) or higher
- Axillary (armpit) temperature: 99°F (37.2°C) or higher

Parents often use the term low-grade fever to describe temperatures below these cutoffs. Sometimes they believe their child tends to run a low temperature, so if it's normal, that's a fever for her. It's not. Remember, a normal temperature goes up and down during the day anyway. Your child may be getting sick and may feel warm, but until her temperature goes above those values, she does not have a fever, at least not yet.

Newborns can be too cold as well as too warm. A rectal temperature below 97.7°F or 36.5°C suggests a serious bloodstream infection; babies with this temperature need urgent medical care.

when to worry

Assuming you've identified a fever in your child, the next step is not to panic. (Unless the reason she's hot is that the house is on fire; that would be a major exception.) Remember, fever is not a disease—it's just a sign of a disease. The next 4 questions to ask are 1) How old is your child? 2) How high is the fever? 3) How long has she had the fever? and 4) How does she look?

You would imagine if being sick gives you a fever, then the sicker you are, the higher your fever would be. Unfortunately, it's not nearly that simple. For the most part, the height of a child's fever tells you almost nothing about how serious her illness is. That said, most viral illnesses cause temperatures between 100°F and 104°F.

when to call the doctor

If your baby is younger than 3 months and has any fever at all, get her to a doctor immediately! As a rule, any fever in a newborn buys that baby a major medical evaluation in the hospital. Not only are newborns especially susceptible to serious bacterial infections, but they don't display the signs doctors normally use to tell when a child is critically ill. Meningitis, for example, causes a stiff neck, but not if a baby's neck muscles are too weak to stiffen it. An infant younger than 3 months may continue to look normal up until the moment the infection is too far gone to treat, so doctors usually presume any fever results from a life-threatening infection until laboratory studies are back proving otherwise. Once your baby turns 3 months old you can relax a little about fever, although you should at least call the doctor's office about fever until your child turns 6 months old.

Here's a fun bet: ask your buddy how high a fever has to be for it to cause brain damage. The answer is around 108°F; you can decide what your buddy is going to do for you when he loses. Fortunately, the body's thermostat doesn't allow for temperature to get this high from illness alone. Temperatures in this range result from a child being left enclosed in a car on a summer day or from a football player being made to run up and down the field in August without enough access to water. Some people with a rare genetic condition called malignant hyperthermia generate these temperatures in response to certain anesthetics or antipsychotic medications. But your child, no matter how warm she feels or how sick she is, will not get a fever high enough to hurt her.

when to call the doctor

If your child's temperature is above 104°F, her doctor is probably going to want to get a look at her within 24 hours to make sure she just has a virus. For temperatures above 105°F, you should have her seen more urgently, again to determine the cause of the fever.

In many cases, doctors care more about the duration of the fever and other symptoms than how high the child's temperature is. Between the ages of 3 and 24 months we only allow a child 1 day of unexplained fever before we want to see that child and figure out what's going on. A surprising number of unexplained fevers at this age result from kidney infections; untreated, these infections can damage the kidneys permanently. Once children turn 2 we relax a little. Children this age can have an unexplained fever as long as 3 days before we need to figure out what's causing it. Often by the third day, these kids will develop a viral rash and their fevers will resolve.

when to call the doctor

As a rule, fevers from most viral illnesses last 3 days at the longest. Once your child's fever lasts 4 days or more, her doctor will probably want to examine her to determine the cause. In some cases it may still be a virus, but by that fourth day ear infections, sinus infections, and pneumonia all grow more common. Fevers that last longer than 5 days always deserve further investigation. A fever that goes away for 24 hours and then returns also worries us; it suggests that what started as a viral infection has progressed to a bacterial one. Some inherited conditions cause fevers that cycle at predictable intervals. If your child has an unexplained fever every 2 weeks, for example, her doctor will probably want to investigate.

If you call your child's doctor to report a fever, be ready to answer the question, "How does she look?" (*Hint:* Look at her first.) Some signs are predictable with fever—your child's heart rate and breathing will speed up, and she may seem uncomfortable. She may shiver and look pale when her temperature is going up, and when her temperature is coming down her skin will look flushed. You'll want to be on the lookout for signs of more severe illness like difficulty breathing, poor feeding, not waking up easily, a blue color to the lips, or blood-colored spots on the skin. These are all nature's way of telling you to get your child to a doctor now! Other very alarming signs include a bulging soft spot in a baby or confusion or difficulty moving or speaking in an older child. Any baby who simply won't stop crying needs evaluation, as does any child with fever and pain when she pees. If your child has a chronic illness like sickle cell disease, immunodeficiency, or cancer, her doctor will want to hear immediately about any fever. Finally, keep track of how much your child is peeing. If it's less often than every 8 hours, she's probably getting dehydrated.

feed it, starve it, what?

You're a guy. You fix stuff. So when you see your child shivering and pale and you feel her face and think, "I couldn't fry an egg on her forehead, but I could maybe poach one," you'll naturally want to step in and make things better. Chances are your parenting partner will be equally eager to intervene. Remember, however, that fever is not going to hurt your child, and it may even help her fight off an infection. There's nothing wrong with trying to make her more comfortable, but you want to make sure the cure isn't worse than the disease.

For temperatures below 102°F, there's really no need to give any medicine at all. For higher temperatures, only a couple of medications are safe to use for childhood fevers. Acetaminophen (eg, Tylenol) is approved for babies as young as 2 months. Ibuprofen (eg, Advil, Motrin) provides an alternative for infants 6 months and older. In general, both drugs work equally well, although ibuprofen lasts a little longer, 6 to 8 hours instead of 4 to 6 hours. Otherwise, some children seem to respond better to one drug or the other, but neither one seems better overall. You may still see bottles or boxes labeled "Children's Aspirin." They lie. Aspirin can cause a deadly disease in children called Reye syndrome. Unless a doctor has prescribed it to your child to treat a specific disease (usually Kawasaki), never give her aspirin.

Just because a medication is sold over the counter does not mean it's completely safe. Ibuprofen and acetaminophen carry risks, especially in overdose. Acetaminophen overdoses cause permanent liver damage and, in severe cases, death. Ibuprofen causes stomach upset and ulcers when overused, and it can damage the kidneys. The child's weight determines the safe dose of both drugs, which is why for children younger than 2 years, the bottles and dosing guidelines all say, "Call your doctor." Recently, the manufacturers of acetaminophen simplified dads' lives by making infant drops and children's syrup the same concentration; older bottles of infant acetaminophen are more concentrated, so make sure you tell the doctor what concentration you're using before you give the medicine.

In the past, some doctors would instruct parents to alternate acetaminophen and ibuprofen in an attempt to make sure that when one drug wore off, the other would still be in effect. It turns out that alternating drugs increases the risk of overdose ("Honey, did you just give the purple one or the red one?!") and may not relieve symptoms any better than picking one and sticking with it. I suggest parents do their best to reserve one to use only for breakthrough symptoms. Remember, fever doesn't hurt children—medication overdoses do.

A fever is going to bounce up and down as your child's body responds to her illness and environment. Don't put too much stock in whether your child's fever goes away when you give her acetaminophen or ibuprofen. In general you can expect her temperature to fall 2°F to 3°F with treatment. It doesn't mean she's sicker just because her fever doesn't break, and it doesn't mean she's less sick because it does. On the other hand, if your child seems uncomfortable, don't avoid treating her just so she'll have a fever when she gets to the doctor's office. Pediatricians in general are very trusting people. If you say she had a temperature of 103.8°F at 2:00 am, we'll believe you, even if she's 98.6°F in the office at 11:00 am.

If you want to cool a child down, it makes sense to put her in a bath. There's nothing wrong with this approach if it seems to make your child more comfortable, but remember, your only goal is to make her more comfortable. Make the bath tepid, not warm but not cold either (85°F–90°F) (29.4°C–32.2°C). If your child's lips are turning blue, chances are good you are not making her more comfortable. Never put rubbing alcohol in bathwater or use it to sponge your child's skin. Children can absorb enough alcohol through the skin this way to poison them. Really.

Children with fevers lose more water through sweat and rapid breathing, so they need plenty of fluid to stay hydrated. Make sure your child has something to drink at all times. Provide her enough clothing and blankets to be comfortable, but don't overdo it. Bundled babies cannot take off their clothes when they get overheated, and they may suffer heat stroke or sudden infant death syndrome. There's no reason to keep a child in bed just because she has a fever, although she probably should avoid vigorous exercise and very warm conditions.

seriously, dude, if my child has a seizure...

A small number of children between the ages of 6 months and 5 years may have a seizure as a result of fever. This condition, called febrile seizures, runs in families. If this does happen to your child you will be frightened because, you know, it's a seizure. But you will not panic because you realize that these seizures are not dangerous. They usually last 5 minutes or less and do not cause brain damage, nerve damage, learning disabilities, or intellectual disability. Children who have had febrile seizures have a minimally elevated risk of suffering other seizures by age 7.

During a febrile seizure your child will become unresponsive. If she was sitting or standing, she will fall to the floor and you may see her eyes roll upward. Her head may turn to one side, her body will stiffen, then both arms and legs will shake rhythmically. If you can, try to note the time the seizure begins. It will seem to go on forever, but most febrile seizures last less than 5 minutes. If possible, place your child on a surface where she's not likely to hurt herself, such as a carpeted floor or bed, and turn her head to one side in case she vomits. Do not put anything in your child's mouth during the seizure; it is physically impossible for her to swallow her own tongue, no matter what that kid told you at summer camp.

when to call the doctor

You do not need to call emergency medical services (EMS) (911) for a febrile seizure unless your child is having difficulty breathing or the seizure lasts more than 15 minutes. You should, however, contact her pediatrician once it's over for further instructions.

A child who has had one febrile seizure stands about a 30% to 50% chance of having another one before she turns 6 years of age. Seizures almost never occur within 24 hours of each other, so while you're likely to be as anxious as a long-tailed cat in a room full of rocking chairs, there's little to worry about. Once your child has experienced a febrile seizure, it's easy to become paranoid about fevers, but she can have a seizure just as easily with a low fever as a high one; giving fever-reducing medications earlier or more often does nothing to cut her chances of having another seizure.

it will only be a minute

Just because fever due to an illness cannot get high enough to injure a child doesn't mean heat cannot harm children. Every summer newspapers feature a rash of tragic stories about children who die from heatstroke. Most of these deaths occur in vehicles. Cars heat up fast, as much as 20°F in 10 minutes, even when windows are cracked, and even when it doesn't feel all that hot outside. Babies and children are especially prone to heatstroke, so don't leave them unattended in the car, even if you think you'll only be gone a short time. As impossible as you might think it would be to forget a child in a car seat, once they're asleep and you're distracted, it can happen. One idea is to keep a stuffed animal in the front seat with you whenever you're traveling with your baby or toddler as a reminder to check the car seat when you get out.

Adolescents and older children risk heatstroke when they exercise outdoors. Check to make sure they have plenty of water available to drink. If they're training with a team or as part of a sports camp, don't be shy to ask the coach what measures are in place to avoid heatstroke. *Hint:* Hot people sweat. When the sweating stops, that's a bad, bad sign. Being tough is great, but there's nothing tough about training through a headache, dizziness, nausea, vomiting, confusion, or feeling faint. Those are all signs of approaching heatstroke; the next signs are unconsciousness and death.

when to call the doctor

If you suspect your child is on the verge of heatstroke, move her to the coolest possible location, even a cool bath. If she is alert and responsive, she should drink cool fluids, but if she is out of it, she may choke while drinking. In this case, it's time to call EMS (911).

You are now prepared to take charge of almost any situation involving a child who seems too warm. As for the levitations, fiery eyes, and bottomless backyard chasms, you'll have to await my forthcoming book, *Exorcist to Exorcist.*

13

ear, ear: how to tell if your child has an ear infection and what to do about it

if one day someone were to invent a reliable, inexpensive device to identify and treat ear infections at home, I might have to retire from medicine and follow my dream of farming avocados in the San Joaquin Valley. Imagine it—acres of guacamole, as far as the eye can see! The irony is that at this very moment, somewhere in California, an avocado baron is pining to spend his days peering in screaming kids' ears.

Ninety percent of children in the United States suffer at least one middle ear infection by the time they turn 2 years old. Acute otitis media (AOM) is the most common bacterial infection in childhood, accounting for more than 20 million antibiotic prescriptions and more than 24 million office visits every year in the United States, with annual costs estimated at up to $5 billion. Learning to diagnose AOM is one of the greatest challenges for pediatricians in training, requiring hundreds to thousands of ear examinations to master. I suppose for now my dream is on hold, but still, all those beautiful Hass….

journey to the center of the ear

If some dad tells you his kid has an ear infection and you want to get all smart with him, just ask, "What do you mean by ear infection: otitis externa, otitis media, or labyrinthitis?" Then tell him you got that out of some book and you were just messing with him. The ear consists of 3 distinct parts, and each one gets its own kind of infection. The outer ear starts at the cartilaginous shell that sticks out on the sides of our heads, called the pinna. The little button-shaped piece in the front of that is called the tragus. Next is the external auditory canal, which is everything from the hole down to the outer surface of the eardrum (tympanic membrane). The outer ear is the part that becomes inflamed when your child has swimmer's ear, or otitis externa.

On the other side of the tympanic membrane is a chamber called the middle ear. This chamber houses 3 bones that carry sound vibrations from the eardrum to the nerves of the inner ear. Normally the middle ear is filled with air and the air pressure stays just a little lower than the pressure outside the body. Tiny tunnels called eustachian tubes connect the middle ears to the inside of the nose, allowing air to pass when there's too much difference in pressure between the middle ear and outside world. The eustachian tubes also drain fluid that may collect in the middle ear. When most people talk about an ear infection, they mean a middle ear infection, AOM.

Beyond the middle ear lies a snail-shell–shaped organ called the cochlea, along with 3 loops of tissue called the semicircular canals (guess what shape they are!). The cochlea turns sound vibrations into nerve signals the brain can process. The semicircular canals function as the body's gyroscopes, telling the brain which way is up and what direction the head is moving. These organs are all filled with fluid, and when this fluid becomes infected (usually by a virus), it's called labyrinthitis.

a cute otitis media

Your child is likely to be among the 90% who suffer at least one middle ear infection, most often between the ages of 6 and 18 months. There are several reasons this is the golden age of the earache. For the first months of life, mom's antibodies protect babies from many infections. Mother's milk also contains additional antibodies that protect breastfed babies, making them less susceptible to ear infections, among other diseases.

Getting an ear infection before age 6 months suggests a child is at risk for more frequent, more severe ear infections in the future.

Younger children's eustachian tubes are shorter, straighter, and narrower than those of older children, giving bacteria an easy shot from the nose into the inner ear and making it harder for fluid or pus to drain out. Infants' and toddlers' immune systems are also still developing, and they're less able to fight off some infections than older children. Add to these risks the fact that toddlers average around 8 colds a year and you have an ear infection waiting to happen. About 20% of children suffer recurrent ear infections. Don't despair if your child is among them; by age 8 almost all children will outgrow any problems they had with ear infections.

Any condition that interferes with eustachian tube function can predispose a child to getting ear infections. Children with Down syndrome or cleft palate, for example, are more prone to AOM. Cigarette smoke causes chronic airway inflammation, so smoke exposure causes AOM. When babies lie down to drink from a bottle, formula can irritate the eustachian tubes and cause AOM. Children with gastroesophageal reflux disease, allergic rhinitis, or disorders of the immune system all face increased risk as well. Child care exposes children to more colds and therefore to more ear infections.

Irritants like a cold, allergic rhinitis, or gastroesophageal reflux inflame the eustachian tube. The eustachian tube swells, allowing fluid to collect in the middle ear. That fluid provides a perfect environment for viruses or bacteria to grow, especially if they're already hanging out in the nose during an upper respiratory infection. Ear infections are most common around the third day of a cold. The body reacts to the infection with inflammation; pus collects behind the eardrum, causing often intense pain. It's times like these you should be happy you don't speak baby. You wouldn't like what you hear.

What you see may also gross you out, but play it off like it's no big deal. In 5% to 10% of cases the eardrum actually ruptures, allowing pus to leak out of the ear canal, sometimes mixed with blood. While a draining ear looks really bad, perforation often provides instant pain relief. Eardrums heal rapidly in most cases, with the hole closing up on its own within 2 to 3 days.

Infections in the middle ear result from viruses or bacteria; which one matters, because while antibiotics may help cure bacterial infections, we have no effective treatments against most viruses. Numbers vary, but cultures of ear fluid grow bacteria between 50% and 90% of the time. That means right off the bat that a certain number of ear infections are not going to respond to antibiotic therapy, as they're caused by viruses.

Even if your child is acting just like he did last time his ear was infected, remember that unless pus is dripping from the ear canal, there are no surefire signs a child has an ear infection. Pain is most common; children may cry, feed poorly, or wake up from the discomfort. Infants who can reach their ears (around age 6 months) may pull at them or poke at the ear canals, but many infants also pull or stroke on their ears for comfort, so it can be hard to tell when that behavior means they hurt. Ear pain may also result from a sore throat or uninfected fluid in the middle ear. Every week I see some child whose parents and I are all sure has an ear infection only to look in the ear and find a perfect eardrum. I also see happy, well-appearing babies whose wellness examinations turn up raging otitis media.

Fever is another suggestive but unreliable symptom. About half of children with AOM have fevers, but so do many children with colds and healthy ears. Fevers are more likely to come from an ear infection when they last more than 3 days or when they occur after the first few days of cold symptoms.

Other symptoms of ear infections are more subtle and may overlap with lots of other illnesses. Infants and toddlers may vomit or have diarrhea; they may appear to have sore throats because of discomfort associated with swallowing; or they may become dizzy or unstable when they walk. The bottom line is that until the doctor sees that eardrum, no one knows if the ear is really infected.

Of course, getting a look at an eardrum isn't always easy. Small ear canals, wax collections, drainage in the ear, and excessive squirming all stand between the doctor and a decent examination. Here's where you come in—an older infant or toddler will often do best sitting in your lap right up against your chest. This position keeps him calm and prevents him from whipping his head around. Some children will cooperate, but others need help keeping their hands away from their ears, usually in the form of a firm, loving hug. The doctor can then help the child turn his head to the side. You'll see the doctor pull back gently on the outer ear with her free hand; this straightens out the ear canal to afford a better view of the eardrum. In many cases you'll notice a little tube attached to the otoscope.

By squeezing a rubber bulb or puffing into this tube, the doctor can see how well the eardrum moves in response to changes in air pressure. This maneuver often makes the difference in diagnosing borderline cases.

If wax is blocking the canal, the doctor may try to remove it with warm water or with a little scooper called a curette. Even under the best conditions, the tender tissue of the ear canal may bleed a little during this process. Some kids just make a lot of earwax, but the best way to avoid this potentially difficult ordeal is to never use a cotton swab to clean ears. Swabs just shove wax further into the canal. Often when I examine an ear, I'll see a column of wax with the perfectly concave impression of a cotton swab.

Technology can help diagnose middle ear infections as well. A handheld instrument called a tympanometer measures how well the eardrum moves in response to sound waves or changes in air pressure. A diminished response suggests the middle ear is full of fluid, but it doesn't tell the doctor whether that fluid is infected.

You might think once the doctor has seen the eardrum that it's simple—get an antibiotic and call it a day. But is anything really simple? The first step is to determine that the middle ear really is infected. Sometimes the doctor simply can't see the eardrums well enough to tell, and he has to make a guess based on other symptoms and findings. Kids get fluid behind their eardrums with colds and allergic rhinitis all the time, but if it's just fluid and not pus, antibiotics offer no benefit and quite a lot of potential harm. Likewise, all sort of things can make eardrums look red on examination, from the cold itself to the child crying. If a doctor wants to give your child antibiotics because "his eardrums look a little red" or "he might be getting a little ear infection," go ahead and ask if the prescription is really necessary. When used appropriately for AOM, antibiotics can hasten recovery and prevent complications, but their use also risks allergic reactions and bacterial resistance, so it's important to reserve them for the right occasions.

Sometimes, even when your child clearly has AOM he does not need antibiotics. Most children older than 2 years will get better just as quickly without taking antibiotics. Many pediatricians offer parents of these children a safety net antibiotic prescription to fill only if the child still has fever or ear pain 2 days after the office visit. Younger children, on the other hand, face higher risks for complications, so they still require treatment every time. Children with complicated infections, high fever, or other risk factors may also warrant more aggressive therapy.

At least once a week a parent tells me, "Amoxicillin doesn't work for my child." Indeed, the last time that child was treated for an ear infection, he may have needed a second antibiotic. Any antibiotic stands about a 10% chance of failing, between the presence of antibiotic-resistant bacteria and the fact that some ear infections are viral in the first place. But let's be clear: it's the infection that's resistant to the antibiotic, not the child. If more than a month has passed since he has taken that antibiotic, his chances of antibiotic failure the next time are the same as anyone else's.

When hunting bacteria you want to use a rifle, not a shotgun. The idea is to take out the bad guys with minimal collateral damage. For children without a penicillin allergy our rifle is amoxicillin, a form of penicillin that, given in a high-enough dose, kills most of the bacteria that cause AOM without wiping out all the good bacteria in the body.

when to call the doctor

Your child may not feel at all better in the first 24 hours of treatment. If he still has fever more than 48 hours after starting the medication, or if his ear pain or discharge lasts more than 72 hours after his first dose, it may be time to choose a different weapon. For children who are vomiting or have failed oral antibiotics, sometimes an injected antibiotic (ceftriaxone) is a better choice.

Out of the millions or billions of bacteria causing a given infection, there will always be a handful that, thanks to genetic mutations, eat your drug of choice for breakfast. As long as there are not too many, the immune system can take care of them, but if they multiply the infection may get worse. One way to avoid resistance is to give the medication as directed for as long as directed. Antibiotics vary; some require 3 days of therapy to work, others 10 days, but stopping too early allows the resistant bacteria to flourish before your child's immune system can knock them out. Also never, ever grab some old antibiotics from a family member or a prior infection and start giving them to your child. First of all, you don't know what you're treating or if you're using the correct dose. Second, antibiotics degrade with time, and the best way to create a resistant infection is to give weakened antibiotics. Save yourself from temptation by disposing properly of any unused medications as soon as the treatment course is complete.

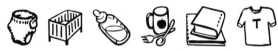

what you can do

Arguably the most important part of treating acute otitis media is pain control. You can use acetaminophen (eg, Tylenol) or ibuprofen (eg, Advil, Motrin) for infants older than 6 months. If the infant is younger than 6 months, just use acetaminophen. In addition to these medications, your doctor may prescribe numbing drops to put in the child's ear. If he has a ruptured eardrum, using these drops may not be safe, but if he doesn't have drainage you can use them as often as every 2 hours to help with pain. If you don't have these drops, putting a few drops of olive oil in the ear may soothe the pain a bit and shouldn't hurt anything. A cool or warm compress applied to the ear for 20 minutes may also help, but be careful not to let him sleep on an electric heating pad; he could suffer an accidental burn.

There are some things you don't have to worry about. Swimming with a middle ear infection is fine; the water can't get to where the infection is unless the eardrum has perforated, and in that case swimming probably isn't a good idea until it's healed. You don't have to cover or plug the ears either; a little wind isn't going to hurt anything. Don't stuff a cotton ball or anything in the ears; if there is drainage it may actually increase the child's risk of developing an outer ear infection. Your child can also fly in an airplane safely, although you might want to give him a dose of pain reliever about an hour before takeoff. Your child may also safely return to school once the fever is gone for 24 hours. Ear infections are not contagious, although the colds that cause them are. But don't worry—all the other kids in child care already have that cold.

After about the third ear infection parents always ask me, "Is there anything we can do to prevent him from getting all these ear infections?" Of course there is. The first one goes all the way back to birth—breastfeed. As a dad, of course you yourself cannot accomplish this, but your support is critical for successful nursing.

The single most important thing you can do to prevent ear infections is to get your child immunized completely and on time. Vaccines, especially those against *Haemophilus influenzae* type b and pneumococcus species, have revolutionized how ear infections are treated. Before we had these vaccines, ear infections were much more likely to progress to more serious infections, like meningitis. In the developing world, complications of AOM continue to kill around 50,000 children a year!

Next, keep your baby and cigarette smoke as far away from each other as possible. Naturally you would never let anyone smoke in your home or car, but you can even encourage smokers to wear a special coat or shirt when they're smoking that they remove before they hold your baby. We now know that even this "thirdhand smoke" that lingers on smokers makes kids sick. Bottle-propping also invites ear infections; it's really cute to see your baby lying there holding his own bottle, but he should be at a 45° angle so formula doesn't run back into his eustachian tubes. That cuteness wears off fast once the screaming starts.

Attending child care is another risk factor for ear infections, but most families with children in care have little choice about the matter. Don't feel too guilty, though. Kids in child care only get about 20% more colds than those at home, not the 200% you might think! Another risk factor is uncontrolled allergies. If your child constantly has a runny nose or itchy, dry skin, his doctor may want to consider treating or testing him for allergies.

If your child has more than 3 cases of AOM in 6 months or more than 5 in 1 year, you and his doctor may want to discuss having him evaluated for pressure equalization (PE) tubes. These are tiny rubber or plastic tubes an ear, nose, and throat surgeon inserts into the eardrums to drain fluid and prevent future ear infections. Getting these tubes may seem like another no-brainer if your child suffers from frequent bouts of AOM, but what did we say about stuff being simple?

Remember that kids tend to outgrow ear infections over time, so even if a child meets basic criteria for tube placement, his doctor may want to try a longer course of antibiotics or, if summer is coming, see how things go for a few months before committing him to even minor surgery. Children who have fluid behind the eardrums may benefit from tubes, even if that fluid is not infected. Those children should have their hearing checked first, however, because the fluid doesn't always make it hard for them to hear, and if they don't have hearing loss for at least 3 months' duration, there's usually no point in placing the tubes. On the other hand, if your child has specific risk factors for hearing loss or ear damage, he may benefit from earlier surgery.

Most PE tubes fall out of the eardrums on their own within about a year of insertion. Some tubes, however, are designed to stay in until the surgeon removes them. When a child has been sick enough to need 2 or more sets of PE tubes, surgeons will also often remove the adenoid, glands in the upper airway that may block drainage from the eustachian tubes. Adenoidectomy helps prevent recurring ear infections in these kids, but if the doctor also wants to remove the tonsils, ask why. There are some good reasons to remove tonsils, but taking them out does not do anything to prevent ear infections.

If your child already has PE tubes, you're probably a pro at taking care of them. Follow his doctor's instructions on water exposure, but you don't have to be paranoid if he swims without earplugs; a little water isn't likely to hurt anything. When he does get an ear infection you should see lots of goo coming out of the ears, at least if the tubes are still in place and not clogged. Often these kids respond to antibiotic eardrops and don't need to take medicine by mouth.

give that swimmer back his ear

Nothing stinks more than planning your vacation around, say, a water park, and then your child can't swim because of ear pain. Because really, how much miniature golf can you play? Your child doesn't have to swim to suffer from swimmer's ear, but it helps. That's because water trapped in the external auditory canal creates a friendly environment for bacteria to invade the vulnerable tissue lining the outer ear.

Normally, ear canals do an impressive job of protecting themselves against the onslaughts of the outside world. Earwax is not just a hygiene nuisance; it's an amazing substance. Cerumen, as doctors call it, not only serves as a barrier against moisture and insects, it also has a slightly acidic chemistry that suppresses the growth of bacteria and fungi in the ear canal. Unless you cram it back into the ear with a cotton swab, the wax usually rides out on a miniature conveyor belt, as the skin of the ear canal grows outward. Jaw movement from chewing and talking speeds the process. Some people have dry, flaky ear wax and others have gooey wax;

you inherit your earwax from your parents, along with the tendency to grow hair in your ears once you become a dad.

The skin lining the ear canals is relatively delicate; it's not meant to stand up to the same sorts of abuse as the skin on your elbows. If something (like a cotton swab) damages that tissue or if water gets trapped in the ear canal, bacteria can enter and cause an infection. These infections are seriously painful, especially if anything touches the outer ear, putting traction on the tissue of the ear canal. Sometimes looking at your child's ear you can see the hole is swollen or red, or you might notice watery drainage.

A variety of antibiotic solutions treat swimmer's ear. Some of them are combined with topical steroids like hydrocortisone, but there seems to be little difference in how well they work. If your child ends up needing drops for swimmer's ear, have him lie on his side or put his head in your lap, pull back gently on the outer ear (if this doesn't cause too much pain), and put 3 to 5 drops into the canal. If you want to make bomb-falling sounds while you do this, it's your prerogative. If the swelling is too severe, your child's doctor may have to introduce a cotton wick into the ear canal to help the antibiotic drops get all the way inside. Rarely, the infection is so bad doctors prescribe oral antibiotics to go with the drops. Ideally your child won't go back into the water until the infection clears up, usually in 5 to 7 days. This may be the only reason people try to hit golf balls under little windmills.

As much fun as it is to put medicine in a miserable child's ears, you'd probably be better off avoiding the situation. When you're packing for the water park, you can buy a commercially prepared ear solution, or just look in your pantry for white vinegar and isopropyl alcohol and make a 1:1 solution. After your child gets out of the lazy river, have him shake his head to each side and towel off well, especially around the ear canals. Then put a few drops of the solution in each ear and let it drain back out. Another strategy is to use a hair dryer on its lowest setting and dry the ear canals after each swim, taking care to keep a good distance between the hair dryer and ears. While this technique does work, it may also prove way too boring to continue.

say what?

Otitis media and swimmer's ear can reduce hearing, but they are hardly the only causes of childhood hearing loss. Genetic conditions, tumors, and loud noises, including those from headphones and live concerts, can all rob children of their hearing. Some signs of hearing loss are obvious—your child starts shouting at you; he sits too close to the television; or he cannot hear what you say. Parents are always tempted to assume their children just aren't paying attention, and sometimes they're not, but without examining the ears and taking hearing tests, that's not a safe assumption. Ringing in the ears is one subtle symptom of hearing loss you don't want to ignore.

when to call the doctor

A child who suddenly shows difficulty keeping his balance might have labyrinthitis, but he might have a brain or nerve problem as well, so he should see a doctor immediately.

As many as 1 in 250 babies are born with hearing loss; at some point before your newborn leaves the hospital, the nurse will whisk him away for a hearing screen. Don't be alarmed if the first screen comes back abnormal; most of these babies will do fine on repeat screening. It's critical, however, to identify hearing loss early because the sooner you treat, the better you can help preserve language development.

Later signs of hearing loss in infancy include failure to startle with loud noises, failure to turn toward the sound of your voice by age 4 months, or difficulty learning to speak. Your child's doctor should screen for speech and language development at each well-child checkup and arrange for follow-up if there's a problem. Pediatricians begin office hearing screenings at 4 years of age, but audiologists can test hearing even in newborns. Of course, if everything checks out fine, maybe it's time to work on your Daddy Voice. Remember, it comes from the diaphragm.

You now know more than any other dad on your block about childhood ear problems, unless of course you live next door to an ear, nose, and throat specialist. As long as children have ears it looks like doctors who take care of them will have work to do. In the meantime, I've heard there's a bed-and-breakfast in Sonoma where you can pick your own avocados in season.

14

food fight:
why your toddler won't
eat anything

have you ever seen one of those cute photos of a toddler with a bowl of spaghetti upside down on her head, where she's looking all pleased with herself while noodles and sauce run down her face? I've never really appreciated the charm of those pictures, but now that I'm a parent I see them in a new light. I now know that just before that photo was taken, the toddler's dad put the bowl on her head in hopes that at least some of the pasta might end up in her mouth.

Among the challenges of fatherhood no one seems to warn you about are the galactic battles that center around food. There will be screaming fits, thrown plates, and endless frustration, and that's just while you and your parenting partner discuss feedings! Understanding your toddler's needs will help ease a lot of the pressure and help you establish healthy eating patterns that will last a lifetime. But first you have to go pick up that plate.

your toddler: a bromeliad?

You know bromeliads, those tree-dwelling plants that get all their nutrition and water from the air? Sometimes it can seem like your child, once ravenous, has become like one of those plants. (*Hint:* If she sprouts thick, spiny leaves, be sure and mist her once a day.) What has really happened is that her growth rate has slowed. She just doesn't need as many calories as she did during the first year of life, now roughly 1,000 calories a day. We like to think she'll consume these calories in the form of 3 small meals and 2 snacks a day, but you've probably noticed by now that toddlers don't always do what we think they should. In reality, your child's eating may vary dramatically from one day to the next, even from one meal to the next! It may help to think more like her body does, in terms of weeks rather than hours. If you put too much stock in whether she eats any given meal, much less one particular food, you will make yourself crazy, and then you'll end up with a bowl of spaghetti upside-down on your own head, posing for a photo. Don't go there.

Compared with the mounds of food that pass for adult portion sizes these days, toddlers' portion sizes are quite small, roughly one-fourth the volume of an appropriate adult serving (or one-20th of what the guy in front of you just put on his plate at Golden Corral). A serving of vegetables is only around 1 or 2 tablespoons. A serving of meat is about the size of your child's palm.

It also helps to think of your toddler's food choices in the long term. She's likely to go on eating jags, enjoying one food several days in a row and then suddenly deciding that particular flavor has all the appeal of old oatmeal (it may in fact be old oatmeal) and picking a new favorite. Assuming you're providing her healthy choices, she's likely to average out her nutrients over the course of the week such that she's actually consuming a very balanced diet. Of course she'll have growth spurts as well, and some days she'll be more active than others, so her food intake may vary dramatically.

Your child's scheduled wellness examinations should reassure you about her eating as well. Her doctor should measure her weight, length, and head circumference at each of these visits and show you how her growth compares with other children her age. If she is growing normally, you know your toddler is getting all the food she needs.

Kicking the Bottle

It's hard to overstate what an amazing invention an infant bottle is. For the most part, liquid stays in it until the baby sucks it out, making bottles darned convenient for the baby on the move, not to mention her dad!

Many toddlers find bottles comforting and familiar, and they don't all take quickly to drinking from other containers, like sippy cups. For these reasons you might be tempted to let your toddler keep using a bottle until her husband starts making fun of her.

In fact, if the bottle contains water, your child is welcome to take it to graduate school. If, on the other hand, it contains any liquid with sugar in it (for example, milk), the bottle poses a major threat to healthy teeth. Infant bottles deliver a steady stream of sugar to the teeth, especially the ones in the front of the mouth. Bacteria on the teeth convert the sugar to acid, which eats away at the enamel, causing cavities. Toddlers who sleep with a bottle of milk or juice in the bed are especially susceptible to this tooth decay because the bacteria have all night to do their dirty work. For this reason, you're going to want to help your toddler graduate to more tooth-friendly drinking technology around her first birthday.

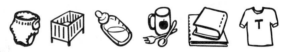

what you can do

Like everything else, drinking from a cup requires a little practice to master (there are days I still have trouble with it). You don't have to wait until your child's first birthday to start. By 6 to 9 months of age, she should be developing the motor skills to drink from a straw or sippy cup. Start at that age, putting formula, expressed breast milk, or water in the cup. As she gets the hang of it you can use the bottle less often, so that by 12 to 15 months of age, she's no longer using bottles at all. If she drinks milk before bedtime, make sure you clean her teeth afterward to protect her from tooth decay.

Toddlers being what they are, don't be surprised if your child doesn't embrace this plan enthusiastically. She may push the cup away or even throw it across the room. Some toddlers seem content to drink water or juice from a cup but insist that milk come from a bottle. There's nothing wrong with giving your toddler a few months to transition, but if she's still being stubborn by age 15 months (and does not suffer from some developmental delay that impairs her ability to drink), it may be time to help her out a little. Pick a day when all the bottles will disappear. If you are the charitable sort, you might donate them to another family or a shelter. Alternately, you can prop them on a fence and use them for target practice.

Either way, prepare your toddler by letting her know that she's a big girl now and big girls drink from cups. Then, on D-day (drink day), she won't have a choice. So long as she has demonstrated the skill to obtain fluid from a cup, you can rest assured she will not allow herself to become dehydrated, although she may throw a world-class fit that leaves you both a bit thirsty. Many parents worry their children won't get enough milk during this transition. She may indeed go on a milk strike for a week or so, but toddlers have short memories. Soon she'll forget bottles ever existed, at least until she has a younger sibling. By age 2 or 3 she should be able to drink from an open cup reliably, spilling her drink only rarely.

Parents also fret about what their toddlers are going to drink. If your child is nursing, she is welcome to continue doing so as long as it makes her and mom happy. There are, however, some precautions to take. Nursing after bedtime, just like sleeping with a bottle, puts her at risk of tooth decay. By 12 months of age, she should be sleeping through the night in her own crib or bed without waking up to feed. Also by this age, most of her calories should be coming from food, not breast milk, cow's milk, juice, or other fluids. If your toddler is nursing so often she's not interested in eating, it's probably time to cut back.

Do not introduce cow's milk to your toddler's diet until she turns 1 year old. Unlike cow's milk, formula and human milk contain plenty of iron, which your baby needs to make red blood cells. By 1 year of life your child should be getting enough iron from other sources to tolerate the transition, but starting cow's milk before then puts her at risk of anemia. Once you do start, choose whole milk. Older children and adults may benefit from a diet low in diary fats, but during the second year of life your toddler should still be getting around half of her calories from fat. This fat helps her brain and nerves develop. After her second birthday you can reduce her fat intake to account for about one-third of her calories.

There is no reason not to transition directly from formula or breast milk straight to whole cow's milk. If your toddler doesn't seem to like the flavor of milk, you can transition by mixing milk and formula for a while. Manufacturers market a variety of formulas for this second year of life, but if your child has a healthy diet she really shouldn't need these products. In some cases, if a child isn't gaining weight normally, her pediatrician or dietitian may recommend a supplemental formula, but parents' perceptions of a normal weight vary based on their own experience and culture.

when to call the doctor

If you're worried your child is too thin, have her doctor plot her growth before you take it on yourself to fatten her up.

Parents often worry that their children are not drinking enough milk, spurred on by people dressed as milk cartons or celebrities wearing white mustaches. Milk is a great source of calcium, vitamin D, and protein, but it is not the only source of any of these nutrients. In general we recommend children consume 3 servings of dairy a day, and yogurt does count. In fact, there is such a thing as too much milk. Consuming more than 24 to 32 ounces of milk a day can cause iron deficiency anemia and constipation. Children who drink too much milk may also eat fewer solid foods and risk poor weight gain.

On the flip side, don't worry if your child just isn't a big fan of the moo juice. Unless she's drinking 32 ounces of milk a day, she should be taking a daily vitamin D supplement of 400 international units (IU) anyway. Calcium comes from all sorts of foods, especially meats, dark-green vegetables, and dried beans. All of these foods also double as rich sources of protein and iron!

Juice marketers target parents hard, trying to make us view their products as essential to child health. "Wow," they want us to think, "look at all that vitamin C! Not to mention the colorful, user-friendly packaging!" But honestly, unless your child has scurvy, she's getting all the vitamin C she needs from eating fruits and vegetables. What juice has more of than anything else is sugar. Think of it as liquid dessert. Like dessert, a little is fine, around 4 to 6 ounces a day. When you do serve juice, look for 100% real fruit juice. (I've never seen a "juicy" orchard.) Many parents water juice down when they give it, which is fine, but keep track of how much you've poured out of the bottle. You can easily wind up giving your child 16 ounces a day of juice combined with water.

Speaking of water, you'd be amazed how well it quenches thirst. There was a time not so long ago when people, even children, drank water regularly. Most municipal water supplies are perfectly safe without any special filtering or other preparations, but if it makes you feel better to buy your toddler bottled water, go for it! Beyond her 16 or so ounces of whole milk and 4 ounces of juice a day, water should provide all her other fluid needs. Water lacks only one thing for perfect child health—fluoride, a chemical critical to healthy tooth development.

Most municipal water supplies have fluoride added, but if you have a well you'll want to have your water tested for fluoride content. Depending on where you live, your well water may or may not have adequate fluoride. The way dentists learned about fluoride in the first place was by examining dramatic regional variations in cavities. It turned out that people whose water supply was naturally high in fluoride had much better teeth. Regular water filters don't remove fluoride, but if you have a reverse-osmosis filter (one where you have to add salt to the tank), your child will need a supplement. Just as children can get too little fluoride, they can also get too much. Ironically, excessive fluoride intake can damage teeth just as badly as inadequate intake. If your child is on fluoride-deficient well water or drinks exclusively spring or distilled water, her doctor can prescribe fluoride supplements. Alternately you can purchase nursery water or infant's water, which is like any other bottled water except that it has adequate levels of fluoride. Children younger than 3 years should not be using fluoride toothpaste or dental rinse because they may swallow too much of it.

why toddlers hate everything

To understand why toddlers are so hard to feed, it helps to take a trip back in time several thousand years, to a period in human evolution when the term baby carrier referred to a person's arm. The world at that time was strewn with poisonous mushrooms, toxic berries, and mastodon poop. If toddlers ran around eating everything they could grab, the human species would never have survived long enough to read books on child care. Instead, our toddler forebears evolved to be highly selective, trusting only those foods their parents gave them repeatedly. At the same time, prehistoric children were often quite hungry, and food choices were limited to whatever their parents happened to forage for or kill that day. There is a reason most primitive languages don't have a word for picky eater.

Let's return to the modern day, when even a small grocery store confronts parents with a dizzying array of food choices, many of them involving both macaroni and cheese. The same selectivity that saved our ancestors' children from poisoning themselves now just looks like willfulness. On top of that, modern toddlers eat in high chairs using utensils, cups, and plates, all of which are great fun to throw around the houses in which we now live. It's not that your child is determined to make mealtime an ordeal, it's just that toddlers are little cave people.

what you can do

One choice is to move your family into a tent, but there are other, less dramatic strategies to cope with the historical mismatch described above. It's kind of a no-brainer to use unbreakable cups, plates, and utensils and to feed your toddler over a washable surface, but we're guys, so I'll say it anyway. If your child seems more interested in the ballistics of her food than the flavor, she may just not be hungry right now. Try putting any thrown utensils back where they belong a few times and telling her "No," but if this isn't working, it's OK to put her down and try again at her next mealtime. You'll notice your toddler is picking up eating skills quickly at this age. She'll begin with an ambition to feed himself that far outstrips her ability to keep food on her spoon. By 18 months, however, she'll be getting the food to her mouth most of the time, at least when she wants to.

Here's another chance to win a bet with one of your buddies: ask how often a toddler needs to experience a new food before she comes to accept it. The answer is 10 to 20 times. You're welcome. Remember, she doesn't know it's OK to eat unless you show her. Until then, as far as she's concerned, it's mastodon poop.

Some foods tend to go over better than others. Certain vegetables like broccoli, asparagus, cabbage, and brussels sprouts contain a bitter-tasting chemical to which some toddlers are particularly sensitive. These may just not fly (or more accurately, they may go flying) even after 20 attempts. Carrots, squash, and sweet potatoes, on the other hand, are popular toddler foods due to their sweetness. Avoid spicy foods; toddlers' palates are very sensitive to salt, pepper, and spices. If your toddler doesn't seem so excited about vegetables, try fruits instead; dietitians don't care whether we call something a fruit or a vegetable so long as it comes from a plant and it's not a french fry. When introducing new foods, try pairing the novel flavor with something your toddler already enjoys. If broccoli is friends with pears, how bad can it be? Also try introducing the newer food early in the meal, when your child is hungriest.

In providing food choices, try to vary the food groups between proteins such as meats, fish, poultry, and eggs; dairy products; fruits and vegetables; and carbohydrates such as whole-grain cereals, breads, pasta, rice, and potatoes. If your toddler turns down one healthy choice, feel free to substitute another healthy choice. Do not, however, let her fill up on junk

what you can do

Even toddlers who have tons of teeth use their teeth differently than we do, and not just to bite their playmates. Until age 4 they chew in an up-and-down motion rather than a side-to-side grinding motion, which means they're more susceptible to choking. Even if your child seems to be a good eater, you'll want to cut her food into small pieces, ideally smaller than the tip of her pinkie. Practice your *Top Chef* skills by cutting hot dogs and carrots first in quarters lengthwise and then in small bites crossways. (If it helps, while you do this, pretend to berate your line cooks.) Grapes and cherry tomatoes should get a similar treatment. Peanuts and other whole nuts, and even fat chunks of peanut butter, can become lodged in your child's airway and choke her. Other notorious choking hazards include popcorn and candies like gummi bears or jelly beans. Also, take time for your toddler to sit down and eat. Eating on the run or, worst of all, in a moving car increases her risk of choking. You don't want to crash while trying to reach in the back seat to perform the Heimlich maneuver. Follow these rules throughout the second year of life; "She hasn't choked to death yet" is not a solid rationale for putting her at risk.

foods and sweets after she has turned down a variety of better options. Hungry children eat; a child who is only hungry for dessert isn't really hungry.

Food is supposed to nourish your toddler, not harm her, so it's worthwhile to emphasize a few safety tips. Microwave ovens are miraculous machines for heating up food, but remember that even the ones with turntables heat food unevenly, leaving hot spots in unpredictable places. When you pull a food out of the microwave, be sure to mix it up well and let it sit a minute for the heat to even out. It's a good idea to check the first bite with your finger or, better yet, your tongue, to make sure it's not too hot.

food-o judo: winning the food fight

As guys we like to confront problems head on, wrestle them to the ground, and defeat them by sheer force. If you watch enough martial arts films, however, you'll realize it's often better to take a more subtle approach. Studies show that when parents try too hard to force their children to eat, those kids actually end up eating less. Likewise, parents who are highly restrictive about diet may end up with kids who overeat. You'll want to approach mealtimes less like a linebacker and more like a judo master.

Start by readying the battleground for victory. If you love to prepare some exotic dish guaranteed to offend small children, save it for date night and go for something more child-friendly. Preschoolers get persnickety about foods that are mixed up, so some comfort foods like chili and lasagna often end up bombing with young children at the dinner table. Try making things where different foods don't have to touch each other.

If your child digs in her heels and refuses a meal, offer a reasonable, simple substitute. The alternative choice should still be healthy. This is where a lot of parents get into trouble, allowing themselves to become short-order cooks. Don't prepare one meal for the family and then make your preschooler chicken nuggets every single night. A cup of yogurt, bowl of whole-grain cereal, or turkey sandwich should do. Under no circumstances should you force your child to join or even apply for the Clean Plate Club. Preserve your child's ability to respond to hunger cues by not making her eat when she's not interested.

Encourage your child to try at least one bite of everything that's offered. She will never learn to enjoy new flavors if she doesn't try them. After this bite, however, the fight is over. You don't want to find yourself forcing a child to eat something that makes her gag or vomit. If you think about it, you're going to be on the losing end one way or the other. If your child turned green last time she had a bit of liver and onions, save yourself the drama, not to mention the cleanup.

Mealtimes should be pleasant in general, which means conversation about food should be mainly of the "Mmm, that's great!" variety. You already aren't forcing your child to eat something she doesn't like, so there's no need for her to complain. If she continues to whine after one warning, she can leave the table so everyone else can enjoy their meal in peace. This strategy, however, works both ways. If you spend your dinner begging, threatening, and cajoling your child about food, you've just wasted an opportunity to have a pleasant evening. Likewise, don't stretch mealtime out too long. If your child needs an extra 5 minutes to finish eating, don't sweat it. But there's no reason to make her sit there another half hour. If she's hungry at bedtime, allow her a small, healthy snack before she brushes her teeth.

Using food as a reward is one of the hardest temptations for any parent to avoid. After all, it works with the dog; why not try it on the kid? There are 2 problems here. The most immediate is that when you reward one food with another, the child comes to perceive the reward food as being even more desirable and the food she has to eat in return as even less desirable. There's no better way to make your child love ice cream than to make it the reward for eating broccoli. But then most kids already kind of like ice cream.

The other problem is that food rewards set up an unhealthy relationship with food. When food becomes the way we reward ourselves, we tend to stop paying attention to whether we're hungry and start eating for other reasons. Naturally, most reward foods are loaded with sugar, fat, and salt. A healthier approach to dessert is to agree that some nights are dessert nights and others are not, regardless of what your child eats. A little dessert from time to time isn't going to hurt anyone, especially if some of those desserts are fruits.

When it comes to peaceful, healthy meals, the television is your enemy. The more television children watch, the more commercials they see for unhealthy foods. These commercials have an enormous effect on children's food choices, which is why advertisers pay tons of money to air them. Studies show that children's television viewing hours predict whether they'll be overweight. Even more interesting is that when those same children reduce their television time, their weights improve! Think about it—how many televised characters shout at your children about food? Toucan Sam, Tony the Tiger, Cap'n Crunch, Ronald McDonald, the Trix Rabbit, the Keebler Elves, Cheesasaurus Rex…sure they seem all friendly, but they are not to be trusted. They are like the Legion of Doom, just without the scary masks.

who needs food when you have vitamins?

The thing that gets me about vitamins is that even people who claim to be skeptical of medicine seem enthralled with the idea that you can put good stuff in a pill and give it to a kid to make her healthy. I love parents who say, "Oh, I never give my child medicine, just these 7 nutritional supplements every morning!" The only difference between prescription medicine and those pills is that the Food and Drug Administration actually monitors prescription drugs for safety and efficacy.

There is one and only one vitamin for which most children need a supplement, and that is vitamin D. Vitamin D, also called ergocalciferol, is critical in helping bodies absorb and use calcium to make things like teeth and bones. It also plays a key role in the immune system; people with low levels of vitamin D seem more prone to autoimmune diseases like type 1 diabetes and multiple sclerosis. To understand why we would give kids vitamin D, you have to return once again to cave times.

Sunlight exposure provides a critical step in the body's manufacture of vitamin D. For most of human evolution, adequate sun exposure was a given because we didn't have houses or wear much in the way of clothes. People who lived near the equator evolved to produce more melanin to protect them from skin cancer, and those who lived farther from the equator tended to be paler so as to allow more sunlight into their skin. The one food naturally rich in vitamin D is oily fish, a staple in the diets of most cultures that developed in darker climates.

Since that time, however, we built houses, learned to sew, and stopped eating herring for breakfast, lunch, and dinner. In the meantime we released Freon and chlorofluorocarbons into the atmosphere, blowing a big hole in the ozone layer that used to protect us from the sun's most harmful rays. Today we focus on protecting our children from skin cancer, which, if we are doing it right, means they often are not making enough vitamin D. The bottom line is that children today require a supplement of 400 IU of vitamin D daily.

Vitamin D–fortified milk and dairy products can provide some vitamin D, but a child would need to drink 32 ounces of milk a day to get enough of it, at which point she would be at risk of iron deficiency anemia, not to mention wicked constipation. Instead we start babies at birth with a liquid vitamin supplement such as D-Vi-Sol. Once your child is not at risk of choking, she can move up to 1 chewable vitamin or 2 gummy vitamins a day, usually around age 3.

One supplement your child might need is iron. During infancy, children should get adequate iron from human milk or formula. After that, meats, eggs, dried beans, dark-green vegetables, and molasses can all serve as rich sources of iron. Children whose diets are deficient in these nutrients, however, may require a daily iron supplement. Your child's doctor should screen her for iron deficiency by checking her hemoglobin level at her 12-month wellness examination.

Children who follow a strict vegetarian or vegan diet risk a number of vitamin and mineral deficiencies. Fish and fortified dairy products provide the only dietary sources of vitamin D, so for children who eat neither of these foods, vitamin D supplementation is especially important. They may also need a multivitamin containing riboflavin, vitamin B_{12}, and calcium.

As for all those other vitamins, there's nothing wrong with a child taking a daily multivitamin, but no pill will make up for a diet completely devoid of fruits and vegetables. Some parents believe that vitamins will help increase a child's appetite, but only a couple of medicines actually have that effect, and neither of them are vitamins. Megadoses of vitamins can be just as dangerous as overdoses of any other medication. No good science supports using high doses of dietary supplements to treat conditions such as autism, attention-deficit/hyperactivity disorder, or the common cold. At best these substances are eliminated by the kidneys and liver, and at worst they cause life-threatening complications.

You are now fully armed to raise a child who embraces healthy food choices, even if she only embraces one of them at a time. When you post that photo of her with the bowl of spaghetti on top of her head, be sure the caption mentions those are whole-grain noodles sliding down her face.

15

it's my potty: when changing diapers just isn't fun anymore

....

dad tip

Don't assume your child's potty has to go
in the bathroom. If he has a spot he always goes to
when he needs to go, put it there!

....

when parents ask me about teaching their children to use the potty, I recommend the technique I learned living among the Digo tribe of East Africa. Starting at a few weeks of life, keep the baby in touch with your body at all times, ideally without a diaper. You will soon develop an acute sensitivity to the physical cues that tell you he is about to poop or pee. At that point, quickly put your child between your knees over the ground or a potty, make a gentle whooshing sound, and use the emotional power of touch to aid and reward the process. By age 6 months your baby will have almost no accidents! Then I laugh and admit I never lived among the Digo. It was the Igbo, and it sometimes took as long as 8 months.

There are, in fact, people who pursue the Digo way; if you're interested in this approach there are Web sites to help you along, and the methods they describe are actually quite reasonable. Most dads, however, will find this approach a bit labor-intensive and inconvenient for a world where it seems like everywhere you look there's carpet. Assuming you're one of those dads, keep reading. Otherwise, what are you waiting for, man? Pick up that baby and get ready!

are we there yet?

In America today most children learn to use the potty consistently around age 2½ to 3 years, although it's not unusual to take longer. In past decades, kids did learn significantly earlier, around 18 months of age, but there was no Internet, so what else did people have to do? A couple of factors went into this earlier toilet use. For one thing, in the 1950s you couldn't just run to your local big-box store and pick up the 132-pack of disposable diapers. Diapers were rectangles of cloth, and even if you could afford a diaper service, they still required a certain amount of cleaning. As you might imagine, parents had an incentive to move things along.

Second, parents back then relied on somewhat different methods to teach their children to potty. Some of them might be familiar to the Digo, such as paying close attention to the child's elimination cues and getting him on the potty before he actually used his diaper. Another trick was to put the child on the toilet after meals to take advantage of his reflex to empty the colon, and then hold him there until something happened. The after-meals part might still be acceptable, but modern pediatricians find the forced-sitting-there thing cruel and unnecessary. Other accepted techniques of the day included enemas, punishments, shaming, and strapping the child to the potty. Today we know these techniques by the name child abuse.

Currently we define successful toilet use as the point at which a child can recognize that he needs to go, get himself to the potty, undress, use the potty, and dress again with little help. When you think about the skills involved from start to finish, you realize it may take a while for any given child to be up to such a challenge. Just as with anything else, different children are going to develop these abilities at different rates. But some parents can get competitive about these things, which doesn't make sense to me because now we have the Internet—don't they have better things to do? Don't sweat it if your child is a little slower to get the hang of things. I'm pretty sure that regardless of whether he's applying to Harvard, Juilliard, or the US Olympic soccer team, no one is going to be asking at what age he could tinkle in the potty.

When trying to figure out if your child is ready to start using the toilet, it helps to break down the skills he'll need. First he'll need to know when he needs to pee or poop. An infant's brain is working hard to organize all the various sensations that assault it all the time. Among these sensory inputs are those from receptors in the walls of the bladder and colon.

When tissues down there get stretched out by stool or urine, nerves carry signals to the brain to make us aware. Scientists' best guess is that most babies learn what these feelings of fullness mean around 12 to 18 months of age.

You can use language to help your child identify these feelings and their consequences. Of course, to do that, you're first going to have to pick some words for the relevant body parts and what comes out of them. This part can be harder than you'd think, as even many adults still feel embarrassed talking about this stuff. The simplest thing is probably just to go with the straightforward penis, vagina, buttocks, and anus. If you use cruder terms, your child risks offending people when he's just trying to convey information. If you choose made-up words, people outside the family may not get what your child is trying to tell them, and you're still going to have to teach him the correct terms pretty soon. At worst you could run into the situation my children faced, where the family word for vagina had a very real and innocuous meaning in Yiddish. To this day they giggle uncontrollably at friends' Passover celebrations.

Like the Digo, you'll quickly notice facial expressions or postures that telegraph your child's need to eliminate. You can take a moment to tell him, "It looks like you need to poop now," which is the first half of the sentence that will soon end, "Would you like to try using the potty?" By age 2 your child is going to press the issue by taking inventory of his parts, asking questions about them, and running around naked more often than you might think socially acceptable. Not only will he talk about his own stuff, but he'll want to discuss what's going on with you and your parenting partner as well. This provides you not only an opportunity to talk about elimination but to model using the potty. Your child is going to want to see what's going on, which means that if you get most of your reading done on the john, you may temporarily fall behind in book club. Be prepared to give simple, clear answers about the differences between boys and girls. Remember that whatever you tell him, by the next week he's likely to repeat it to dinner guests.

Another awareness that dawns on children around age 2 is some discomfort with having a wet or soiled diaper. Modern disposable diapers do such a good job of binding water that pee may only leave the diaper feeling a bit bulky. But stool never feels good, and its odor is harder to ignore. Toddlers and preschoolers already have a fear of contamination, so there's no need to use language to reinforce that poop or pee are unpleasant.

Once your child learns to sense when he needs to potty, he will need to develop the thinking skills to make it happen. Since you've been using the toilet successfully for a while now, you probably don't think twice about all the steps involved, unless for some reason you have to wear a tuxedo regularly, in which case you may still have to struggle to undress yourself. First your child has to be able to envision actions in his head, a process called symbolic thought. Once he realizes he needs to eliminate, he has to imagine finding the potty and using it. This process involves memory— where is that potty, and how does he get there from where he is now? It also involves sustained focus. Your child's internal dialogue will often go, "I need to go to the potty, which is in the bathroom way over there. Oh, look, kitty cat! Now I'm wet." This is where your attention and guidance can come in really handy.

There are also some physical skills your child will have to master before he can reliably use the potty. The most obvious is getting his clothes and diaper off. Many toddlers master the secrets of Velcro around 15 to 18 months of age, which is great if they're running around without pants on or in a dress. But if your child wears anything over the diaper, he's going to have to figure out how to escape from it in the limited window of time between realizing he needs to go potty and not being able to hold it. Overalls, shirts that snap at the crotch and jumpers may all pose insurmountable barriers to successful potty use, at least at first. To make using the potty easier, you'll want to remove as many of these barriers as possible, ideally when your prude in-laws are visiting.

There is another set of physical skills, however, that are more hidden. Muscles in the bladder and anus control when urine and stool stay inside the body and when they come out. Newborns have no control over these functions. Just as babies learn with time how to control their hands and legs, they learn to exert conscious control over their eliminations. Think for a moment how often your toddler falls down or knocks his cup over. He has comparable coordination when it comes to his bladder and bowels. Like every other skill, he will have to build his abilities with frequent practice and positive reinforcement. He will easily be 5 before he can fart to get a laugh, usually when your prude in-laws are visiting.

Not all the readiness for potty use rests with your child. You too will need to be prepared to commit to the process. Changing diapers may not be the most pleasant job, but to some extent you can pick when you want to do it. If you're on the phone, finishing dinner, or waiting for the commercial break during a game, you can put off the diaper change for a few minutes, depending on how sensitive you are to certain odors. Once you decide to start your child on the potty, you'll need to be responsive to his needs in short order, ready to help him get on and off the potty and praise him for any success he has. Expect to be working at it pretty intensively for between 6 weeks and 3 months once you start. Know that in many cases, the earlier you start, the longer it will take, as you wait for your child's skills to mature.

The home environment also matters. Life stressors have a big effect on a child's readiness to potty. Don't plan on starting the week you're, say, moving into a new home. Expect to lose ground with the birth of a new sibling, as your child sees the sort of attention one can earn for simply being incontinent. A separation or divorce is likely to distract your child from less pressing concerns like where to pee, even if it seemed like he was getting the hang of it.

So when is all this potty stuff supposed to happen? Not, as you may fear, never. Some children are ready to start as early as 18 months of age. Many start showing some interest in the potty around age 2. Many experts feel there is a "golden age" of opportunity for many kids between ages 2 and 2½. Some children don't develop all the necessary skills until around ages 2½ to 3. It's true what they say—girls do learn on average before boys. By this age, children are mastering a variety of physical skills, including those involving clothes and body parts. They are developing complex thought, planning skills, prolonged attention, complex language, and memory. They are interested in solving problems, from how to fit differently shaped blocks into holes to how to keep themselves dry and clean. Last but maybe most important, they are becoming deeply interested in earning your approval.

let's do this thing! and that other thing!

The time has come. Your child seems aware of when he needs to pee or poop. You know this because he told the checkout lady at the grocery store. He even has a ritual, hiding behind the couch to have a bowel movement so that the guys watching the game with you think perhaps you've done something rude. He is able to remove his pants and diaper undetected during worship services. He knows what happens in the bathroom as a result of flinging the door wide open, often without warning. He is eager to make you proud, showing off the drawing he scribbled on the living room wall and waiting for applause. It's go time, so to speak.

The next most important step is to acquire a potty. You may balk at bringing one more colorful piece of plastic into your home, and some parents choose to just prop a child's seat on the rim of an adult toilet. In some cases toddlers are so eager to imitate their older siblings that they only want to use the big commode. Think, however, about what it feels like to be a toddler. How comfortable would you be using the bathroom if you had to climb a ladder and sit on a huge, cold ledge over a whooshing whirlpool that goes who-knows-where with your feet dangling in the air? Adult potties can be scary, and not just because they're so high. Your toddler does not yet have fixed ideas about the physical properties of the world. It may be obvious to you that even a small human cannot be flushed down a commode, but watch how your child pretends Barbie is riding in a matchbox car and you'll get a sense of how real that fear might be for him. If you do teach him on an adult toilet instead of a child's potty, be sure he has a nice, wide footstool to prop his feet on.

Getting a potty chair also provides your child a sense of ownership of the process. Whether you buy one at the store, borrow one from a relative, or pick one up at a garage sale, try to bring your child along and make a ceremony of it. Write his name on it, let him decorate it with stickers, and surround it with his favorite books and toys. After all, chances are you have a small library, television, or smartphone handy near your own throne, and you've been using the bathroom on your own for years!

Don't be afraid to think outside the bathroom when you decide where to put the potty. If your child always goes behind the couch to have a bowel movement, that might be the natural place for it. The kitchen, his bedroom, or the playroom are other options. Remember, this thing is not a permanent fixture; it's light and easily moved. (My son's potty actually went to the soccer field in the back of the minivan, possibly justifying the existence of minivans.) Once he gets the hang of what he's doing, you can move the potty to its proper location.

You'll also want to involve your child in selecting big-kid underwear or training pants (eg, Pull-Ups). If he has a role model, such as an older sibling, a cousin, or a friend who already uses the potty, point out that soon he'll be "just like" that person! You can even find books and videos on learning to potty, often featuring his favorite characters. With each step you're helping him invest in this tremendous accomplishment he is working toward. Think of all the ways adult society rewards and encourages achievement! Your child should feel like he's receiving a huge honor—the Pulitzer of poop, the Emmy of elimination, the Oscar of excrement, the…OK, you get the idea.

Once your child has a place to potty, he's going to need to get familiar with it. He might start just by sitting there and playing or looking at a book. He may not even want to remove his diaper at first. Don't rush it. You want the potty to be a happy place, not a traumatic one. When your child soils his diaper you can have him walk over to the potty with you and make a ceremony of putting the poop where it goes, so he begins to associate the potty with its function. If he is willing to sit on it without his diaper at some point, he's likely to poop or pee just by random chance. You can improve the odds of this happening by having him sit there right after meals, when his colon is going to want to make room for the incoming food.

If your child happens to have some success, go ahead and make a big deal of it! You don't have to hire a clown or magician or anything, although clowns need the work. Nothing will make a bigger impact on your child than your joy in what he has accomplished. People use all sorts of rewards as positive reinforcement for their children's success. Stickers or gold stars may do the trick for some kids; others might enjoy adding nickels to a jar. Older preschoolers may enjoy working toward a larger reward, such as a toy or an outing, but toddlers and young preschoolers respond better to rewards that are immediate. The biggest reward you can give, however, remains your own hugs, kisses, and praise. Don't forget to trumpet your child's big accomplishment to other family members, too! Still, let your child be the one to tell the cashier at the grocery store.

Another technique that helps motivate children is to tell them about your own experience. If you have no memory of learning to use the potty yourself, it's OK to fudge a little, or you can call your parents and ask how you did. (Be prepared to learn some stuff you may not want to know!) If your parents tell you they used enemas and strapped you to the potty, you should probably just make up a better story.

Also, don't be afraid to leverage the power of play. There is a whole company that manufactures water-resistant housefly stickers to put in public urinals. Being a dude, you know why—guys aim for the fly, and the bathroom cleaning bills go down. You can do the same for your son or daughter with a simple scrap of toilet paper. "Let's see if you can get this one wet! Ten points!" Or, alternately, "Bombs away!" Going potty can be fun!

It's OK at the same time to make diaper changes a little less fun. You never want to punish or scold your child for using his diaper; he's still learning. But if the changing table used to be a place where you sang songs, played games, or had a tickle battle, you may now want to make it more of a workbench. Get the job done quietly and efficiently with a minimum of positive reinforcement. So long as they don't involve a struggle, trips to the potty should become routine, occurring after each meal, before bed, and any time your child shows signs he needs to use it.

If you feel like your child is ready to make the leap, you might scrap diapers altogether and go to training pants. While some training pants are really just disposable diapers kids can pull up and down easily, less absorbent ones provide immediate feedback when a child doesn't make it to the potty in time. For children used to disposable diapers, the feeling of wetness may be a surprise. "Oh, that's how it feels when I pee!"

Depending on how you define it, success may not come for months. This is, after all, a complex set of skills your child is trying to learn. Consistency and practice are key to learning anything, from a golf stroke to parallel parking to using the bathroom. You'll keep your part of the bargain by reminding your child every time he might need to go potty, by jumping up to help him as soon as he expresses the inkling to go, and by maintaining whatever reward program you agreed to. He does his part by being willing to sit on the potty at the times the 2 of you have agreed to.

As for whether children learn first to pee or to poop in the potty, it depends on the child. Pee is easier to get out, so it's likely to be the first thing your child successfully aims into the toilet. Poop, on the other hand, is easier to hold in, so it may be the type of accident that is first to disappear. Even children who learn quickly and easily to pee in the potty in the daytime may not remain dry at night for years. Most pediatricians don't even consider nighttime wetting (enuresis) an issue worth addressing until children turn 6 years old, and even then around 15% of children struggle to remain dry overnight.

Try not to get discouraged if your child has a setback. Even the best professional golfers hit a ball into the rough every now and then, so why shouldn't your child have the occasional accident? Recalling how much planning and memory your child needs to potty successfully, it won't surprise you to learn that distracting situations pose a high risk for toileting accidents. If your child is playing outside, not only is he absorbed in whatever he's doing, but the potty is that much farther away! If you're out of the home at a restaurant, friend's house, or hotel, he may have no idea where to go. At those times you'll want to be a little more vigilant about reminders. Your child may not want to interrupt his activity, but go ahead and encourage him to take a break every now and then and lead him to the potty "just to try and see if you can go."

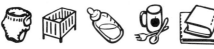

what you can do

Expect your child to need at least 6 months to get really proficient at using the toilet. Because accidents are bound to occur, it helps to have a plan for dealing with them. Never leave the house without at least one change of clothes and some wipes, no matter how eager you are to retire your man-purse. Wherever you are when an accident happens, play it off all cool. Just help your child clean up and say, "You had an accident this time, but next time I know you're going to make it to the potty!" You're not only expressing your confidence in your child, you're helping him envision what success will look like. When accidents do happen, your child should participate in cleaning up, even if he expresses some reluctance. You should never yell at or punish him for an accident, but it is his mess after all, and helping clean up will help reinforce how nice it is to have a potty to use.

Your child, of course, is not the only one learning in this situation. You too are figuring out what works best for this child in this situation. You may have another child who learned at a certain age in a certain way, and you just figured you'd repeat whatever worked last time. Good luck with that! Each child is bound to be different. While one likes to potty in the middle of the living room while the family watches television, another may insist on privacy. You may find that stickers are the perfect reward for one child while another wants to get that big-kid underwear as soon as possible.

Watch your child's responses and be willing to change up your game if a particular strategy seems not to be working.

If your child has a sudden setback in using the potty that does not seem to be a result of some external situation, don't jump to the conclusion that he has just become lazy or stubborn. Remember, he may not have the words to tell you something is uncomfortable or painful. Yeast infections are common in girls at this age and in uncircumcised boys. Strep infections of the anus or irritation from poor hygiene can lead to painful stools and constipation. Girls may suffer a condition called vaginal adhesions in which a thin layer of scar tissue seals the lips of the vagina, trapping urine inside and interfering with urination. Girls and boys can get urinary tract infections or even kidney stones. If potty training suddenly runs off the rails, don't be afraid to take a look down there and see if something is amiss, and have a low threshold to bring your child to the doctor for an undercarriage inspection.

you don't tell my butt what to do!

There are a decent number of preschoolers who are content to pee in their potties all day long, but when it comes time to poop insist on using a diaper. You control almost every aspect of your child's life, from when he wakes up to what he eats to whom he plays with, but there is one thing you cannot do no matter how hard you try, and that is make him poop in the potty. If you find yourself facing this problem, it's time once again to pull out the old dad-jitsu.

Your first job is to try to figure out why he won't poop in the commode. He may be afraid of the bathroom or the toilet itself, fearing he'll be flushed down the pipes. If he seems afraid try to reassure him, even showing him how large objects won't go down the tubes. Alternately, his bowel movements may be painful because of irritation or constipation. Or he may have just decided that this is the place where he's going to make his stand (or squat, so to speak). Interrogating a toddler or preschooler isn't always the easiest job, but if you're pretty sure you're dealing with that last one, there's only one thing to do—beat a strategic retreat.

It takes 2 to fight, so if you walk away from the battle your child is likely to forget pretty quickly why it was he was refusing to poop in the potty. Continue to have him join you as you dump his stools in the toilet to show him where they are supposed to go. He may continue to participate in cleanups as well. But otherwise, whatever word you use for stool shouldn't pass your lips unless you hit your thumb with a hammer, and even then you have other, more colorful choices. Don't ask if he has pooped in the potty, don't remind him to do it, don't urge him to go, don't tell him how wonderful his life would be if he would just for gosh sakes take a dump in the commode! Once there is no point in resisting, your child will figure out soon enough that life feels better when his bottom is clean. When he finally does use the potty, let him know how proud of him you are using means including, but not limited to, interpretive dance.

the constipation situation

You may feel like you already have enough crap to deal with in your life, but when your child stops pooping for a day or two, you've got a problem. Learning to potty seems to back up the pipes in some kids. The colon and rectum do a critical job in the digestive process—they wring as much water as possible out of waste products and consolidate them into a neat package the body can eliminate when the time and place are appropriate. If stool stays in there too long the colon may do its job too well, drying and con-solidating the poop until it's really hard to get out. Fiber in our food helps keep stool soft and moving along; dairy products tend to do the opposite. Sometimes constipation starts as a vicious cycle—one painful bowel move-ment causes the child to hold his stool in, and the next time he goes it hurts even more.

You can sometimes break the cycle of constipation by giving your child more fruits and vegetables to eat, getting him to drink more fluids, and cutting back on the dairy. If these measures fail, you may need to add a stool softener like polyethylene glycol (eg, Miralax) as well. If the problem doesn't improve or seems to come back frequently, you'll want to make a plan with his doctor.

when kids work blue

Your preschooler will quickly learn what every touring comedian knows: potty humor kills (stand-ups call this working blue). Whether you're on-stage at The Improv or in circle time at child care, mention elimination or private parts and you're going to get a laugh break. The difference is at The Improv they don't send a note home to your parents (only at Laugh Factory). As bathroom use and body parts occupy a large part of your child's thoughts at this age, you'll inevitably notice him using his newfound vocabulary for entertainment value.

Rather than blowing up when you hear this, use your dad-jitsu and ask him more about it. "So that word sounds pretty funny, huh?" You might even find he has some more questions he needs answered. Then you can let him know that using these words in this way is likely to get him in trouble with a lot of adults, and remind him not to do it. You can even leverage his desire to be funny by teaching him a joke that plays to a family audience: "Knock knock." "Who's there?" "Ice cream." "Ice cream who?" "Ice cream if you don't let me in!" It's no "poopy-head," but delivered with the right bugeyes and vaguely foreign accent, it will have them rolling in the mulch at recess.

the boys' room

Public restrooms provide great adventures in potty use. The toilet is too high, the seat is too big, and depending on the location, you often have some cleaning up to do before you'll let your child get anywhere near the thing. I remember one roadside filling station where I actually had to go the register and buy a pack of sanitary wipes to clean the potty for my kids, a surefire money-maker and labor-saver for them, no doubt. If you leave the house with your child, it's only a matter of time before you'll find yourself crouched on the floor of a bathroom stall helping him stay on the seat and learning more than you ever wanted to know about public restroom hygiene.

If you have a daughter, at some point you're going to wonder how long she can keep going with you into the men's room. Sometimes you luck out and find yourself at a mall, airport, or department store that has a family restroom, but most of the time you'll have to make a choice. Usually around age 5 girls become more embarrassed about going in the "wrong" restroom and more capable of dealing with toileting on their own.

At this point it's appropriate to let her start going to the ladies' room while you stand outside trying to look the opposite of how you think a pervert might look. Feel free to call in there periodically, "Are you OK, honey? Do you need any help?" Chances are a good number of the other people in that restroom are mothers, and in most cases they will be all too happy to lend your daughter a hand, especially if they see the awkward expression on your face as they open the door. Of course, you could always choose instead just to simplify your life, move to East Africa, and live among the Digo.

16

time-out:
rules of the game

chances are you're coming into fatherhood with some pretty strong preconceived notions about discipline. You might look in the mirror and think, "I turned out so awesome myself that whatever my parents did must have been perfect! I'm going to make sure my child has a chance to be as incredible as I am!" On the other hand, you might think, "It's amazing I am a functional member of society given the miserable job my folks did of raising me. I'm never going to do that stuff to my kid." Regardless of which way you feel, you have an advantage over your own parents—you can rely on a whole generation's worth of research on what does and does not work in child-rearing. No one can tell you exactly what's right for you and your family, but there are some general guidelines on what works best. Who knows? As awesome as you are, it's just possible your child could do even better!

the right stuff

Experts divide parenting styles into 4 basic categories based on 2 questions: how much do you expect of your child, and how responsive are you to your child's needs? Then they look at what parenting styles produce the best real-world outcomes. While this kind of research might seem squishy, the outcomes we're talking about are anything but soft. Which kids do best in school? Which ones are at risk for mental illness, depression, and suicide? What children end up using drugs, committing crimes, or becoming pregnant as teenagers? This stuff matters. Let's review the 4 categories and you can guess which one works best.

You might envision the *neglectful parent* as the dad sitting in his recliner, scratching his belly, and yelling periodically for the kids to bring him another bag of cheese doodles. This father has low expectations of his children and tends to ignore their needs. If the kids stand in front of the television complaining they're hungry, he might throw them some cheese doodles and let them have a sip of his soda. This parenting style remains popular due to how little effort it requires.

You could think of the *permissive parent* as the hippie dad letting his children run around the yard naked and feebly chastising them when they trample the organic wheatgrass. This father is tremendously sensitive to his children's needs, but his expectations are low and he sets no limits. If they want to stay up all night watching television and drinking juice until their teeth rot out, that's fine, so long as it makes them happy. This parenting style is great for those who fear conflict (wheatgrass sold separately).

The *authoritarian parent* lives in the popular imagination as the drill sergeant. This father has a cross-stitch on the wall that says, "Spare the Rod, Spoil the Child," and a T-shirt that reads, "Because I Said So, That's Why!" His favorite quote is, "While you live in my house you'll obey my rules," followed closely by, "The truth? You can't handle the truth!" This dad may get pushed around by other people in the adult world, but once he comes home, he's the boss! His expectations of his children are very high, but if they have needs, he can't hear them over the sound of his own yelling. This parenting style is popular among men who fear seeming weak and those who look good in camouflage.

The *authoritative parent* is the family's chief executive officer. When there is a conflict, he first asks everyone to calm down, then hears each side and negotiates a solution that doesn't leave any party feeling too hurt. If a child's actions are not in line with the family mission statement, he re-aligns the incentives to help bring that kid back on task. He is not one of those executives who sits in a glass-walled office behind a big mahogany desk. He is one of those hardworking startup types, the kind who paces the workshop floor with his sleeves rolled up, uncovering problems as they arise and helping parties arrive at a creative work-around. His expectations of his children are high, but he also hears their needs and responds to them. This style appeals to men who understand that anything worth doing is worth doing well, even if it takes a little more work.

So then, which parenting style do you think leads to the best outcomes for kids? Should you strive to be neglectful (gotta love those cheesy puffs!), permissive (love means never saying no), authoritarian (who put the "tator" in "dictator"?), or authoritative (thanks to all your cooperation and hard work, it's been another banner year for the family)? OK, I may have tipped my hand a little. Parents whose approach fits the authoritative model tend to have kids with the best outcomes, but you already guessed that.

Assuming you decide to follow that model, here's the catch: no one will tell you how well you're doing. There are no grades or performance reviews in parenting. You just do it. Some days you feel like you've earned your #1 Dad coffee mug, while others you wonder if you shouldn't just rip up your license to parent. You will, however, get feedback in less formal ways. Most directly you'll see if what you're doing is working. It may take a while for consistent discipline to have the desired effect, but if your child's behavior seems to be heading in the wrong direction, it may be time to reassess your approach. Second, you'll see how well your child is thriving in the world. If she seems loving, outgoing, and cheerful much of the time, you can probably feel pretty good about your parenting. Third, your child's doctor is a resource to give you guidance and feedback. If your child is demonstrating a particularly difficult behavior, don't be afraid to bring it up with the doctor. She may recommend a new approach, or she might find a medical or developmental problem underlying the behavior. Sometimes you just need to hear you're on the right track.

So this authoritative parenting thing sounds good in theory, but how do you do it? Can you really learn to be a good dad? Of course you can! But here's the thing—you being a good dad may not look exactly like anyone else being a good dad. It may not even look the same with one child as with another. Each child has her own strengths and weaknesses, her own personality. So does each dad. This doesn't mean some approaches don't consistently work better than others. There is no combination of father and child that makes spanking or demeaning a child OK. But as you apply discipline techniques you'll be learning as well as teaching, achieving the balance that best helps your child succeed.

disciplinary action

When we think about discipline we often go straight to the idea of punishment—if my child does something "bad," what am I going to do? For this reason, pediatricians prefer talking about *behavior* more than discipline. From the moment she's born, your child is looking to you to reinforce behaviors that will help her thrive in the world. She needs your guidance to know what to eat, how and when to sleep, how to avoid danger, and how to behave around other people in such a way that they're happy to meet her physical and emotional needs. Discipline is not just about getting a child to avoid certain behaviors that you deem inappropriate. It's about helping her learn to make the thousands of choices each day that will help her grow into a healthy, happy adult. But hey, no pressure.

Parents often ask at what age they should start disciplining their children. The answer is if your child has been born, you're already doing it. Your child begins life primed to respond to your cues, positive and negative. From the first time she sees you smile she wants to do whatever will make you do it again. If she perceives you're unhappy with something she has done, she will try to avoid that behavior in the future. If you have a preschooler or teenager you may find this hard to believe, but even when your children are expressing anger or frustration with the limits you impose, they still want to make you happy. Think about it for a minute. You have a dad. Do you want your own father to be proud of you? Even if the 2 of you have a difficult relationship, you know there's some part of you that wants to make him happy. Your child feels the same way, even if you can't always tell.

what you can do

If you're focusing all your efforts on the negative side of discipline, you're missing way more than half the picture. Every hug, smile, and compliment is an opportunity you have to show your child you appreciate her behavior. Even at the most trying of times, chances are good your child does more to make you happy than she does to make you unhappy. Try to never miss a chance to let her know. If your child is happy, secure, and eager to make you proud, your job becomes a whole lot easier when she displays a behavior you want her to change!

Like it or not, the day you became a father you also became a role model. This is not one of those jobs you have a choice about, like, say, whether you want to mow the lawn today. This job is hardwired into the human species. You may feel like you want to run from it, but in the very act of running away you will be teaching your child that's what dads do, so you may as well stay in there and give it some effort. Part of this job entails modeling appropriate ways of dealing with anger and conflict. In case you were wondering, that's not one of the easy parts.

Just because you're a dad doesn't mean you're not allowed to be angry. In fact, having a child opens up whole new frontiers of anger, kinds of anger you never even knew you could have! Each time you get angry, however, your child is learning from you how to deal with it. The most important lesson you can teach her is not to use violence. There are many reasons not to spank a child, and we'll get to the others later, but this is a big one. If you model violence to your child, you can trust she'll prove a quick study.

Second, you can teach her to focus her anger on a situation or an occurrence, not on a person. It's hard to overstate the difference between, "I'm upset with what you did," and, "I'm upset with you." Remember, children believe whatever you tell them, especially if it has to do with them personally. So if you tell your child she's "bad," don't be surprised when she decides you're absolutely right! You may not like what your child did, but you know she's a good kid. When you say she's bad, you're telling her something you don't believe yourself.

Take time to comment if you see your child dealing with her own anger or frustration well. "Use your words" has become a parenting cliché, but there's a reason it's such a popular sentence. Anger and frustration make us want to use our bodies to solve conflict, but learning to live in civilization involves substituting words for fists. Growing up is mostly about learning impulse control. If you see your child balling up her fists and getting ready to strike, step in ahead of time and remind her she can use language instead. You can teach her to say "No," walk away, or tell the other person what she wants. When you see she's successful at this, let her know you're proud of her and start saving up for her law school tuition.

Men in general are notorious for not talking about our feelings. (Personally, I talk about my feelings all the time; honestly, I think the dog is getting tired of hearing it.) Your child, however, is still learning to name her emotions, and you can help by acknowledging what you see, even if it seems obvious. "You're kicking the wall really hard, there, sport," you might say. "You must be really angry." You can also try, "I see you're crying. Are you sad your friend is leaving?" You don't have to lower your expectations of your child's behavior just because she has feelings, but it may help her to cooperate to know you're aware of her emotions.

laying down the law, then picking it up and laying it down again over there

You're probably thinking, "We're going to have to have some rules around here." You're right, but it's not always easy to decide what those rules should be. Having the wrong rules is guaranteed to make you crazy, and you might already feel like you're crazy enough. You don't want to do anything to make it worse.

The mistake most likely to threaten your sanity is to make rules that are not appropriate for your child's developmental level. By 9 months of age most infants understand their names and the word "No." By 15 months of age most toddlers can understand and follow a simple command. This means you can begin teaching children this young how to interrupt inappropriate or dangerous behavior, but they're going to need a lot of help learning to control their impulses. Your toddler may, for example, stop pulling on the dog's tail when you tell her to stop, but unless you move her away from the dog, you can expect the pulling to resume shortly. It's not that your child is poorly behaved, it's just that at this age she has neither the memory nor self-control to stop for long. What you'll see instead is that with repeated reminders over weeks to months she'll become more reluctant to pull the dog's tail, or at least stop and look around before she does it.

Around age 15 to 18 months your child may start biting and hitting, often when she's upset. You can and should tell her, "No, we don't hit," and isolate her for 2 minutes. She does not, however, know that biting or hitting hurts you any more than it would hurt the kitchen table. Nor does she have the intellectual capacity to grasp a long lecture on the inappropriateness of violence in resolving human conflict. She will instead learn that hitting and biting get her removed from where she wants to be and don't get her what she wants.

Expecting your 5-year-old to help clear her dishes after dinner will teach her to do her part in helping out and will provide her with pride at having a grown-up job to do. Try giving your 3-year-old the same task and you'll want to have a mop handy. Your expectations, in other words, will have to grow with your child. This rule also applies to the home environment. If you have a priceless Ming vase on the coffee table within reach of a 2-year-old, you'd better have good insurance on that thing! If you have a white sofa, maybe it's time to reconsider that vinyl slipcover. Do your best to structure your household in such a way that minimizes hazards and temptations. Otherwise, when something happens, whose fault is it, your child's or yours?

Another way to make yourself nuts is to have too many rules. Look around—do you have an official Policies and Procedures Manual posted near the family break room? If so, it's probably time to simplify. Some rules are based in your own family's individual culture, but there are a handful of rules that are universal. The most important involve safety. In addition to, "Don't pull the dog's tail," you'll probably want to include, "Don't run out in the street," and, "Don't pull on electrical cords." Teaching children not to endanger themselves is possibly our most critical job as parents.

A second nearly universal rule is, "We don't hurt other people." Hitting, biting, scratching, choking, and throwing sharp objects at others should all result in a firm "No" and an immediate period of isolation. Hopefully you'll recognize the irony of responding to violence with more violence. If you spank your child, smack her, or for gosh sakes bite her (people do!), you'll be teaching a very different lesson—the one who can be the most violent wins. Even if this is the way you were raised, remember that you now have an opportunity to do even better.

A third common rule is, "We treat each other with respect." Notice the words "we" and "each other" in that sentence. If you're not modeling appropriate language and behavior, your child will learn not that humans interact respectfully with one another, but that bullies can do whatever they want and everyone else just has to deal with it. If you call your child names or belittle her, you've made yourself more childish rather than helping your child become more mature. Being a dude, you're probably already childish enough.

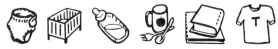

what you can do

You can demonstrate constructive communication just in the way you let your child know what you need her to do. Sometimes you have no choice but to resort to short commands like, "Get away from that rattlesnake!" For less time-sensitive issues, however, try a 3-part request that includes your "ask" along with a positive and a negative consequence. If there's room, you can even sandwich in the rationale for what you're asking. The result would sound something like this: "It's getting close to your bedtime, so please turn off the television and brush your teeth. If you do it now, we'll have time to read a story. If you don't, you'll have to go straight to bed." Is it longer than "Get upstairs and brush your teeth"? Yes, but the request carries a lot more information, too.

With time you may want to tack on a few more rules involving, say, property damage or behaviors that are important to your own family's culture. Whatever you do, however, try to keep the rules as simple as possible. You might insist your child address you with a tone of voice you deem respectful, for example, but are you going to try to police facial expressions as well? Your child is trying to keep track of a lot of stuff already, and you want to pave the way for her to succeed.

so now what are you going to do?

As with so many parts of a dad's life, discipline boils down to having the right tools for the job. Your solution to a given discipline challenge will depend on all sorts of factors, from your child's age and developmental level, to whether she is in immediate danger of physical harm, to whether you're at home or out shopping for groceries. You wouldn't attempt to teach your child appropriate behavior with only one technique any more than you'd undertake major household repairs with just a Phillips screwdriver (just trust me on that one). So let's look in your toolbox and see what you've got.

We already mentioned one tool for pretty much every job, which is to set a good example. Given how powerful an influence you are on your child's behavior, this one bears repeating. The old, "Do as I say, not as I do," line is too lame to impress even a small child. No matter how hard you try, you probably won't behave perfectly in all situations. Then it's time to model another important behavior—admitting and learning from your mistakes. "Back there, when Daddy cursed at that referee? I shouldn't have done that. I needed to speak respectfully to the man in the black and white stripes. Next time I won't yell like that, and we'll get to watch the whole ball game. Are you going to finish that popcorn?"

We've also already mentioned positive reinforcement. This tool works especially well when you can "catch your child doing good." Surprise her regularly with your all-seeing gaze: "I really like the way you shared your truck with your brother just now," for example. As your child grows older there are times you may want to give rewards that are more concrete than a smile and hug. Tasks like potty training or sharing with a sibling, for example, may warrant a sticker chart or nickel jar. In general, we discourage using food rewards to avoid reinforcing a relationship between good behavior and the high-fat, salty, sugary foods usually used as rewards.

As your child gets even older you may decide to establish longer-term rewards, such as a special outing in return for getting good grades or a weekly allowance for completing certain chores. You may find that if you make the system too complicated, it becomes difficult to keep track of what your child has earned. You'll also want use such material rewards sparingly, lest your child decide every good thing she does deserves a reward. No matter what you come up with, it's critical you keep your part of the bargain. Break your promise one time and you can kiss this tool good-bye.

We also already touched on the universal tool of removing your child from a troublesome situation. This one is essential during the first 2 years of life, when your child's self-control hasn't developed to the point where she can limit much of her own behavior. But don't put this tool away just because your child turns 2. There are times that physically taking your child somewhere else is the only way to interrupt behavior that has gotten out of hand.

Another tool, actively ignoring, is more of a specialty item. This approach is useful when your child is using an inappropriate communication style, such as shouting, throwing a fit, or posting unflattering photographs of you on the Internet. As opposed to the passive-aggressive silent treatment, you begin actively ignoring by explaining what you're about to do and what your child must do to make you stop. "I'm not going to answer you until you address me respectfully," is one way to put it, although there's also the ever-popular, "I don't speak Whine-ese. When you stop whining I'd love to hear what you have to say." If you are in fact of scholar of Whine-ese, there's no reason your child should know.

Another special-use tool is called natural consequences. This is useful at times when you know what's going to happen next, but your child needs to find out. If she's throwing her cup to the floor, for example, it may just stay there. Eventually she can have more to drink, but if she's clearly more interested in exploring basic physics than drinking, it's time she discover that objects at rest remain at rest. Likewise, if she treats a toy truck violently and breaks it, she will learn facts about the world that will be critical should she choose a career driving tractor-trailers. Natural consequences, of course, need to be relatively harmless. This is not the tool to use, for example, when teaching your child not to run into traffic.

A related tool is called logical consequences. The only difference between natural and logical consequences is that you have to step in and provide the outcome that should follow an action. Say your child is banging his truck on the coffee table. You might say, "Please stop banging your truck, you're going to scratch the table. If you stop banging you can keep play-ing with it, but if you don't stop I will take it away for the rest of the day." Here's the important part: one more bang and you absolutely must take that truck away! For the rest of the day. Really. Your child is likely to cry or even throw a tantrum, but she will learn facts about the world that will be critical should she choose a career refinishing furniture damaged by people who drive tractor-trailers.

Next up in the same tool drawer is withholding privileges. This tool works just like logical consequences, except that in this case you'll have to get more creative about the consequences. The thing you take away should be something extra that the child enjoys, not something she really needs. Making her turn off the television, for example, is a great use of this tool, especially since she probably should be watching less of it anyway. Taking away dinner, on the other hand, is a horrible idea, as food is lumped in there with water, shelter, and clothing on the short list of must-haves. Taking away a toy works well, but try not to take away your child's trea-sured transition object, whether it's a stuffed animal, blanket, or robot. She's going to need something to comfort herself, after all.

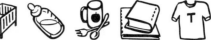

what you can do

One of the most flexible of discipline tools is allowing limited options. Children enjoy feeling like they have some control over their environments, and there's no reason they shouldn't. Take every opportunity to lay out a small number of acceptable choices. "Would you like to brush your teeth first or take your shower first?" "Eat green beans or broccoli with your meat loaf?" "Pick up your toys now or after you eat lunch?" By granting your child some control, you lessen her need to fight you. At the same time, if you offer too many choices she may find it overwhelming to pick one; 2 or 3 should do. She may want to add another choice of her own, but you can decide whether her idea should be on the menu. Green beans, broccoli, or carrots may be great. Green beans, broccoli, or chocolate cake, not so much.

the use and maintenance of time-out

Of all the discipline tools available to a father, time-out may be the most misunderstood. I hear parents say all the time, "I tried using time-out, but it never seems to work." Just as with any other tool, the key is to use it properly.

Time-outs are really an extension of the removing-your-child-from-the-situation tool. The idea is get your child away from a situation that has spiraled out of control and give her time to collect herself. Additionally, there is a punitive element—no one enjoys forced isolation. Time-out tends to work best during the preschool years, but even a toddler can spend a couple of minutes in time-out and, as we'll discuss later on, older children and teens may respond to a variation on the technique. At moments when you're so upset you think you might do emotional or physical harm, you may even need to put yourself in time-out until you can cope with a situation constructively.

Your child should know ahead of time what behaviors will earn a time-out. Preschoolers are likely to need a lot of repetition before they really get the picture, so if you see a time-out behavior creeping up, remind your child what may come next. One warning, however, is enough. Giving multiple warnings turns a reliable consequence into a gamble. You'll want to choose a time-out spot that is away from other people and is not a lot of fun, like a chair in the corner. If your child's time-out spot is in front of a video game, for example, she's probably missing the point. One of the advantages of time-out is that you can impose it nearly anywhere that's safe, from a restaurant to the grocery store to a friend's house. I have yet to figure out how to impose time-out in a moving vehicle.

Establish the duration of the time-out ahead of time. As a rule of thumb, most people use the child's age plus 1 year, but for an especially patient or stubborn child you might have to use a different rule of thumb, like your age minus the age of your car. Whatever the time is, try to set a timer. That staves off the question, "Can I come out of time-out yet?" If your child hasn't heard the timer, she knows the answer. Speaking of questions, time-out is not conversation time. You should let your child know why she's in time-out when you're putting her there. Once she's there, it's not time for a long discourse on the nature of her actions and their consequences. Conversation is a form of attention, and as such it sort of blows the whole time-out concept. Your child may yell, scream, or even throw a tantrum while in time-out. Unless she is a danger to herself or others or is doing property damage, let it pass without comment.

If your child tries to leave time-out early (as she inevitably will at least once), return her there and let her know her time-out is starting over and will every time she leaves. You may end up needing to hold her gently and firmly in place, letting her know you are doing so because she tried to leave. You may have to add a backup consequence for leaving time-out (see your other tools described previously). On the flip side, sometimes you just need your child to get her behavior under control. Especially with older children you can offer an open-ended option: "You can come out of time-out as soon as you feel you can control your behavior."

How you behave before, during, and after time-out can be just as important as how your child behaves. There is some chance that by the time you get to imposing a time-out you'll be angry yourself. You should be firm and gentle in placing your child in time-out; if you feel like you want to hurt her, put yourself in time-out first. One way to ensure a smooth transition to time-out is to use it early and often. Rather than waiting for a behavior to reach crisis level, put your child in time-out as soon as the behavior begins.

Like with all your discipline tools, you'll want to be consistent in using time-out. If hitting her brother gets your child a time-out sometimes and not others, she never knows when it's OK to slug him! After time-out, let your child know if she's done a good job. She has served her time and doesn't need a lecture or to be forced to apologize now. Imagine you've hit the reset button on the day. If you notice your child seems to be getting a lot of time-outs, think about showing her more affection and attention when she's not misbehaving. She may have decided that misbehaving is the only way she can get your attention.

consistency, consistency, cons...

Now that you have a box full of tools, you'll want to wield them properly. Just owning a Phillips screwdriver does you no good if you're using it to bang nails in the wall. Let's talk about some ways to make sure these tools do the job you need them to do.

Immediacy is critical for discipline until children are well into their school years. Think about your own discipline challenges. Have you ever had too much to drink despite the certainty you would suffer a hangover the next day? Do you sometimes stop for donuts knowing you'll have to munch celery sticks for days to stick with your weight-loss goal? Do you look at your credit card bill and wonder what you were thinking last time you went shopping? When a significant amount of time separates actions from their consequences, even adults tend to make poor choices. For children the situation is even worse, because in a child's mind a day lasts, like, forever. The best discipline tools are those you can use right away. Threatening a preschooler in the morning with taking away her dessert at dinner is like telling her she won't get into a good college. To the extent it's practical, do something the moment you see the behavior.

Next, don't make idle threats; you'll just turn your child into a gambler. Think—why do people buy lottery tickets? If they were likely to win, the lottery wouldn't make any money. People know they're more likely to lose, but there's always the chance that they might win. If you threaten your child with a consequence and don't carry out that threat immediately, it's like offering her a lottery ticket. Sure, she might end up facing a consequence, but then again, she might not! There's only one way to find out.

That means the consequence has to be something you can live with and something in your control. I remember dining outside with my daughter when she was a preschooler. We were right next to an ice cream place, and I told her if she threw one more rock we wouldn't go get ice cream. She threw the rock. I missed dessert. That would have been a good moment for a time-out. My biggest pet peeve as a pediatrician is when I hear a parent tell a child, "If you don't behave, that doctor is going to give you a shot." He is now, is he? And when I don't give that child a shot, what has she learned about her parent's truthfulness? Whatever you threaten needs to be something you can really do, right now, every time.

Assuming you share child care duties with any other people, you'll want to make sure everyone is pretty much on the same page when it comes to discipline. This holds true whether your child is going to her grand-parents' house or to visit your ex-spouse. When children have wildly different sets of expectations in different places, they have a really tough time adapting. If your child learns she can talk one caregiver into allowing behaviors that the other doesn't, she will naturally do so, leaving the 2 of you to fight it out afterward. The best way to avoid this situation is for caregivers to decide together ahead of time what the rules are and how consequences are to be enforced. Especially when parents are separated or divorced this type of cooperation can falter, but in those cases you can at least establish consistent expectations within your own household.

Fathers, I suspect, are especially reluctant to discuss the sense of guilt that can accompany discipline. It's fun to make children happy; it stinks to make them cry. Just because we're dads doesn't mean we want to be mean. At the same time, good, consistent discipline is part of showing your child love. Children, even 2-year-olds and teenagers, feel deeply insecure if they cannot rely on their parents to keep them safe and under control. They are guaranteed to vent their anger at you when you set limits, and your job is to be the grown-up and take it, so long as those expressions of anger stay within the guidelines of respect you've estab-lished. There are times you will enforce a consequence and feel like abso-lute garbage. There is no need to share those feelings with your child. If you demonstrate doubt about your discipline, your child will begin to wonder whether the rules and consequences you've set are valid.

That's not to say there may not be situations in which you have to admit your own errors and apologize. You might punish your child for some-thing and then find out she didn't do it after all. You may lose your cool and say or do something you realize afterward was way out of line. There's nothing wrong with showing your child you can admit it when you make a mistake. But establishing age-appropriate boundaries and consequences is not a mistake. It's parenting, and it's your job.

spare the rod. seriously, spare it.

If spanking worked, I would be all for it. The fact is, while you may get it to work once or twice, if you spank your child with any regularity you'll quickly find you're using the wrong tool for just about any job you can name, except perhaps "making your child more aggressive." It does work well for that.

There are plenty of adults who were spanked as children and never did get arrested for anything, but on average children who are spanked are at higher risk when they grow up for depression, alcohol use, anger issues, criminal behavior, and violence within and outside the home. If your goal as a parent is to set an example of how your child should behave and you don't want your child to hit people in anger or to control their behavior, it doesn't make any sense to spank.

Spanking also can put you on a slippery slope toward causing your child more pain than you had intended. If for some reason you feel the need to spank your child, at least protect her in the following ways: First, don't use any foreign object, be it a spoon, switch, or belt. Your hand has nerves, which tell you how much force you're using. Foreign objects are real tools, lever arms that increase the force of your blows and give you no feedback. Once you apply a lever arm to the situation you've lost physical and emotional control. Second, never spank in anger. Have your child wait in time-out while you calm down, and if you haven't thought better of it, administer the spanking quickly and calmly. Third, just don't do it! If you couldn't get any of those other tools to work, chances are your child has a behavioral problem that needs a doctor's attention or you weren't using them right, which suggests you're not going to have any more success with this one. Before you spank your child, talk to her doctor and see if there's something you could be doing differently.

big-kid discipline

Just because your child is tall enough to look you in the eye doesn't mean your job is over when it comes to discipline. Given the risks to teenagers' safety, health, and future success, discipline is, if anything, more important than ever. That said, you're going to have to adapt your tools to the job at hand.

Many of the same tools you used for younger children still work. There's more room than ever, for example, to model appropriate behavior. Praise remains a powerful tool; your kid may duck down in the car when you drive past the mall, but she still wants your affection and approval. Actively ignoring remains a useful tactic; more than ever she wants to be heard, but for you to listen she'll have to speak respectfully.

Even time-outs can evolve into the teen years. You might point out that your teen is upset and needs some time to gather herself. Suggest 15 or 20 minutes of time to calm down so the 2 of you can resume a more constructive conversation. Your adolescent can choose between various methods of sulking, from drawing to playing guitar to surfing the Internet, as long as she isn't posting unflattering pictures of you.

Natural and logical consequences remain useful as well. The natural consequence of not studying, for example, is to make a lousy grade. The logical consequence of making lousy grades may be to lose video game privileges for the next grading period. Loss of privileges may include use of the car, time spent with friends, or shopping opportunities. You also have the option of adding household responsibilities. My own parents could get me to do pretty much anything with the mere threat that I might have to mow the lawn. Come to think of it, that still works.

One advantage of having a teenager is that your child can take an active role in determining what the consequences of her actions should be. Go ahead and ask your teen to propose a consequence after she breaks an established rule in the house. You may find her sense of justice is actually harsher than your own! You may be the one arguing for a more lenient sentence. Because the consequence is her idea, she's more likely to comply.

You can also use this approach in establishing what the rules of the house should be. You might negotiate a list of chores, an academic goal, or a curfew that everyone finds satisfactory. You're transitioning your teen into the adult world, where we're all bound by contracts, usually by mutual agreement, and where we often face consequences of our own making.

Now you have a whole shed full of tools to help your child learn appropriate behavior, and you know how to use them, from the simple #2 Phillips screwdriver to the 12-point ⅜-inch left-handed gear-driven socket wrench. You can roll up your sleeves and set about your job as chief executive officer, at least with the advice and consent of your family's board of directors. Go ahead now and pick up that bag of cheese doodles. You've earned them, and you'll need the energy.

17

snot funny:
colds, allergies, sinusitis,
and who nose what else

before i became a dad I remember seeing kids in the grocery store
with snot dripping from their noses and wondering what kind of parent
lets his child out in public that way. "For heaven's sake, would you please
wipe that child's nose?!" I wanted to shout. Now that I've had my own children, I get it. Sure, you start with the nose-wiping, but at some point you
just have to get on with your life! You could come to the grocery store
with a box of tissues and a trash bag, but you'd have to buy more before
you made it down the cereal aisle! Now I'm just thankful when the store
has those sanitary wipes you can use on the grocery cart handles before
you put your own hands on them. I think if you have a toddler you should
mount a box of those puppies right by your front door. "Oh, these? Johnny
has another cold. I'd grab a big handful in case you have to touch anything.
Won't you come in?"

Runny nose is a sign of many of the most common illnesses your child is
likely to have, from colds to sinus infections to allergic rhinitis. Depending
on what else is going on, telling the difference between these illnesses
may be straightforward or pose a challenge, even to pediatric specialists.
The situation is complicated by the possibility that your child may suffer

any combination of these illnesses in sequence or all at the same time. Fortunately, there are some basic clues to help you tell the difference.

baby it's cold inside

I think it's about time for you to win another bet with your friend. (That is, unless he's gone out and bought his own copy of this book, in which case…awesome!) Ask him how many colds a normal toddler or preschooler gets in a single year. Chances are good he won't guess the real average, which is 8. If he does, you can tell him around 15% of children will get 12 colds a year, so that's still technically normal. Because children this age get sick more often in the winter, they may seem to have a runny nose almost all the time during the cooler months. If you have a preschooler and you feel like he's always sick, rest assured it's not your imagination. Doesn't that make you feel better?

You might have noticed your child has had more colds since he started child care. You're not imagining this, either. Kids in child care catch around 1½ to 2 times as many colds as children who stay at home. All 3 of my children attended child care, and I'm still waiting for my thank-you note from the makers of Kleenex.

If you or someone you live with smokes cigarettes, it just makes matters worse. Children exposed to cigarette smoke get sick much more often than children who breathe clean air. Because tobacco smoke is such a powerful toxin to the human respiratory system, it doesn't take much exposure to do the trick. That person who swears she only smokes in the bathroom with the fan on is still leaking enough fumes into the house to make the kids sick.

Just what is a common cold, anyway? The name dates back to the 16th century, when people noticed the relationship between cold weather and cold symptoms. It took until the middle of the 20th century for scientists to isolate some of the thousands of different viruses responsible for cold symptoms in humans. Once doctors knew what caused colds, we predictably took a disease with a simple 4-letter name and renamed it a viral upper respiratory infection, or URI for short. There, doesn't that sound more, uh, science-y?

A group of viruses called rhinoviruses cause about half of all colds (rhino is the Greek root for nose). But rhinoviruses don't have to do all the work; they enjoy the company of multiple other virus classes during the cold season, including adenoviruses, enteroviruses, respiratory syncytial virus, coronaviruses, and influenza viruses. Your child never seems to develop immunity to the common cold because the cold he had last month probably resulted from a wildly different virus than the cold he has this month. His immune system builds defenses against each virus he contracts, but there are thousands more where that one came from.

It seems obvious that sneezing clouds of virus-laden fluid into the air would infect other people, but it turns out few colds are spread this way. Instead, most people contract a cold virus from the hands of someone who is already infected. The virus particles move from that person's hand (or grocery cart) to the victim's; then, when the victim touches his own eyes or nose, the virus infects its new host. This is why careful hand-washing or using alcohol-based hand sanitizer is so critical to preventing the spread of colds. It also explains why we now teach children to cough into the crooks of their elbows instead of into their hands. It's less important to muffle the cough than it is to keep the hands clean. And if there's one thing young children are known for, it's for the cleanliness of their hands!

One thing that does not cause colds is exposure to cold air. While colds are indeed more common in winter, their spread has nothing to do with whether the victim wears a hat, covers his ears, or zips his jacket. Emotional stress and inadequate sleep, on the other hand, do make it easier for people to catch colds. So if your kid won't zip up his coat on a freezing day, don't fuss at him too hard; he might stay awake worrying about it, and then he will catch a cold!

Once a cold virus gets into a child's body, the virus itself is not terribly destructive. Instead, as the infection spreads up and down the airway, the body's immune defenses cause all the symptoms we associate with colds. Cold symptoms often begin 1 to 2 days after exposure to the virus with a scratchy throat, headache, and fatigue. Fever is common at the beginning of a cold but usually lasts only around 3 days, and the temperature rarely rises above 104°F. Blood vessels in the nose and upper airway swell and leak fluid into surrounding tissues, closing off nasal passages. Mucous-producing cells inside the nose and sinuses start working overtime, with the resulting snot dripping out of the nose and down the back of the throat. Often the inflammation extends down into the larger breathing tubes of the lungs (bronchi). The cough with colds results not only from this inflammation, but from mucous dripping down into the lungs from the nose. Inflammation may make the eyes red and watery and cause a sore throat or hoarseness as well, along with plenty of sneezing.

Let's talk about snot, or mucous. (Go ahead and put down your sandwich.) Our bodies secrete mucous in all the moist parts that have contact with the outside world. Mucous protects us by trapping dirt and infectious organisms. Normally this is a good thing, but you've heard the phrase, "Too much of a good thing."

Brace yourself—I am about to reveal the best-kept secret in all of pediatrics: snot color means nothing! Doctors could care less whether it's clear, yellow, or green (although if it's plaid, your child may be Scottish). Depending on the water content and activity of the immune system, mucous may be clear and watery, white and cloudy, or yellow to green in color. Colored mucous does suggest your body's immune system is working to fight something off, but it doesn't tell you whether that something is a virus or bacteria. During the normal course of a cold, mucous tends to start clear and watery, then get thicker and more colorful around the third or fourth day; by around day 10 it goes away for the most part.

While the color of the mucous doesn't tell doctors much, we do care how long it sticks around (so to speak). Nasal discharge that lasts more than 10 to 14 days suggests a bacterial sinus infection. So please, never bring your child's doctor a tissue so he can see the color of the mucous (it happens!), but do make a note on your calendar of when your child first became ill. That's something the doctor really will want to know!

In case you were wondering, there still is no cure for the common cold. There are, however, some things you can do to help your child with cold symptoms, and many of them don't even require a trip to the drugstore.

To start, let's get back to the problem of nasal congestion and snot. The simplest solution, especially for babies and younger children, is to mix a half teaspoon of table salt in 1 cup of water to make normal saline. You can also buy saline nose drops if you want to have a bottle to keep them in, but at 2:00 am you'd probably rather peek in your pantry than grab your car keys. To better dissolve the salt you can bring the solution to a boil, then cool it to room temperature. Put just a few drops in each side of your child's nose and wait a minute while your child screams like you're trying to drown him. Don't worry, this part won't last long. Then use the little blue or red rubber suction bulb from the hospital to suck out the now-loosened secretions. If you lost the suction bulb you can buy a new one at the pharmacy, but then you're back to needing your car keys. If you're going out anyway, you can pick up a cool mist humidifier, which may also help loosen dried secretions.

The best-known cough therapy also lives in your pantry, not your medicine cabinet. If your child is older than 1 year, you can use a half to a whole teaspoon of honey. Children younger than 1 year are vulnerable to deadly botulism from honey, so for infants substitute corn syrup. Honey actually worked better than the common cough suppressant dextromethorphan in a large, well-controlled study, proving your grandmother is smarter than many giant, multinational pharmaceutical companies.

If your child has a fever you may want to give him acetaminophen (eg, Tylenol) or ibuprofen (eg, Advil, Motrin) for comfort. A child should turn 6 months or older before taking ibuprofen, 3 months or older to take acetaminophen. Remember, any fever in a child younger than 3 months deserves a doctor's immediate attention whether or not the child has a cold.

Say you locate your car keys and get to the pharmacy to pick up a humidifier, a new suction bulb, and some acetaminophen. You find yourself standing in front of a vast array of children's cough and cold medicines, each promising to relieve the very symptoms your child is suffering. Shouldn't you just buy one and see if it works as well for your child as for the adorable, pitiful-looking kid on the box? That depends very much on how old your child is and what's in the bottle. Of the more than 600 cough-and-cold products for sale in the United States, they all share only a handful of active ingredients, and few of those have ever proven to do what they claim.

First, ask yourself whether your child is younger than 6 years. If so, unless his doctor has specifically told you to get one of these medicines, don't. In 2008 the Food and Drug Administration (FDA) counseled parents not to use over-the-counter cold medicines for children younger than 4 years, and many manufacturers voluntarily stopped labeling their products for children younger than 2 years, when kids are at highest risk of serious overdose. But even for older children, products like dextromethorphan (cough suppressant), guaifenesin (expectorant), pseudoephedrine or phenylephrine (decongestant), and diphenhydramine, chlorpheniramine, or brompheniramine (antihistamine) have never proven useful in fighting symptoms caused by a viral URI in children. Save yourself the money and buy an extra suction bulb instead.

There are a couple of products on that shelf that may be helpful in a limited way. One study of Vicks VapoRub showed it was moderately better than placebo at relieving stuffy nose. Whether further studies will confirm this finding remains to be seen. Nasal decongestant sprays like oxymetazoline (eg, Afrin) do indeed relieve nasal congestion but at a cost—if you use them more than a few days in a row and then stop, congestion often returns with a vengeance. We generally don't recommend using them at all before a child turns 12. Ipratropium, a prescription nose spray, relieves the runny nose from colds; it is FDA approved for children as young as 6. It does nothing for sneezing or congestion, however, and I almost never see it used.

when to call the doctor

Colds, while pesky and hard to treat, are usually benign infections, with 2 exceptions. When babies younger than about 3 months get colds, they may develop fever or serious breathing problems (see Chapter 9 for a full discussion), both of which deserve immediate medical attention. Influenza may also share some features with the common cold, but flu often also comes with muscle aches, vomiting, diarrhea, and severe headache, all unusual with the common cold. If you suspect your child has influenza, he should see his doctor within the first 2 days of symptoms.

Most colds resolve without any problem, but a viral URI sometimes sets the stage for a more serious bacterial infection. About 5% to 10% of colds progress to bacterial sinusitis, and among toddlers and preschoolers up to 30% of colds usher in middle ear infections. While we have no effective treatments for the common cold, bacterial ear and sinus infections may respond to antibiotics, so it helps to know when your child has crossed over from one illness into the other. Fortunately, we have some pretty good signs to tell us.

that's cold...not!

Bacterial sinus infections and colds share many symptoms—fever, runny nose, stuffy nose, cough, throat discomfort, and headache. That's because both are infections of the nasal cavities and sinuses, just with different agents. The only surefire way to know whether these symptoms result from infection with a virus or bacteria is for a surgeon to insert a needle into a sinus cavity, suck out some fluid, and send it for culture. Fortunately, researchers have studied enough of these cases of confirmed bacterial sinusitis that you can know what signs suggest sinusitis without having to use any objects sharper than your own mind.

Most people know the sinuses have something to do with the nose, but at least where I live folks use the term sinuses to refer to anything that causes a runny or stuffy nose. The sinuses are actually air-filled cavities within the skull that help sound resonate and make our heads lighter (even your thickskulled boss has them). There are 4 pairs of these spaces: the maxillary sinuses are in the cheekbones just beside the nose; the frontal sinuses are in the forehead above the eyebrows; and the ethmoid and sphenoid sinuses are deeper in the skull. All 4 sets of sinuses drain through tiny tubes into the nasal cavities. Cold viruses often cause inflammation and fluid collection in these spaces, but most of the time those problems go away when the cold does. In some cases, however, bacteria from the nose invade the now-inflamed sinuses and set up shop.

Babies come into the world with only 2 of these pairs of sinuses, ethmoid and maxillary. Frontal and sphenoid sinuses don't fully develop until age 12. For this reason, if your child is complaining of a frontal headache, chances are it's not his sinuses. Younger children may report pain in the cheeks when their maxillary sinuses are infected, but this is also a pretty rare complaint, usually heard only when the infection is severe. Older children may also complain of pain behind the eyes, which is especially concerning if they say it feels worse when they bend over.

So if pain isn't the most common symptom of childhood sinus infections, what is? The 2 best signs we have that it's time to pull out the antibiotic big guns are prolonged fever and prolonged symptoms. Viral URIs often cause fever, especially in the first few days. Most of the time temperature remains below 102°F, and these fevers should generally go away after 3 days. Fevers that last 4 or more days or fevers that go away for 24 hours and then return are reliable signs that your child has a bacterial infection. Of course, that infection doesn't have to be in the sinuses! The ears and lungs are also vulnerable. The only way to know is for a doctor to examine your child.

The runny, stuffy nose from a viral URI should get better after 7 to 10 days, 2 weeks at the outside. If your child's nose is still running after a couple of weeks or if it starts to improve after a week and then acutely worsens, chances are good he has a bacterial sinus infection. Cough, on the other hand, can last much longer with a cold. It often takes 2 or 3 weeks for the cough to resolve, even when the child has nothing more than a virus.

when to call the doctor

Chest pain, shortness of breath, and wheezing are never normal. Those symptoms deserve a doctor's attention immediately.

Antibiotics remain the cornerstone of therapy for bacterial sinusitis, although how much they help remains a matter of some debate. Studies in adults have repeatedly failed to prove that antibiotics alter the course of acute sinusitis. In children the results look a little better. Amoxicillin is still the best choice to start with, unless the child has a penicillin allergy or just finished a course of amoxicillin. Some parents urge doctors to prescribe "something stronger," or believe "amoxicillin never works for my child." Amoxicillin, when given at the right dose, is plenty strong to kill the vast majority of bacteria that cause sinusitis while doing less damage to the good bacteria that, say, keep your child from having diarrhea. Antibiotic resistance is a property not of the child but of the infection. Just because amoxicillin didn't seem to cure a previous infection doesn't mean it will fail this time. There are a variety of reasons your child's doctor may

when to call the doctor

One potential complication of colds and sinusitis is worth mentioning just because it's so dangerous. If you notice one or more of your child's eyelids are bright red or swollen, get him to the doctor immediately. Infection can spread from the nose or eyes to the skin of the eyelids, and from there it can progress rapidly to involve the tissue behind the eyes, even the brain. This infection, called *periorbital* or *orbital cellulitis*, requires immediate and aggressive antibiotic therapy.

choose a different antibiotic, but don't worry that amoxicillin is somehow inferior to other medications; it's popular because it works.

Once your child starts taking antibiotics he should feel better pretty quickly. If he has facial pain, it should improve after the first day. Fever should get better after a couple of days, and his nose symptoms should start getting better within 2 or 3 days. Your child is also welcome to return to school as soon as his fever goes away, unless he seems too sick for some other reason. He is no more likely to infect his classmates than all those other children running around with snotty noses. Come to think of it, maybe you'd better send him back with some of those sanitary wipes.

hay fever: not the best disease name we've ever made up

There are reasons other than viral or bacterial infections to have a runny nose. Let's look at your child and run through a quick checklist: is he playing outside in cold air, eating a jalapeño pepper, or missing a bead, bean, or other small, nostril-sized object? All of the above can cause a watery runny nose, although when you address the underlying cause it usually goes away. On the other hand, he may just be among the 40% of American children who suffer *allergic rhinitis,* what most people simply call allergies or hay fever.

Allergic rhinitis is just one type of allergic disease, or *atopy.* All these diseases result from certain parts of the child's immune system mistaking benign allergens like pollen, dust mites, mold, or animal dander for more dangerous invaders. The immune system cranks up inflammation trying to fight off the imaginary attacker and, depending on where the inflammation is the worst, the child may have any number of symptoms. In allergic rhinitis, inflammation causes sneezing, runny nose, nasal congestion, nasal itching, and postnasal drip. Often children with allergic rhinitis will also suffer redness, itching, and watering of the eyes, called *allergic conjunctivitis.*

Asthma results when inflammation occurs in the lungs, causing coughing, wheezing, and shortness of breath. Eczema is a skin allergy that causes itching, scaling, and rash. Food allergies in the intestines may cause diarrhea and vomiting, and allergies against foods, insect stings, and medications may lead to symptoms ranging from hives to wheezing, low blood pressure, even death. Compared with some of those possibilities, that runny nose is starting to look pretty good, right?

Children with one type of atopy often have other types. If your child has allergic rhinitis, for example, he's at increased risk for asthma as well. Allergies tend to be inherited; if both parents have allergies, there is a 60% to 70% chance their children will also have them. The specific type of atopy, however, is not inherited. Just because you are allergic to ragweed, peanuts, or penicillin doesn't mean your child will be. On the other hand, your history of eczema may put him at increased risk for allergic rhinitis or asthma. For reasons that remain elusive, the rates of allergic disease have skyrocketed over the last 3 decades.

What's wrong with calling allergic rhinitis hay fever? The "hay" part actually holds a kernel of truth. Pollen and leaf mold are common triggers for allergic rhinitis, and while hay pollen itself does not seem to cause a lot of allergy symptoms, other plants like ragweed that may bloom during hay season certainly do. The hay harvesting process kicks up plenty of dust, pollen, and mold, and baled hay provides a great environment for more mold to grow. Suffering allergies myself, I dread hayrides. Fever, on the other hand, is never part of allergic disease. Allergies may make your child miserable, but if he has a fever something else is causing it, most likely a cold or sinus infection.

Sometimes it's obvious what triggers a child's allergies; other times it's more subtle. If your child reliably has a runny nose every spring or fall (*seasonal* allergic rhinitis), there's probably a pollen or mold at fault. If he starts sneezing like crazy when he comes near dogs or cats, the cause should be pretty obvious. Other allergens may be harder to detect. Dust mites are a common allergy trigger, but they are invisible to the naked eye. They eat dead skin cells, including those found in feathers and hair. Cockroaches also cause plenty of allergic rhinitis, but unless you go around flicking lights on without warning you may not know you have them. Because these allergens are present year-round, children who are sensitive to them tend to have symptoms all year instead of just during certain seasons (*perennial* allergic rhinitis).

In most cases your child's doctor can diagnose allergic rhinitis without needing to do any tests. The first clue is sneezing, runny nose, or stuffy nose going on longer than the 7 to 10 days usually associated with a cold. Allergies also tend to cause much more itching than a cold or sinusitis. If your child seems to be constantly itching his nose or eyes, you've been given what pediatricians call the *allergic salute*. Feel free to salute back, but wash your hands afterward. When you can identify an obvious trigger for symptoms, the diagnosis is pretty much certain.

Other, more subtle signs emerge when the doctor does a physical examination. Allergic rhinitis typically lends the lining of the nose a pale, blueish, swollen appearance. Your child may also have a crease across the tip of his nose from frequently wiping along with a darkening of the skin under his eyes *(allergic shiners)*. Additionally, swelling of the skin under the eyes may create fine lines *(Dennie lines)*. Looking at the back of the throat, the doctor may see bumpy-looking tissue *(cobblestoning)* resulting from chronic inflammation. Untreated, severe allergies may even affect the growth of the child's face as a result of chronic mouth-breathing. Children with allergic facies have a receding chin, overbite, arched hard palate, and elongated face overall. Just think what effective allergy therapy might save you in orthodontic bills!

Parents often ask if their child needs allergy testing. In most cases the answer is no. A good history and physical examination should nail down the diagnosis of allergic rhinitis almost every time. The exceptions come when a child seems resistant to the usual medications we use for allergies, when he has asthma that is particularly severe or unresponsive to medications, or when you'd give away the dog to make the allergies better. Doctors may also test for allergies when a child has unexplained hives or develops a severe reaction to foods.

Scratch-testing remains the gold standard of allergy diagnosis. Scratch-testing is not, as I used to think, looking to see if your child is clawing at himself. Instead, an allergist scrapes or pricks the skin with purified allergens and looks to see if the child's skin responds with raised hives, a telltale sign of allergic disease. In some cases doctors prefer to do blood-testing for allergies, but these tests are not always as reliable as skin-testing because they don't provide a direct measure of how the body actually responds to certain allergens.

Once you know your child has allergic rhinitis, what are you going to do about it? The first line of defense is to remove the allergen from the environment if you can, although that depends a lot on what the allergen is. For cockroaches, for example, you can clean up the house and call an exterminator. If the family pet is the problem you may face a wrenching decision, unless you never liked Fido in the first place. Note too that any kind of dog may cause allergies, regardless of what the breeder told you.

Not only pet hair but shed skin cells and saliva are all potential allergens, and they are everywhere the animal goes. A dehumidifier may cut levels of mold and dust mites, which rely on moisture in the air to live. Keeping kids indoors with central air conditioning cuts their exposure to pollen and leaf mold, but it's also kind of sad. While down comforters and pillows do provide unlimited food for dust mites, there is little evidence that mite-proof pillow cases or mattress covers actually decrease symptoms in allergy sufferers. Air filters work pretty well to remove some airborne allergens, but dust mites tend to collect on the floor, not in the air, and the filters seem to have no effect whatsoever on cats, except to give them yet another place to nap.

If environmental control measures fail, it may be time to try allergy medication. There are 3 basic classes of medication that help with the symptoms of allergic rhinitis: *antihistamines, inhaled corticosteroids,* and *leukotriene receptor antagonists.* A child can use 2 or even all 3 classes at the same time because each interferes with a different part of the immune system to block allergic reactions.

Antihistamines have been around the longest, and most of them are available without a prescription. Older antihistamines like diphenhydramine (eg, Benadryl) cross from the bloodstream into the brain and may make children sleepy or irritable. Newer drugs like loratadine (eg, Claritin) and cetirizine (eg, Zyrtec) are not supposed to do this. Most antihistamines are safe to use in children as young as 6 months. They are especially good for controlling the itching parts of allergic diseases, to the extent that a child shouldn't take them for a week prior to getting scratch-tested for allergies. They are reasonably good at controlling nose symptoms, but only if you remember to give them. Because allergic rhinitis is a chronic disease, you have to use medicines like antihistamines every day to get good symptom control. *Hint:* If you keep running out of tissues, you may need to give the antihistamine more regularly.

Or it may be that the antihistamine simply isn't cutting it. The single most effective class of medications for allergic rhinitis is the inhaled corticosteroids. These are steroids like fluticasone (eg, Flonase), mometasone (eg, Nasonex), budesonide (eg, Rhinocort), and others that decrease inflammation in the nose. When people hear "steroids" they get worried about the side effects associated with steroids people might take by mouth—poor growth, immune suppression, diabetes, and high blood pressure. Nasal steroids, however, have no such side effects because their absorption into the bloodstream is barely detectable. Some children object to the flavor of these medications, which they might taste as the spray runs down the back of the throat. Steroid nose sprays may also cause nosebleeds in some patients. Other drawbacks are that you must have a doctor's prescription to use them, and none of these drugs are FDA approved for children younger than 2. That said, for children who can use them, this class of medications has the best chance of keeping them breathing through their noses and cutting your Kleenex bill in half.

when to call the doctor

Leukotriene receptor antagonists used for allergic rhinitis include montelukast (eg, Singulair) and zafirlukast (eg, Accolate). These drugs are not terribly powerful on their own, but they have some role as add-on therapy, especially for patients who also suffer asthma. Reports have raised some concerns about mood and thinking disorders associated with these drugs, so if your child is taking them and he starts to act out of character, let his doctor know. It may be he's just crazy like his old man, but the medicine could still be making it worse.

When none of these drugs are cutting it, there is one more option that seems drastic but works quite well. Because of how the immune system regulates itself, repeated exposure to an antigen *(immunotherapy)* has the potential to turn down the allergic response, sometimes eliminating it altogether. Traditionally doctors have used injections (allergy shots) given over a period of months to years to achieve this effect, but newer studies are looking at allergens that might be given under the tongue instead. This sort of therapy should be managed by an allergy specialist, but in the right hands it can have a dramatic effect. You may still find it simpler to give away Fido, but then again, one day that old mutt might just save your life....

Even for pediatricians it can be hard to determine whether a child just got 2 colds back-to-back, caught a cold that progressed to a sinus infection, or has had allergies all along. Hopefully, after reading this chapter you'll be alert to some clues that can help with the case. In the meantime, think about bringing sanitary wipes with you to the grocery store. My kid might have been the last one to touch that cart.

18

how much does it cough? when breathing doesn't come easy

of all the symptoms of childhood illness, cough is most likely to make you crazy. You can control a fever, wipe a nose, clean up vomit, and wait for a rash to go away, but the cough is just…there. And there again. And…wait for it…there! Coughing not only keeps you and your child awake all night, but it makes you worry she may stop breathing. It's a symptom you want to fix before you hear it again…there.

This may explain why so many cough medicines throughout history contained sedatives like alcohol and opiates. If the medicine didn't help the child, maybe it could at least do a little something for dad! Narcotic cough medicines remain popular to this day, but they have a small downside—every now and then they're fatal, especially for young children. There are many ways to address the curse of cough, but stopping the child's breathing altogether is probably a bit extreme. Let's take a look at some less dangerous alternatives.

236

18. How Much Does It Cough? When Breathing Doesn't Come Easy

cough benefits analysis

When your child is coughing nonstop it's easy to view the cough as an enemy that must be defeated. This approach is not only wrong, it's actually backward. Cough is a hardwired reflex, present in pretty much every animal with lungs, and its purpose is to protect those vital organs. Whether the danger comes from something as large as a Barbie shoe or as small as a virus, the cough reflex is designed to get it out. In response to irritation in the lining of the lungs, your child is programmed to take a deep breath; build up pressure inside the chest cavity by tensing the muscles of the abdomen, diaphragm, and chest wall; and release all that pressure at once by suddenly opening up the throat and letting it rip. The resulting burst of air explodes from the lungs as fast as 100 miles per hour. Cough is a deep-seated and unconscious reflex that may come under some voluntary control, but it usually occurs without thought.

The sound of a cough carries some information, but what you learn from hearing it is limited. The easiest element to hear is fluid or mucous in the large airways. People say this kind of cough sounds *productive* or *wet.* Some parents worry that if their child swallows mucous it will make her sick, but swallowing is actually part of our body's defense system—acid in the stomach kills whatever organisms the lungs are trying to expel. We're not usually aware of it, but mucous from the lungs travels up into our throats and down into our stomachs all day long. (Don't think too hard about that.) A wet cough might result from mucous dripping down the back of the throat due to a cold or sinus infection, or it may suggest an infection of the lungs themselves resulting in increased mucous production. It could also mean your child has aspirated some food or beverage into her airway.

A *dry* cough is missing this bubbly sound and suggests some irritation in the airway. Dry coughs are common with colds, asthma, croup, and inhaled foreign bodies. The vocal cords may also contribute to the sound of a cough. A hoarse sound suggests the vocal cords are inflamed, usually because of a viral infection like croup, but chronic gastroesophageal reflux or a small foreign body might also cause this sound. Just coughing repeatedly can inflame the vocal cords as well.

A wheezing sound usually results from inflammation and narrowing in the smallest tubes of the lungs, the bronchioles. Wheezing may result from a viral infection of the lungs like respiratory syncytial virus (RSV) or it may be due to asthma. Whatever the cause, it's never normal.

Don't think your child needs to cough for her doctor any more than she needs to show the doctor her snot or to have a fever at the moment she shows up to the clinic. If you say she was up all night with a wet-sounding cough, I promise her doctor will believe you! On the other hand, don't assume your baby is faking a cough, or doing it to get attention. Young children just don't think that way. If your child is coughing, it's real.

breathalyzer: when a cough is serious

While even a really annoying cough may be a normal part of a cold, there are some signs that should alarm you if you see or hear them. The first one we just touched on—wheezing. Many parents are confused about what a wheeze really is, probably because wheezing is much easier to hear with a stethoscope than with the naked ear (and even harder if your ear wears clothes). When your child has a cold you're likely to hear a coarse, bubbling

when to call the doctor

Wheezing is never normal. It may result from a viral infection or it may be a sign of an asthma attack, but it always deserves a trip to the doctor. Illnesses that cause wheeze are among the deadlier diseases of childhood.

sound coming from her chest as a result of increased secretions in her airway. Doctors call that sound *rhonchi,* and we consider it a normal part of a cold. In contrast, wheezing results from the collected whistling of air moving at high speed through thousands of narrowed tubes deep in the lungs. It's a high-pitched sound and it only occurs when your child is breathing out, not when she's inhaling.

Stridor is another sound that should get your attention. Stridor is the coarse, raspy noise that results when inflammation and swelling of the vocal cords cause them to rub together. Usually if your child has stridor, she also has a hoarse-sounding voice and a barking cough, like a seal. A viral infection called *croup* is the most common cause of stridor; we'll discuss croup more later in this chapter. Stridor may also result from an inhaled foreign body stuck in the airway or nerve damage paralyzing a

238

18. How Much Does It Cough? When Breathing Doesn't Come Easy

vocal cord. You might hear this sound when your child breathes in and exhales. Especially if she has stridor when she inhales, she needs to see a doctor as soon as possible! If she seems short of breath with stridor, you may need to call emergency medical services (EMS) (911).

Grunting is another sound that should have you and your child on your way to the doctor. Infants make this sound when they're having major breathing trouble or are severely ill. To open up the lungs, they hold their breath for a second each time they breathe in, then they let it out with a little "huh." If your baby makes that sound before each exhalation, get her medical care now, by EMS in most cases.

Sometimes when you're worried about your child's breathing, your eyes tell you more than your ears. Pull your child's shirt up and look at her chest. Can you see the skin pulling between her ribs, under her rib cage, or at the base of her throat? Is she tensing her abdominal muscles with each breath to help her get air out? These signs are called *retractions* and *accessory muscle use.* They indicate that your child is working too hard to breathe. If you have an infant you might also see her nostrils flaring with each breath. With any of these signs, call for immediate medical evaluation. In other words, don't spend too long deciding what to pack for your hospital stay. They'll give you a toothbrush when you get there.

Skin color is yet another visual clue that may have you dialing EMS (911). Your child's hands and feet may look a little blue or purple in color when she's developing a fever, but her lips and face should never be blue, unless she just ate one of those blue popsicles from the ice cream truck. Blue lips mean low oxygen, and because oxygen is so useful for, say, remaining alive, you'll want to act quickly to fix the situation.

Another visual clue your child has a serious cough requires a watch. Count her breaths over a period of 60 seconds. Any infant breathing more than 60 times a minute needs to see a doctor quickly. A toddler or preschooler breathing more than 40 times a minute may also be having serious breathing trouble and deserves an immediate examination.

If your child is old enough to talk, listen to how many words she can say in a row without stopping to catch her breath. If she is resorting to short sentences to save air, you know she's in trouble. Likewise, if she seems short of breath with household activities like going up the stairs, you're going to want her to come right back downstairs, get in the car, and go get medical care.

when to call the doctor

Other reasons to seek immediate attention for a cough include chest pain, coughing up blood, and any condition that weakens the immune system, such as sickle cell disease, chronic steroid therapy, or organ transplant.

There are a few other signs that your child's cough might need more than a home remedy. Many illnesses that cause cough also cause a fever, but the fever should not last more than 3 days, and it shouldn't go away for 24 hours and then return. Fever in infants younger than 3 months always deserves immediate medical attention, but you were probably already calling the doctor anyway because of the cough. A cough with a cold may last as long as 3 weeks, but if it hasn't gone away by then it may be something more serious.

when to call the doctor

Infants younger than 3 months have very small airways and are at high risk for breathing trouble. Babies this young should see a doctor whenever they start to cough.

cough links: some common causes of cough

By far the most common cause of childhood cough is viral cold, which doctors call an upper respiratory infection (URI). Colds (see Chapter 17) cause coughing in a couple of ways. First, mucous from the nose and sinuses drips down into the lungs, where it has to be coughed back up. Second, many cold viruses actually infect the linings of the airway. It may take the lungs up to 3 weeks to clear these infections, which is why cough is the last cold symptom to go away.

You have several options for treating the cough associated with a URI. A cool mist humidifier may loosen secretions and help keep the upper airway moist. Honey is a more effective cough suppressant than over-the-counter cough medicines—and it tastes better, too! As long as your child is older than 1 year, you can give her ½ to 1 teaspoon of honey as often as she seems to need it. Babies younger than 12 months should use corn syrup

240

18. How Much Does It Cough? When Breathing Doesn't Come Easy

(eg, Karo) instead because traces of botulism in honey may prove deadly at that age. Children older than 6 years benefit from cough drops or hard candies as well; younger children risk choking on these candies, especially when they take a deep breath to cough! Feel free to try a cough drop or two yourself, just to make sure they're OK. Warm fluids like tea, apple cider, or chicken soup also help soothe the airway and help your child feel better.

You might notice I haven't mentioned any medicines for cough. That's because there are no cough medicines proven to work for children. The one most commonly sold over the counter is dextromethorphan, the active ingredient in hundreds of "cough suppressants" on drugstore shelves. In 2008 the Food and Drug Administration declared it was not approved for children younger than 4 years and not advised for children younger than 6, although there's no reason to think it works any better for older children. The other widely sold cough medicine is guaifenesin (eg, Mucinex), labeled "expectorant" on most bottles. Guaifenesin is supposed to loosen mucous and make it easier to cough out, although definitive studies are lacking. Guaifenesin at least seems harmless. Narcotic cough medicines like hydrocodone and codeine, on the other hand, are not safe or effective for children. I scratch my head whenever I see a remedy that contains guaifenesin and dextromethorphan. What is the child supposed to do, cough more or cough less? Do the 2 medicines just get in there and slug it out?

Bronchiolitis is a special kind of viral infection. It causes cold symptoms like every other URI, but the virus also infects the smallest airways in the lungs, the bronchioles. Older children and adults tolerate bronchiolitis without any trouble, but in younger infants it cause life-threatening wheezing. The best-known cause of bronchiolitis is RSV, but plenty of other viruses can cause the same symptoms. For a full discussion of bronchiolitis, check out Chapter 9.

People often confuse bronchiolitis and bronchitis, but despite the spellings they are actually very different illnesses. *Bronchitis* refers to inflammation of the bronchi, the larger airways in the lungs. In children this inflammation almost always results from a virus, whereas in adults, bacteria are sometimes the cause. Unless a child has an artificial breathing tube (tracheostomy) or a disease like cystic fibrosis that affects the immune function of the lungs, she just isn't going to get the sort of bronchitis that responds to antibiotics. Adults, on the other hand, especially smokers, may suffer bacterial bronchitis that responds to antibiotic therapy. One day I hope to start a nonprofit, the Bronchitis Is Not a Disease of Children Foundation (BINADOCF), unless that one is already taken. Hopefully together we can stamp out antibiotic use for routine childhood cough. In the meantime, if a doctor tells you he's going to give your child an antibiotic for a cough, feel free to ask him why, and if his answer is "Bronchitis," you might ask a few more questions.

Pneumonia, on the other hand, is a disease of children, and a relatively common one. In pneumonia the infection invades the air sacs of the lungs *(alveoli)*. Pneumonia usually results from infection with viruses or bacteria. Children older than 5 also get pneumonia from a bacteria-like organism called *Mycoplasma pneumoniae*. Because these *Mycoplasma* infections rarely require hospitalization, they're nicknamed *walking pneumonia*. (I was relieved to learn it's the victim, and not the disease, that walks.) Rarer causes of pneumonia include tuberculosis and even some fungi. In the days before antibiotics, pneumonia was a frequent cause of childhood death. Now it's rarely dangerous when treated appropriately, but anything that infects air sacs still deserves a little respect.

There are several clues that can let you know your child might have pneumonia. One is fever. If your child has a cough and her fever lasts more than 3 days, she may have a bacterial infection such as pneumonia, sinusitis, or acute otitis media. Coughing may produce pain in the chest wall from muscle strain, but chest pain is always a worrisome symptom. Your child may be old enough to complain of discomfort, or she may just hold her side or brace herself when she coughs or breathes. Either way a doctor should check her out. Shortness of breath is always concerning and never normal. Pneumonia may even cause symptoms outside the chest, like fatigue, stomachache, and poor appetite. A cough that starts with a cold but fails to improve within 3 weeks may also suggest pneumonia.

when to call the doctor
Fever from colds usually stays below 102°F; any temperature above 104°F that lasts more than a couple of hours should prompt you to call your child's doctor.

242

18. How Much Does It Cough? When Breathing Doesn't Come Easy

Doctors often diagnose pneumonia based on history and physical examination alone. Pneumonia creates a handful of unique sounds doctors can hear while listening to the child breathe, even if she's crying at the time (the child, not the doctor). In cases in which the diagnosis is unclear or the child seems especially sick, a chest radiograph can help determine treatment, but your child doesn't necessarily need an x-ray just to confirm she has pneumonia. In fact, doctors sometimes hear pneumonia before it gets bad enough to show up on x-ray film. Likewise, if your child's symptoms improve, she should not need an x-ray just to prove she got better. Blood-testing may be helpful in the most severe cases, usually those requiring hospitalization. For less ill children, the only point of a blood test may be to look for evidence of infection with *M pneumoniae*.

Doctors treat pneumonia based on what they think is causing it. Influenza is the only virus for which we have any effective therapy; if your child has a viral pneumonia she may take medicine for influenza, or she may take nothing at all. Children younger than 5 years with bacterial pneumonia often respond to good old amoxicillin, as long as the dose is high enough. Children aged 5 years or older may also get a type of pneumonia caused by *Mycoplasma*. It's difficult to tell by history or physical examination when *Mycoplasma* is the problem, but for children in this age range, doctors

what you can do

You might read all this stuff and think, "Pneumonia sounds bad. I hope my child doesn't get it!" While you can't protect your child from all types of pneumonia, you do have the power to keep her from getting 2 of the worst kinds—influenza and pneumococcal pneumonia. Children vaccinated against pneumococcus enjoy protection from severe infections and hospitalization (see Chapter 7 for more information). Likewise, most deaths from influenza result from pneumonia, and an annual influenza vaccine provides strong protection against this complication. If you're one of those dads who envisions protecting your child from harm, getting her these vaccines is one of the easiest ways to do it. It's up to you whether you choose to wear tights and a cape at the time.

will often add azithromycin (eg, Zithromax), erythromycin, or clarithromycin (eg, Biaxin) to try and treat it. In more severe cases of pneumonia, children may require hospitalization for intravenous antibiotics, oxygen, and careful monitoring.

Croup is one of the most frightening causes of cough in young children, usually striking between the ages of 3 months and 3 years. Croup occurs when a virus (most often parainfluenza) infects the vocal cords and causes them to swell. Because vocal cords serve as the double door to the lungs, you can imagine what happens if they get too inflamed. Right—it's a bad thing. Croup begins with a hoarse voice and distinctive barking cough. How distinctive? Let's just say when seals are teaching their babies to talk, they tell them to make a sound like a human child with croup.

As the vocal cords continue to swell, a child with croup will begin to have stridor as we discussed previously. At first you might only hear stridor when the child is crying or shouting, but if you start hearing it when she's at rest, you know she's getting behind the 8-ball. You'll want to be extra vigilant in the early morning hours, when croup always seems to get worse. There are a couple of things you can try to help her feel better. If it's cool outside, taking her into the air may help. Alternately, you can steam up the bathroom and bring her into the humidity.

when to call the doctor

Whatever you try to treat croup, only give it about 15 or 20 minutes; if your child still has stridor, get her medical care immediately. If she is struggling to breathe, looking blue when she coughs, unable to speak, or excessively sleepy, call emergency medical services (911).

Two medicines form the cornerstone of therapy for croup. Doctors can treat children with an inhaled mist form of the medicine epinephrine, which helps open the airway. Epinephrine, however, wears off after a couple of hours. Corticosteroids like dexamethasone often cure the symptoms in about 6 to 8 hours. Depending on how sick your child is, the doctor may want her to stay in the office, emergency department, or hospital until she's clearly better.

Whooping cough (pertussis) is a special kind of infection that seems to be making a resurgence, especially among children who are not vaccinated

244

18. How Much Does It Cough? When Breathing Doesn't Come Easy

against its cause, a bacteria called *Bordetella pertussis.* This disease causes severe, prolonged coughing spells that may cause the victim's skin to turn blue from lack of oxygen. Affected children may make a classic whooping noise as they try desperately to inhale between coughing spells. Symptoms often last for months, and many children with pertussis also contract pneumonia. Antibiotic treatment may help some kids with pertussis if it's caught early, but by the time many children are diagnosed it's too late for medicine to do much good. Immunization provides excellent protection from the disease, but many adults' childhood pertussis immunizations have worn off. If you're expecting a child or if you have a baby in the house, make sure all the adults who regularly care for that child have gotten updated vaccines against pertussis to protect your baby.

cough control measures: mastering asthma

Asthma should be at the top of your mind when your child's cough just seems to have gone on too long. While asthma is famous for causing wheezing and shortness of breath, a surprising number of children with asthma just cough. They might be wheezing too, but remember, wheezing is hard to hear without a stethoscope, so you could have missed it. Children with chronic asthma might not even realize they're short of breath! After all, if you never can get a good breath, you just assume what you're feeling is normal. Look for a cough that lasts more than 3 weeks, that gets worse at night, and that occurs whenever your child exercises or gets excited. If your child is having these symptoms, there's a good chance she's among the 6.2 million American children with asthma.

Most people know asthma affects the lungs, but beyond that the picture often gets sketchy. Asthma is one form of allergic disease, related to eczema and allergic rhinitis (see chapters 6 and 17). Asthmatics' immune systems respond to perceived threats by inflaming the airways of the lungs. Muscles around the bronchioles contract, narrowing these tiny airways in a process called *bronchospasm.* Mucous-producing cells in the airways also work harder, blocking the breathing tubes with excess secretions. With repeated bronchospasm the muscles around the bronchioles grow bigger, just like any muscle that gets enough exercise, and the tubes become chronically narrowed. When a patient with asthma inhales, the bronchioles open up just a little, and when she exhales they close even more, trapping air in her lungs. Some children with asthma have symptoms all the time, while others only seem to cough or wheeze in response to a trigger like a cold or cigarette smoke.

As a dad you might worry that if your child has asthma, she'll never be a great athlete. The best reason to diagnose and treat asthma early is that with effective therapy, almost every asthmatic child can breathe normally and participate fully in the activity of her choosing. Professional sports and Olympic teams are so loaded with competitors with a history of asthma that it doesn't even warrant a mention during the pregame commentary, unless of course the commentators just run out of stuff to talk about, but when does that ever happen?

Diagnosing asthma is sometimes easy but not always. Much of the diagnosis depends on your report of how often your child is coughing and at what times.

what you can do

If you've scheduled your child a doctor's visit for asthma, try keeping track of how many nights in the prior couple of weeks you hear her cough, how often she coughs with exercise, and what other triggers seem to make her worse. Does she reliably start hacking when she goes outside, pets the dog, or walks past someone smoking? If you can answer questions like those, her doctor is likely to think you're a genius. While you're earning your genius badge, ask around the family and find out which close relatives have asthma, allergies, or eczema. If you, her mom, or her siblings suffer allergic diseases like these, it's more likely your child has asthma.

The physical examination is also critical for diagnosis. Your child's doctor will look at her nose and eyes for signs of allergies, and of course he'll listen carefully to her lungs. When children are old enough to cooperate, usually around age 5 or 6, doctors can test their breathing to look for signs of asthma. The best test uses a computerized device called a spirometer that measures airflow at every part of the child's breath. Not all doctors' offices are equipped with these devices, which can be expensive and tricky to maintain and use. A fast-and-dirty test, somewhat less accurate, uses a handheld *peak flow meter*. The peak flow meter is a plastic device with a little arrow on it that measures the fastest speed the child can exhale.

246

18. How Much Does It Cough? When Breathing Doesn't Come Easy

Because asthma traps air in the lungs, children with asthma have trouble expelling air as fast as children without the disease. Your doctor may even prescribe a peak flow meter your child can use at home to monitor her symptoms.

Children with asthma don't necessarily need allergy testing, but testing can help guide therapy. If you discover, for example, that your child is allergic to the cat, you might finally have an excuse to give the creature away to a good home (the cat, not the child). When dust mites are the problem you might install hardwood floors, replace a down comforter with a synthetic one, or invest in a dehumidifier. For a child with harder-to-treat asthma, an allergist may be able to use regular injections *(immunotherapy)* to help her immune system react less violently to certain triggers.

One trigger you should control whenever it's an issue is cigarette smoke exposure. Mothers who smoke during pregnancy are more likely to have children with asthma, and it doesn't get better from there. Children who grow up exposed to cigarette smoke are more likely to develop asthma, and children who have asthma are more likely to suffer asthma attacks if they are around smoke. Unfortunately for the smoker, just keeping the smoke in one room or smoking with the door open is not good enough. Cigarettes need to stay outside the child's house and car the entire time they're lit, period. You can accomplish this by asking the smoker to go outside to indulge or by immediately throwing any lit cigarettes out the window. Because clothing can carry cigarette smoke, smokers should ideally have a special smoking jacket that doesn't come into the house. Sometimes having a child in the home is just the incentive a smoker needs to finally quit for good.

Asthma medications confuse more people than medicines for any other condition. The problem is that while a lot of them look alike, what they do is fundamentally different. Asthma is a chronic condition—it's always there, and many children with asthma need to take one or more medications every day to keep the chronic inflammation at bay. When asthma symptoms suddenly flare up, other medicines help relieve those symptoms in the short run. These rescue medicines don't do a thing to fix the underlying problem, inflammation of the airways. They just help the symptoms of wheezing and coughing for a little while. Using rescue medicines without controller medicines is like bailing out a leaking boat—things seem better temporarily, but you haven't fixed the problem.

Let's start with the rescue medicines. There are 2, albuterol (eg, ProAir, Ventolin) and the nearly identical levalbuterol (eg, Xopenex). Pharmacists call these medications *bronchodilators* because they open up the airways, or *short-acting beta-agonists* because they target beta adrenaline receptors in the lungs. Levalbuterol lasts a little longer, but the differences between them are generally negligible. Children use these medicines when they start to cough or wheeze, and some kids need a dose before they exercise.

There are 2 ways to get these medicines into the child's lungs, where they open up the airways for a period of 4 to 8 hours. Infants and young children often use *nebulizers,* machines that create a fine, breathable mist from liquid medicine. Children breathe the mist through a mask or plastic mouthpiece over about 5 minutes. Toddlers and older children can use a metered dose inhaler (MDI), the classic L-shaped pump you might have seen. While children can inhale directly from the MDI, they get much better drug delivery when the inhaler is attached to a wide plastic tube called a spacer that holds the medicine and gives it a little room to spread out. By attaching a mask to the other end of the spacer, parents can give MDI medicines even to very young children. The MDI/spacer combination works just as well as the nebulizer for most children.

If your child has an asthma attack that doesn't respond quickly and completely to rescue medicines, she will probably also need to take a corticosteroid like prednisolone (eg, Orapred, Prelone) or prednisone. These medications calm down the immune system hyper-response that drives asthma. In most cases, corticosteroids are the only medicines that have the power to reverse a serious asthma attack. Corticosteroids do carry side effects, some of them a bit unpleasant. Children taking them may become hyperactive, irritable, or unusually hungry. They may have temporary weight gain and increased blood sugar levels as well. All these symptoms go away shortly after the child stops taking the medicine. Most children with asthma only need to take steroids for about 5 days, too short a period to worry about other side effects like slowed growth and a weakened immune system, but children who have to take steroids for weeks or months may face these issues. If your child has taken steroids for more than a week, she will need to taper off them slowly rather than stop all at once.

Children with very mild asthma may need nothing more than a rescue medicine now and again when they catch colds, but many children with asthma benefit from using daily controller medications. If your child is

248

18. How Much Does It Cough? When Breathing Doesn't Come Easy

using her rescue inhaler more than twice a month or waking up from coughing more than twice a week, she probably needs one of these medicines. Asthma controllers have revolutionized asthma care in the last generation, turning it from a disease that limited many children's activity to one that most sufferers barely notice. I had asthma as a child, and if we'd had these medicines back then I might have been a major league baseball player, if only I'd also been taller and better at throwing, catching, and hitting balls.

Two things get in the way of parents using controller medications properly. First, except for color, they often look the same as rescue medicines, leading to lots of confusion. Second, you have to give your child these medicines every single day, *even when she's not having symptoms*. It's easy to remember to give a medicine to a child who's coughing, wheezing, and struggling for breath. It's much harder to remember to medicate a child who looks fine. After all, if she's breathing so great, why does she need the medicine? *Because the medicine is the reason she's breathing great!* No medicine, no breathing great, but it's very hard to remember day in and day out. I encourage parents to keep controller medicines next to the child's toothbrush to remember to do both twice every day. Of course, if they're not brushing the kid's teeth twice a day….

The most potent of asthma control medicines are *inhaled corticosteroids.* Examples include budesonide (eg, Pulmicort), fluticasone (eg, Flovent), beclomethasone (eg, Beclovent), and triamcinolone (eg, Azmacort). Most are available as MDIs, just like albuterol. Budesonide can also go in a nebulizer, and many come in dry-powder delivery devices shaped like silos or flying saucers. Unlike corticosteroids children take by mouth, these medicines have minimal side effects because they stay mostly in the lungs, entering the bloodstream only in minute quantities.

In cases in which high-dose inhaled corticosteroids alone are not helping, there are a few other classes of medicine to add. Children may use *leukotriene receptor antagonists* like montelukast (eg, Singulair) and zafirlukast (eg, Accolate), given by mouth in chewable pill, non-chewable pill, or granule form. Some inhalers combine corticosteroids with longer-acting bronchodilators (eg, Advair, Symbicort). Medicines like cromolyn and nedocromil help control allergic reactions when inhaled, although they are not as powerful as steroids for this purpose. In rare cases, doctors may still prescribe a relative of caffeine called theophylline.

Because pretty much everyone finds asthma control confusing, your child's doctor should give you a written asthma action plan listing every medicine your child has and when she should take it. The plan also guides you through handling an asthma flare, including when to call the doctor's office and when to seek emergency care. If your child is on asthma medicines, go ahead and bring them with you to all her doctor's appointments so you're not stuck trying to remember what color MDI you're using when. If your child attends school or child care, a copy of the action plan should also be kept on site.

Hopefully this chapter has given you plenty to think about next time your child won't stop coughing. Remember, that cough is probably helping her lungs clear out some gunk that really shouldn't be there. Get her some warm fluid and honey or corn syrup, and turn on her cool mist humidifier. If she's not better, reread this chapter for ideas, by which time you'll probably be asleep or in the emergency department. I hope for your sake and your child's that you're drooling on this page.

19

i don't feel so good: vomiting, diarrhea, and bellyaches

you may feel like you're already a man, what with the whole becoming-a-father thing and all. Perhaps you thought you transitioned to adulthood when you graduated school or got your first job or married. But among the tribe of fathers there is a special coming-of-age ritual into which you may not have been initiated—you are not really a man until you've cleaned up your child's vomit and/or diarrhea. The strongest warriors among us have cleaned these things off of ourselves. It's up to you whether you choose to observe a period of fasting as part of this ritual, but many men do, at least for 10 or 15 minutes afterward.

Vomiting, diarrhea, and tummy pain are universal experiences of childhood. Arising separately or together, they can challenge parents and pediatricians too. To this day I feel a little spasm of anxiety when I first face a patient with these problems. Then I take a breath and remind myself that while there are tons of possibilities, some of them quite frightening, there are ways to tell them apart, and most of them get better on their own. So let's work our way through tummy trouble—that is, if you're man enough.

quit your bellyaching. please?

The belly (we doctors prefer the word tummy or, alternately, abdomen) is full of stuff, and all of it might hurt. In addition to the stomach, small intestines, and large intestines, there's the liver, gallbladder, spleen, pancreas, kidneys, urinary bladder, and in girls, 2 ovaries and a uterus. Sometimes the source of abdominal pain isn't even in the belly! Abdominal pain may come from the lungs (pneumonia), esophagus (gastroesophageal reflux disease [GERD]), throat (strep pharyngitis), bloodstream (lead poisoning, sickle cell disease), scrotum (incarcerated inguinal hernia), or brain (migraines, anxiety).

Several features of abdominal pain can make it difficult to guess the cause, even for experienced doctors. Part of the problem has to do with how nerves carry signals from the body's organs to the brain. The nerves of our skin and muscles are like ace reporters, bringing us very precise information about what's going on and where. The nerves that supply our insides, on the other hand, tend to carry vague and misleading messages…more like politicians. When an internal organ like the appendix becomes inflamed, the pain often involves the whole abdomen, localizing only when that inflammation involves more sensitive surrounding tissues. Nerve signals may even tell us that pain from the lungs or testicles arises in the abdomen. No one knows, for example, why strep throat infections often cause tummy aches.

It would take a whole book (and has) to run through all the various causes of abdominal pain and how to tell them apart, so instead let's focus on the questions every parent wants answered: What are the most common causes of tummy ache? How do I know when it's something bad? Will I ever get to use the bathroom in peace again? OK, that last one is more of a general question, but admit it, you want to know!

In Chapter 5 we discussed colic, crying in infants that seems to come from abdominal pain but remains a medical mystery. In Chapter 11 we reviewed vomiting in infants. The good news is that as your child grows, he is able to tell you more about what's bothering him, which can help you with decision-making. Of course, even when your child can talk, it may not be obvious what's going on. It takes a while, for example, for children to learn that hunger might cause abdominal discomfort. Hunger pangs usually strike in the upper part of the abdomen. Fortunately for you, there's a simple home test to determine if your child is suffering hunger pangs—feed him. If the pain goes away, that's probably what it was. On the other hand, irritation of the lining of the stomach (*gastritis*) also sometimes gets better with eating, so if symptoms persist or worsen over days to weeks, you'll still want to have a doctor check your child out. Just as eating too little can cause tummy pain, overeating may also cause discomfort. This pain, too, should resolve quickly on its own, so long as your child stops eating.

While most of what kids call a stomachache arises in other organs, the stomach itself certainly can hurt. Sometimes the pain comes from acid or medications like ibuprofen irritating the lining of the stomach, a condition called gastritis. These cases often respond to antacid medicines like ranitidine (eg, Zantac) or omeprazole (eg, Prilosec), both available over the counter.

Peptic ulcer disease is related to gastritis but is more severe. Whereas gastritis irritates the lining of the stomach, an ulcer is an actual hole forming in the stomach or the very first part of the small intestine, the duodenum. Pain from ulcer disease tends to be more severe and persistent, and it may worsen after a child eats. Antacids often provide some pain relief, but they may not cure the condition. Much of adult ulcer disease stems from infection with a bacteria called *Helicobacter pylori*. This infection can strike children as well, but it doesn't explain their ulcers as often as it does in adults. The only reliable way to tell the difference between gastritis and ulcer disease in children is for a specialist to visualize the stomach and intestines with a fiberoptic endoscope (esophagogastroduodenoscopy, or EGD). Therapies differ based on what the specialist finds, but they usually involve strong antacids, with or without antibiotics to kill *Helicobacter*.

Stomachache is sometimes really esophagus-ache, but that's a lot harder to pronounce. Just as excess stomach acid can irritate the lining of the stomach, acid may also wash up into the esophagus and cause pain, a condition called GERD. A child may feel the pain of GERD in the upper abdomen, or he may complain of chest discomfort. Pain often worsens after meals, especially meals that are large or high in fat. Lying down may worsen GERD pain, and taking antacids or drinking milk may help it. Children with GERD often need to use antacids like ranitidine or omeprazole daily for a couple of months to heal the esophagus. In the meantime, encourage smaller, lower fat meals and give your child plenty of time between eating and going to bed.

Mild to moderate abdominal pain that comes with vomiting, diarrhea, and fever often signals that your child has a viral infection that should pass on its own. We'll talk more about vomiting and diarrhea later in this chapter, but the pain with a viral tummy bug should not be terribly severe. Children may complain of discomfort all over the tummy, in the upper part of the abdomen, or at the belly button (umbilicus). If your child is old enough to use such terms, he may describe the pain as "cramping." The more localized the pain, the less likely a viral infection is the cause. Usually abdominal pain from a tummy bug worsens just before the child vomits or has diarrhea and then gets better in between these episodes. If your child starts complaining of vague stomach pain, it's always wise to look around and make sure he has a clear path to a toilet and a bucket nearby.

If diarrhea is a common cause of childhood abdominal pain, so is its opposite, *constipation*. Constipation may cause discomfort anywhere in the abdomen, but the pain often settles in the lower parts. The pain from constipation comes and goes as periodic waves of intestinal contractions *(peristalsis)* encounter the immobile mass of stool in the rectum. While constipation is rare during infancy, it becomes quite common during the preschool and elementary school years. Any stress, from potty training to travel to starting a new school, can back up the works. Dairy products and dehydration tend to worsen constipation; fiber from fruits, vegetables, and whole grains prevent it. In other words, if your child eats 2 cups of yogurt for every apple slice that passes his lips, he's doomed.

Kids don't keep track of when and how they poop, and parents are often surprised to learn that constipation is causing a child's abdominal pain. But really, once he's out of diapers, do you really know the last time your child went, whether it was soft, and if it hurt? If so, you might consider taking up a hobby. That said, if your child is complaining of cramping pain in the lower abdomen that gets worse after he eats, it may be time to start paying attention.

Normal children may have a bowel movement a few times a day or may go every few days. More important than frequency is what sort of stool they pass. A child who potties 5 times a day but passes a few hard pebbles each time is probably getting backed up. A child who has a large but soft bowel movement every few days may not be constipated. Any stool that is large enough to cause pain, bleeding, or plumbing problems probably counts as constipation.

Treating constipation often requires patience and persistence. Mild cases may improve with a cup of apple or pear juice or with a day or two of increased water and fruit intake. Moderate constipation may require a dose of a laxative or an enema to get the first large, painful stool out of the way, followed by a change in diet. Some cases, however, build up slowly over a period of months. With time, retained stool stretches out the rectum, making the nerves less sensitive to the presence of stool and the muscles too weak to push stool out when the time comes. Children with constipation this bad may even leak stool without knowing it *(encopresis)*.

Healing constipation this bad must begin with a cleanout, using a medicine called polyethylene glycol (eg, Miralax) and a stimulant laxative like senna (eg, Ex-Lax) to rid the colon of all retained stool. That's the easy part. The hard part comes in the months afterward, when you must give the child enough polyethylene glycol every day to ensure he has 2 to 3 soft stools. Remember, it took months for this problem to develop, and it will take months for it to improve.

when to call the doctor

If your child seems to have severe constipation, you'll definitely want to work with his doctor on a plan of care.

Constipation and urinary tract infections (UTIs) sometimes come as a matched set. That's because the stool mass that collects in constipation may put pressure on the *urethra,* the tube that carries pee out of the body. Children who are tightening their bottom muscles to hold in stool also sometimes hold pee in the bladder, where it's more likely to become infected. With or without constipation, however, UTIs often cause lower abdominal pain. If the infection spreads to the kidneys it may also cause back or side pain. Children with UTIs don't always complain of discomfort when they urinate; sometimes belly pain is the only clue you have to an infection.

Diagnosing UTIs is as easy as having a child pee in a cup, at least for children who are potty trained. For children who are too young to urinate on command, things get a little harder; the best way to get an accurate diagnosis is to pass a sterile catheter up the urethra and into the bladder, a procedure you can imagine might be a little uncomfortable. Making the diagnosis correctly, however, is critical—repeated UTIs may damage the kidneys, sometimes severely enough to require dialysis or transplant. The good news is that once diagnosed, UTIs tend to respond quickly to antibiotic therapy.

When mild to moderate abdominal pain doesn't seem to have any obvious cause, parents often wonder if it's real. Anxiety, stress, and other emotional problems are common causes of abdominal pain, affecting around 10% of children, especially during the school years. Anxiety may cause loose stools or nausea, but diarrhea, vomiting, or fever suggests something else is going on. Just because the pain doesn't appear to have a physical cause doesn't mean it's any less real. Children are not faking this sort of pain; in fact, they're often more confused than their parents about why they hurt.

Emotional abdominal pain often comes and goes for weeks or months at a time. You may notice your child's demeanor has changed; he may be more withdrawn or seek more attention. Sometimes you might notice an obvious trigger, like going to school or dealing with a parental separation, but the cause is not always so clear.

when to call the doctor

If you suspect your child is suffering emotional abdominal pain, start by asking him what might be bothering him. At the same time, don't just assume his pain is emotional; have a doctor check him out.

In some cases of emotional abdominal pain your reassurance may solve everything. Children often worry about their parents, imagining, for example, that you might be sick or in trouble. In tougher cases, however, a doctor, psychologist, or counselor may need to help him cope with issues that underlie the pain. Childhood may look easy to an adult, but growing up can be a lot to stomach.

Among the more frightening common causes of abdominal pain is *appendicitis*. The appendix is a little worm-shaped organ that hangs off the very first part of the colon. Scientists have determined that the function of the appendix is to provide business for emergency departments and general surgeons; otherwise it seems to have no purpose. If anything blocks off the opening of the appendix, it may become infected, sometimes rupturing and spreading dangerous bacteria all over the abdomen. The trick is that there's no surefire way to guess when that's about to happen.

Children with appendicitis often have fever, vomiting, and diarrhea, and they may appear very ill. Appendicitis is rare in children younger than 3 years and becomes more common during the school years. Appendicitis pain typically starts all over the belly and then gradually localizes in the lower right-hand area. If every child with appendicitis would just follow this pattern, the disease would be simple to diagnose, but is anything ever that easy? Instead, children may suffer vague or prolonged symptoms. When the diagnosis is uncertain, doctors most commonly use a computed tomography (CT) scan to help figure out what's going on. In some cases, even the CT scan doesn't answer the question, leaving exploratory surgery as the only option. In addition to surgery, antibiotic therapy is critical for treating appendicitis; sometimes antibiotics alone may cure it.

So now you know that your child's vague abdominal pain might indicate anything from hunger pangs to life-threatening appendicitis; don't you feel better? It might be handy to review what symptoms should have you on the phone to his doctor and which you can try to handle at home.

when to call the doctor

If your child is younger than 2 years, has pain for more than 2 hours nonstop, or has a temperature above 104°F, you should call his doctor. Pain in the lower right side of the abdomen could always be appendicitis; little else hurts over there. If you have a boy, look for swelling in the scrotum—he might have a hernia requiring emergency surgery. If you have a teenaged girl, never discount the possibility that she might be pregnant, regardless of what you think you know about her sexual activity. Pregnancy outside of the womb (ectopic pregnancy) poses a life-threatening surgical emergency. If you're on the fence about whether abdominal pain is severe, ask your child to jump up and down a few times. Pain that gets worse when he jumps is more likely due to a serious cause, as is pain that makes him bend over or makes it hard for him to walk.

Let's first assume that if your child is not moving or is too weak to stand, you're no longer reading this book but instead you've called emergency medical services (911). Then let's hit some obvious stuff—if your child seems very sick, if his pain is severe, if he has suffered an injury to his abdomen, or if you suspect he has ingested something poisonous, you should be on your way to a doctor with him.

what throws up must calm down

If you stop to think about it for a minute, vomiting is an amazing protective reflex (don't think about it too long). When sensors in the brain detect a potentially harmful substance in the stomach, they work to expel it through the mouth. To do so they trigger the mechanism that usually gets food from the mouth to the stomach to work in reverse, with more force. You have to stand in awe of such a finely tuned defense, although if you are standing in awe right now you might also want to stand back.

We discussed infant vomiting in Chapter 11, so now let's talk about children who are at least 1 year old. Just as with abdominal pain, there are tons of reasons a child might vomit, many of them arising far from the gastrointestinal tract. While childhood vomiting most commonly results from viral intestinal infections *(gastroenteritis),* other causes include food poisoning, constipation, toxin ingestion, ear infections, kidney infections, migraines, meningitis, and coughing. When your child starts to vomit, what are you going to do (after you grab a bucket)?

The first question to ask is whether the vomiting might be due to a serious cause. Part of the answer is to be found in the vomit itself. You're going to have to look at it, something that's hard to avoid if, say, it's on your shirt. Blood in the vomit is often an alarming sign, although in the case of very forceful vomiting it may just come from a small tear in the tissue where the esophagus joins the stomach. When blood spends time in contact with stomach acid it may turn black and granular, like coffee grounds. **If you see bright red blood or coffee grounds, you should get your child to a doctor quickly.**

Bile is another potentially alarming component of vomit. The gallbladder secretes this lemon-yellow– to lime-green–colored substance into the small intestine to help the body digest fats. Vomiting bile suggests a blockage farther along in the intestines, and if you see it you should seek care for your child urgently. Causes of bilious vomiting include malrotation, volvulus, intussusception, and incarcerated hernia, all potential surgical emergencies we reviewed in Chapter 11. In older children, appendicitis joins the list.

Vomit that seems to contain stool may, in fact, contain stool. Vomit like this suggests a child is severely constipated to the point where almost nothing can move forward. Fortunately, constipation this bad occurs rarely.

The duration of vomiting provides another clue to how serious the cause might be. Gastroenteritis and food poisoning, for example, produce similar symptoms. The difference between the 2 is that while gastroenteritis involves an infection in the child's intestine, food poisoning occurs when bacteria secrete toxins into poorly refrigerated food. Most cases of gastroenteritis come with diarrhea, and often with fever as well, while food poisoning does not cause fever.

At the beginning of either illness the child may vomit repeatedly for the first 2 to 4 hours. Often things calm down from there, and after the first 8 hours vomiting should have slowed substantially. Vomiting from gastroenteritis may linger for 2 to 3 days, but it shouldn't be nearly as frequent by that time.

when to call the doctor

If your child vomits at least once an hour for more than 8 hours or if he continues to vomit for more than 24 hours without obvious symptoms of gastroenteritis, you should call his doctor.

Once you've figured out your child's vomiting is not from a dangerous cause, you'll likely want to do something about it. You probably most want to make it stop, but there are few good ways to do that. Doctors use some medicines to keep children from vomiting, but unless a doctor has examined your child and prescribed a specific medication, you shouldn't give him anything. Some medicines that are useful for older children and adults, such as promethazine (eg, Phenergan) and prochlorperazine (eg, Compazine), can have nasty and even permanent neurologic side effects when given to young children. These medications are no longer approved for children younger than 2, and many pediatricians are cautious about using them for older children as well. A different drug, ondansetron (eg, Zofran), seems safer for young children, but the vast majority of children recover from vomiting without any medication at all.

If your child has a high fever (temperature above 102°F), you may want to treat it with acetaminophen rather than ibuprofen, as ibuprofen may upset his stomach. Acetaminophen comes as a suppository for children who are vomiting too much to take medicine by mouth. If your child takes critical medicines for a problem like epilepsy or heart disease, you'll want to call his doctor for instructions as soon as the vomiting starts.

The most important priority when your child is vomiting is to keep him hydrated. The younger a child, the more easily he becomes dehydrated. The good news is that while it may appear your child is about to vomit his toenails, it's impossible for him to completely empty his stomach when he throws up. That means that if you can just keep enough fluid going into him, you can probably avoid hospitalization. The keys to successful rehydration are picking the right fluid and giving it in the right way.

Water is naturally a great choice for hydration. Water can enter the body right through the wall of the stomach, which means it works quickly. Some children prefer ice chips to drinking out of a cup. You're probably willing to carve your child an ice sculpture if it will keep him from spending the next 6 hours in the emergency department! For severe vomiting, an oral rehydration solution like Pedialyte may be an even better choice because the salt and sugar in such solutions helps the water enter the bloodstream without worsening diarrhea the way more sugary beverages can. Again, freezing the solution to make popsicles or ice chips may help it go down. If your child refuses both of these options, you can try a sports beverage like Gatorade diluted to half strength, or you could use half-strength lemon-lime soda such as Sprite or 7Up. The best fluid for rehydration is one the child will actually drink.

When I think about rehydrating sick kids, I like to imagine a leaking pipe. While each drop may be small, together they can fill a bucket in no time. You want to use the same idea when rehydrating your vomiting child. To avoid triggering more vomiting, give only a little fluid at a time, around 2 or 3 teaspoons. But give it frequently, at least every 5 minutes. Don't stop just because your child continues to vomit. If anything, ongoing vomiting makes it more critical you keep fluids going in.

Once your child has gone 4 hours without vomiting, you can increase the amount of fluid he takes each time. If he makes it 8 hours without vomiting, he can try other fluids and even some bland, starchy foods like crackers, cereal, or rice. Within 24 to 48 hours he should be able to resume a normal diet.

There are some signs you can follow to see how well your child is hydrated. The best is urine output, although when children are also having frequent watery stools this one can be impossible to assess. Children should pee at least 3 times a day or once every 8 hours.

when to call the doctor

Peeing fewer than 3 times a day or once every 8 hours should prompt a call to the doctor. Other concerning signs of dehydration include crying without producing tears or a dry appearance to the inside of the mouth. Severe dehydration may lend a child's eyes a sunken appearance or make a child's skin appear loose. At the extremes of dehydration a child may appear lethargic and difficult to awaken. Call emergency medical services (911) if you see any of these signs; they suggest the sort of life-threatening dehydration that can only be fixed during a hospital stay.

pooped out

The fact that we don't have diarrhea all the time is a testament to what an amazing organ the human colon is. Digested food arrives at the colon in liquid form, and as it travels the roughly square path from where the colon starts in the right lower abdomen to where it ends (you know), most of the water has been absorbed back into the body, leaving a waste product that is solid enough to stay together but soft enough to pass easily out of the body. In the meantime, bacteria in the colon manage to eke out a few more nutrients from the food without themselves escaping from the intestines into the body and causing serious infections. Anything that disrupts this finely tuned balance may leave the stool too watery, resulting in diarrhea.

Just as with abdominal pain and vomiting, diarrhea may result from processes within the intestines and far removed from them. The most common cause of diarrhea is, you guessed it, gastroenteritis. The most dangerous viral cause of gastroenteritis, rotavirus infection, has grown much less common with the advent of effective vaccines (see Chapter 7).

Viral infections, however, are far from the only types of infections that cause diarrhea. Bacteria, including *Salmonella, Shigella, Escherichia coli, Campylobacter, Clostridium difficile,* and others can cause infections ranging from mild to life-threatening. Parasitic infections, especially from *Giardia* and *Cryptosporidium* species, may cause prolonged diarrhea in children who ingest contaminated water.

Sometimes diarrhea results not from having the wrong kind of bacteria in the intestines but from having too few of the right kind. If your child is on antibiotics and gets mild to moderate loose stools, for example, the antibiotics may have killed the beneficial bacteria that keeps his colon functioning normally. In these cases it's worth trying a probiotic supplement like some *Lactobacillus* species, *Bifidobacterium bifidum,* or *Streptococcus thermophilus.* These probiotics are found in many brands of yogurt, but dietary supplements may include higher doses. If diarrhea is more severe, contains blood, or comes with a fever, the problem is probably something more serious and deserves medical evaluation.

One common, benign, and easily remedied cause of diarrhea may be something your child enjoys—fruit juice. Sugars in fruit juices escape being completely digested in the small intestine, instead making their way into the colon where they draw water into the stool. Whenever your child begins having diarrhea, an easy first step is to stop giving her juice. Another possible cause of diarrhea and abdominal pain may be in your refrigerator right next to the juice—milk. The sugar in human and cow's milk is lactose; while almost all human babies are born able to digest lactose perfectly well, some children lose this ability in the years following infancy. If you notice that dairy products seem to upset your child's stomach, there's no harm in withholding cow's milk for a week and seeing if he improves. If he does, you can usually find lactose-free substitutes.

Other causes of diarrhea arise far from the colon. Cystic fibrosis, a genetic disease, may cause diarrhea and weight loss. Diseases affecting the pancreas inhibit digestion, causing diarrhea as well. Celiac disease, an immunologic reaction to the protein in wheat, impairs digestion and also causes diarrhea. Hyperthyroidism, while rare in children, may cause diarrhea and weight loss.

There are several signs to look for to alert you that diarrhea deserves a doctor's attention. Blood in the stool usually results from a more severe bacterial infection like *Salmonella* or *Shigella.* Children who have had contact with other infected people or with reptiles like turtles or lizards

what you can do

Treating diarrhea at home is largely about preventing dehydration, using the same techniques we discussed previously. With mild diarrhea (3 to 4 stools a day), dehydration is really not a threat unless the child is also vomiting. With more severe diarrhea (8 or more stools a day), you'll want to be more aggressive with hydration. If your child is not vomiting, there's no reason to stop feeding him so long as you avoid giving him fruits and fruit juices. Bland, starchy foods are probably still a better bet than, say, a big spicy burrito.

are at especially high risk. Some of these infections require antibiotics, while others are best left to resolve on their own, but it takes a doctor's examination as well as stool cultures to know what to do.

The abdominal pain from diarrhea should come and go, usually getting worse right before your child uses the bathroom and then improving afterward. If the pain sticks around for 2 or more hours, he should see a doctor. Viral gastroenteritis often comes with a fever, but any child with

when to call the doctor

Mucous or pus in the stool may suggest a more serious infection; call your child's doctor if you see this.

fever that lasts more than 3 days or a temperature that stays above 104°F more than 2 hours after treatment deserves a medical evaluation. Diarrhea from viral gastroenteritis may linger for as long as 2 weeks, but it should not be severe or frequent after the first day. Diarrhea that lasts longer than 2 weeks suggests a problem a doctor should check out.

You should now be prepared to handle the rite of passage that involves dealing with your child's vomit and/or diarrhea. In many cultures, men who have proven their worth wear some special mark to identify their distinction. Hopefully your badge of honor will come out in the wash.

20

water, water everywhere: is this wetting normal?

As little as people talk about bed-wetting (nocturnal enuresis), you'd think it was something incredibly rare like, say, a fair catch kick in football. The fact is if you're in a room right now with 7 adults, chances are at least 1 of them wet the bed as a child. If those people are really good friends, you could prove this to yourself by going around the room and asking them. If they're not that comfortable with each other, you might just ask if anyone knows what a fair catch kick is.

some enchanted evening

Sleep puts the body and brain in very different states than wakefulness. For this reason nighttime bladder control often lags daytime control by years. While the average American child is potty-trained before age 3, one-quarter of 5-year-olds still wet the bed at night. With every year that passes, around 15% of children gain the ability to stay dry, so by age 7, about 1 in 5 wet the bed, and by age 10 the number is only 1 in 20. Until age 13, boys outnumber girls 2 to 1, but the numbers even out with adolescence. Only around 1% of adults continue to have trouble with nighttime urination, so no matter how bad it is now, you can reassure your child (and yourself) he's almost certainly not going to have this problem forever. Nighttime wetting is so common that pediatricians rarely consider intervening before children turn 6.

Doctors may think differently about children who have always wet the bed (primary enuresis) and children whose bed-wetting starts after at least 6 months of dry nights (secondary enuresis). Children who were previously dry are more likely to have a new problem compared with children whose bodies just haven't mastered the trick of keeping urine in the bladder all night.

understanding bed-wetting...or not

There is a simple answer to the question, "Why do some children wet the bed?" That answer is...we don't usually know. Parents often believe their children just sleep too deeply to wake up when they need to pee, but studies of sleep and bed-wetting have proven that theory just plain wrong. Bed-wetting occurs at all phases of sleep, not just the deepest parts. It occurs in children who are easy to wake up and those who seem dead to the world.

More promising theories involve differences in bladder size and urine production among children. It makes sense that children with smaller bladders can't hold a night's worth of urine as easily as those with bigger tanks. At night hormones tell our kidneys to make less urine, but some people still make more than others. We do know that genetics play a strong role in bed-wetting—if one parent wets the bed, there's nearly a 50% chance a child will, too. If both parents had enuresis, that number goes up to 75%! (These are the things you never think to ask before you have a child with someone.)

To understand what might go wrong with peeing, it helps to know how it works when it goes right. The kidneys filter toxins from the bloodstream all the time, excreting them and any excess water as urine. Increases in fluid or salt intake cause the kidneys to make more urine.

Urine travels from the kidneys to the bladder via 2 tubes, the *ureters*. Once the bladder is full, urine exits the body through the *urethra*. The hole at the very end of the urethra is called the *meatus*. A muscle around the urethra, the *urinary sphincter*, closes to hold urine in the bladder until it's time to pee. A sheet of muscle, the *detrusor*, surrounds the bladder, remaining relaxed until it's time to pee, when it contracts to squeeze out the urine.

There are some medical conditions that may predispose a child to bed-wetting. The most common is constipation (see Chapter 19). Don't assume that if your child had constipation you would know it—kids don't tend to talk a lot about their bowel habits, and once they learn to flush the commode, you're hopefully not thinking too hard about their poop!

If your child snores loudly or seems to stop breathing for brief periods at night, he might have obstructive sleep apnea. Children with this condition may benefit from tonsillectomy or adenoidectomy. In these cases, curing sleep apnea may also cure bed-wetting.

If you really want to freak yourself out, you can start worrying about urinary tract infections (UTIs), spinal cord diseases, or diabetes as causes of bed-wetting. These are rarely the problem, even more rarely in children who were never dry in the first place. If you bring these concerns up to your child's doctor, she should be able to reassure you pretty quickly with a simple history, physical examination, and urine test.

Social and emotional issues also sometimes cause bed-wetting, especially when it starts after a period of dry nights. A child who faces a new stress, such as the birth of a sibling, the death of a relative, or a parental separation or divorce, may start having accidents. If you suspect something like this may be going on, the first thing to know is that your child is not doing it on purpose. Bed-wetting is not something children do to get attention (screaming is much more efficient for that purpose). You may want to consult a doctor, psychologist, or counselor to help your child work through whatever is worrying him.

when to call the doctor
There are a few symptoms that should prompt you to address bed-wetting with your child's doctor sooner rather than later. Wetting that starts in the daytime as well as at night is more concerning. If you notice your child straining to pass urine or if you see that the urinary stream is small or narrow, he may have some sort of blockage. Urine that continues to dribble out after the child is done peeing also deserves evaluation, as does urine with any hint of blood. If your child starts hiding wet underwear or clothes, that's a pretty clear message that it's time to talk about what's going on and see what you can do to help. You might also take a look in your child's genital area for any signs of rash, redness, or irritation that might be interfering with normal urination.

peeking at the pee

If you do decide to talk with your child's doctor about wetting, get ready to spend more time than you usually do discussing pee (unless you repair urinals for a living, in which case I stand corrected, so to speak). The doctor will want to know about any family history of wetting in close relatives (be honest—this means you). She'll ask how often and when your child uses the bathroom and when and where accidents occur. She may ask you to describe your child's urine, including appearance and smell (don't go out of your way to obtain this information, but if you've noticed something, now's the time to mention it). She'll probably also ask about fever, abdominal pain, and any changes in gait, mood, or school performance.

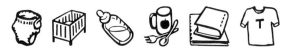

what you can do

You'll want to prepare your child for a physical examination that will inevitably involve the private area. School-aged children often become anxious about letting the doctor check them out, no matter how often they streak through the house naked. Talking about what's going to happen ahead of time helps kids prepare for the examination and reassures them it will be OK. Most pediatricians will keep a parent in the room or have a staff member serve as chaperone during such examinations, and they often preface the examination with a short reminder on appropriate and inappropriate touch. The physical examination should cover not only the genitals but also the back, abdomen, and strength and reflexes in the legs. If the doctor suspects severe constipation or nerve disease, she may even perform a rectal examination (yes, that rectum).

In some cases the doctor will also want to examine the child's urine. An office urinalysis can detect signs of infection, diabetes, and kidney stones. Only a urine culture has the power to accurately diagnose a UTI, and the results often take 2 or 3 days to come back, but treatment can start immediately. Unless the doctor suspects diabetes, blood testing rarely adds anything to the diagnosis.

Other, more specialized tests can provide more information about the kidneys and bladder. A bladder ultrasound, for example, can tell doctors how much urine is left over in the bladder after a child does his best to empty it. Children with frequent or severe UTIs or any boy with a UTI is likely to need an ultrasound of the kidneys and a special kidney x-ray called a *voiding cystourethrogram.*

Doctors who specialize in diseases of the urinary tract (urologists) can perform a urodynamic test. This test uses special equipment to measure urine output as a child empties his bladder. The resulting computer analysis is especially useful to evaluate abnormal structure or function of the urinary system.

turning the tide before you run out of Tide

Knowing that bed-wetting is common and normal probably doesn't make you feel better when you're laundering a load of sheets every day. Fortunately there are a number of interventions that can help your child enjoy dry nights sooner rather than later. Some you can try on your own; others will require a doctor's help.

Most important is to remember that you and your child are allies in this battle, not adversaries. No one likes waking up in wet, smelly sheets. As children start to enjoy sleepovers at their friends' houses or weeks at summer camp, they often feel intense shame and embarrassment about wetting the bed.

what you can do

When you discover a new accident, adopt a casual attitude and enlist your child's help in cleaning up. Remember, this isn't his idea of a good time either! Make sure you tell him directly that you know this isn't his fault and you're not mad at him; otherwise, your child may interpret your frustration as anger. If you yourself wet the bed as a child, let him know; your story may inspire him. There's nothing wrong with rewarding him for dry nights, but punishing him for wet ones accomplishes nothing. Moreover, it makes no sense.

Many experts recommend limiting your child's fluid intake in the couple of hours prior to bedtime. If your child seems to benefit from fluid restriction, go for it, but if it fails after a few nights, don't sweat it. More important than when your child is drinking is what he's drinking. As any devoted coffee drinker (ahem) knows, caffeine makes you pee more. Children metabolize caffeine slower than adults, so there's really no place for tea, energy drinks, or caffeinated soda in a child's diet. Dairy products may also increase urine output, so in the evenings have your child stick with water.

It's kind of a no-brainer to encourage your child to pee right before he goes to bed and again as soon as he wakes up. You might even try setting an alarm halfway through the night so he can pee again then. While the midnight pee strategy seems logical, it remains unproven, so don't get too upset if it's not working.

The single most effective intervention for bed-wetting is the bed-wetting alarm. You have several models to choose from, many of them quite affordable, especially compared with the price of medications. They all have a sensor to detect moisture and a device to awaken your child, using sound or vibrations. To start, you may have to help your child wake up in response to the alarm, but with time he'll probably get the hang of it. Expect your child to use the alarm every night for 3 or 4 months before he's consistently dry.

Bed-wetting alarms enjoy 3 advantages over medications. First, they work better, with success rates of 60% to 70% after regular use. Second, after a month of dry nights, your child may be able to stop using the alarm altogether, whereas medications stop working as soon as you stop using them. Third, bed-wetting alarms have no side effects.

The disadvantage of bed-wetting alarms (aside from that thing where you wake up at night) is that they require regular use over a period of months, which doesn't do your child a lot of good if he has a sleepover tonight. For more immediate relief, medications remain an option. Desmopressin (eg, DDAVP) is the most popular of these agents. It is a synthetic version of the hormone that signals your kidneys to make less urine when you're starting to get dehydrated. Children take desmopressin a half hour before bedtime in the hopes that it will decrease their urine output overnight.

Desmopressin seems to help around 50% to 60% of children with bed-wetting. Some doctors feel you should know pretty quickly if it's going to help your child. The medicine lasts about 9 hours in the body, so it only works the nights you give it. Because kids tend to outgrow bed-wetting anyway, you might want to try stopping the desmopressin every 6 months or so to see if the problem has gone away.

A second medicine, imipramine, can also help with bed-wetting. Originally marketed decades ago to treat depression, imipramine has the useful side effect of making it harder for patients to empty their bladders. Imipramine is less popular than desmopressin in part because it has the potential to affect a patient's heart rhythms. Some doctors screen patients with an electrocardiogram prior to starting this medication. For enuresis, doctors usually dose imipramine at levels far below those once used to treat depression.

Some urologists try combining desmopressin with agents used to treat bladder spasm, such as oxybutynin (eg, Ditropan). This medicine is especially useful in children who also have problems with daytime wetting.

to pee or not to pee: daytime wetting

Daytime wetting *(diurnal enuresis),* while less common than bed-wetting, is still more common than you might guess. Up until age 5, it's not unusual for a child to get distracted playing and dribble a little from a full bladder. At age 7 years, 2% to 3% of boys and 3% to 4% of girls continue to have urine accidents during waking hours. That said, children who have trouble holding their urine when awake are more likely to suffer a medical condition.

when to call the doctor

Daytime wetting that occurs after successful toilet training deserves a doctor's evaluation.

The doctor will start assessing daytime wetting the same way she would evaluate bed-wetting, with a history and physical examination. The doctor will want to know how often the accidents occur and in what situations. She will ask if urine volume is large or small and whether it comes out all at once or constantly dribbles out. She will be curious about bowel habits and any discomfort the child may have when using the bathroom.

She is very likely to order a urinalysis and urine culture. Daytime wetting is more likely than bed-wetting to require the advice of a urologist.

While daytime wetting raises concerns about UTIs, diabetes, and diseases of the nerves or spinal cord, the problem in girls may be as simple as vaginal irritation (vulvovaginitis). This condition often responds to antifungal medicines, improved wiping hygiene (front to back, not back to front!), and avoiding bubble baths.

Constipation is another common cause of daytime wetting. Not only can the mass of retained stool press on the bladder and urethra, but as children tighten their bottom muscles to hold in their poop, they may also tighten the sphincter that keeps urine in the bladder. Over time the muscles involved in peeing (and not peeing) lose the precise coordination that makes everything work smoothly. This condition, dysfunctional voiding syndrome or detrusor sphincter dyssynergia, is more common in girls than boys.

The most important step in treating dysfunctional voiding is to treat the underlying constipation (see Chapter 19). Children also require bladder retraining, starting with peeing every 2 hours whether they feel the need or not. Chances are your mobile phone or sports watch has a timer you can set to go off as a reminder. These children may also need to double void, trying to pee one more time after they think they're done. Children with more severe cases may benefit from biofeedback that helps them control the muscles of their bottoms.

Girls also benefit from sitting backwards on the toilet seat, allowing their pelvises to rock forward and opening up their legs to make passage of urine easier. This same maneuver may cure another common cause of daytime wetting in girls, vaginal reflux. If a girl sits so that her bottom hangs down in the toilet, urine may wash up into the vagina. Then, when she stands, it dribbles back out. (This is one of those problems most dads would just never guess could happen.) Girls with vaginal reflux seem to always have damp underwear, even though they never pee on themselves.

While bed-wetting and daytime wetting pose special challenges to fathers and their children, hopefully this chapter has given you an idea of where to start. With persistence you can usually count on the sort of success Ray Wersching enjoyed in 1976 when, playing for the San Diego Chargers against the Buffalo Bills, he scored the last recorded successful fair catch kick.

21

hard to swallow:
the sore throat

sure, your child may have a sore throat and her tonsils might look enlarged, but chances are she's no Justin Werner. Justin, a 21-year-old native of Topeka, KS, entered the *Guinness Book of World Records* in 2011 for having the world's largest tonsils, with one measured at 2.1 x 1.1 x 0.7 inches! He did have them removed, but it's not clear whether surgery was required to qualify for the record. No comment was available from the previous record-holder, Justin Dodge of Milwaukee, WI. I'm sure your child is headed for greatness in many things, but hopefully she will leave Mr Werner to bask in his fame for years to come. Besides, apparently to hold the record, you have to be named Justin.

Sore throats are yet another ordeal of childhood, and like most such trials, they usually pass on their own. Some of them (but not most) require anti-biotic treatment. Occasionally they even call for surgery, but not as often as people once thought. Very rarely, sore throats can be life-threatening. So let's spend some time thinking about the throat. Open up and say, "Ah!"

no, really, say "ah"

The most important reason doctors ask kids to open up and say "ah" is so that we'll seem more like the doctors on television. But the second most important reason is that making this sound pushes the patient's tongue against the floor of the mouth and elevates her soft palate, allowing a better view of the throat. There's more to see back there than you might think.

Before a doctor even looks at the throat, he's checking out the structures toward the front of the mouth. Does the child have sores on her lips or gums? Does she suffer from cavities? Are there white patches on the tongue or inside the cheeks? The roof of the mouth has 2 parts, the bony hard palate in front and mobile soft palate behind it. Some children are born with openings in these structures, a condition called cleft palate. Cleft palate predisposes children to sinus infections; more subtle cases are not always easy to diagnose.

Babies may have little white bumps at the very center of their soft palates called *Epstein pearls,* after a doctor who apparently couldn't find anything better to name after himself. Older children may have a lumpy-looking growth in the same spot called a *torus palatinus,* another normal if weird-looking finding. At the very back of the soft palate hangs the little punching-bag–looking appendage called the *uvula.* Science has yet to determine if the uvula has a function outside the world of animated cartoons.

The tonsils flank the opening to the throat, looking like 2 fleshy lumps with ridges and pits like a walnut. Tonsils vary in size, often dramatically. Some kids have almost no tonsils at all; others sport real honkers. Tonsil size alone usually doesn't mean much (unless of course you're a Midwestern kid named Justin with dreams of fame), but there are exceptions. Some children with immune deficiencies have minimal to no tonsils. Other children with very large tonsils may suffer *obstructive sleep apnea,* a condition we'll discuss in greater detail later in this chapter. Sometimes minerals collect in the deeper pits of the tonsils, looking like little white rocks. These *tonsilloliths* don't signify any disease, although people sometimes mistake them for pus.

The tonsils actually do have a function, aside from providing full employment for ear, nose, and throat specialists (otolaryngologists). They house concentrations of disease-fighting immune cells, much like the lymph nodes elsewhere in the body. Just like lymph nodes, tonsils often swell in response to infection. The tonsils themselves are not critical to immune function; people who lose their tonsils seem to fight off infections just fine without them.

At the very back of the throat is the area doctors call the *posterior oropharynx.* At first glance it looks like there's nothing to see back there, but this area also hosts rich collections of disease-fighting cells called *lymphoid tissue.* In response to infections or chronic inflammation, this tissue may expand, giving the throat a bumpy appearance. Mucous in the posterior oropharynx can be a sign of a cold or sinus infection.

strep down

All sorts of things make throats sore, including colds, mononucleosis, allergic rhinitis, and gastroesophageal reflux disease. Only one of these causes of sore throat deserves antibiotic therapy—infection with bacteria called *Streptococcus pyogenes,* also known as group A beta-hemolytic strep, or GABHS. Only a minority of children who come to the doctor complaining of sore throat have this infection, and they are the only ones who need treatment. Telling which kids these are is important, but it's not always as easy as you might think.

Strep throat infections almost never strike infants, in part because they still enjoy some protection from their mother's antibodies. Toddlers may occasionally get strep, especially if they live with older siblings who are infected. The infection grows more common between the ages of 5 and 15 years, after which rates taper off, but adults can still catch strep.

Not everyone who has GABHS in the throat actually has a strep throat infection. Around 10% to 15% of children are carriers of strep, meaning they harbor the bacteria, but it's not actually making them sick. These children do not need antibiotic treatment; in fact, their strep seems to return even after therapy.

Strep throat infections can be quite uncomfortable, causing throat pain, fever, runny or stuffy nose, abdominal pain, and rash. While treating strep with antibiotics may shorten the duration of these symptoms by a day or so, that's not really why doctors treat it. The dirty secret of strep throat is that the symptoms will improve in a few days with or without medication. The real reason we find it so important to diagnose and treat strep throat is that it causes another potentially deadly condition, rheumatic fever.

Rheumatic fever results from an interaction between the patient's immune system and GABHS bacteria. The resulting inflammation attacks the heart valves, sometimes causing permanent heart damage, leading to heart failure and even death. Treating strep throat within the first 9 days of infection prevents rheumatic fever, and the disease has grown quite rare in the modern era.

Another complication of strep throat involves the kidneys and is also a result of the immune system's reaction to the disease. This condition, post-strep glomerulonephritis, allows blood and protein to leak from the bloodstream into the urine. Unfortunately, treating strep throat does not prevent children from getting glomerulonephritis if they're destined to do so. The good news is that post-strep glomerulonephritis is relatively rare and usually responds well to appropriate therapies.

Because rheumatic fever is such a dangerous disease, you might think doctors would want to treat every child who has a sore throat with antibiotics. The problem with that approach is that it exposes many children to the risks of unnecessary antibiotic therapy, including antibiotic resistance, diarrhea, and potentially life-threatening allergic reactions. For this reason, doctors focus on identifying which children actually have strep throat infections and which ones will get better without taking medicine they don't need. Fortunately we have some clues to guide us.

Age and exposure history are important in deciding which children may have strep throat. In children younger than 12 months, strep is so rare that most doctors don't even look for it. When one member of a household gets strep throat, there's about a one-third chance others in the house will get it. There's no need to test exposed children without any symptoms of fever or sore throat; even if they test positive, they don't need antibiotics. If, however, a close contact of a strep patient starts to complain of fever or throat pain, a strep test is likely in order.

when to call the doctor

The children whose sore throats most likely come from strep are those with fever, enlarged lymph nodes, and few cold symptoms. A child with a cough or a hoarse voice is more likely to have a cold than strep throat, even if sore throat is among her complaints.

Many children with strep develop a white or yellowish exudate of pus on their tonsils. Exudate, however, is a symptom of viral illnesses as well, including mononucleosis. More predictive of strep infection are the little blood-colored spots called *petechiae* on the soft palate. Often strep patients will notice large, tender lymph nodes in their necks. The most distinct finding of strep is a rash, scarlet fever (also called *scarlatina)*. The rash consists of very fine bumps, like 50-grit sandpaper, on the face, trunk, arms, and legs. Sometimes it's especially dense in the groin. The scarlatina rash usually doesn't itch much, if at all. Rash improves over several days, but as it resolves the child's skin may peel, especially at the fingers and toes.

If your child's doctor suspects she has strep, he will probably order a rapid strep test. You might wonder why doctors don't just test every child with a sore throat, but remember that thing about strep carriers? If we were to test every child who came in the door, up to 15% of them would walk out with an unnecessary antibiotic prescription, so it's safer to test only those children who are likely to have the disease. The test involves rubbing a cotton or Dacron swab across the tonsils and the back of the throat, and then processing it to look for the presence of GABHS. Results usually return in about 5 minutes, and tests identify between 80% and 95% of infected patients.

Throat cultures provide another way to diagnose strep. Just as with the rapid test they start with a throat swab, but the swab goes to a laboratory that actually grows the strep bacteria. This test takes 1 to 2 days to come back, but it's more sensitive than the rapid test, catching the handful of patients the rapid tests miss. Most doctors will send a backup throat culture for patients who have a negative rapid strep test to ensure they don't miss treating anyone.

Strep throat remains among the easiest infectious diseases to treat. Unlike other bacteria, GABHS seems unable to build resistance to penicillins like amoxicillin. If your child is vomiting or cannot take oral medications, she can get a shot of Bicillin, a long-acting form of penicillin. If she has a serious allergy to penicillin, the doctor may choose among several alternatives.

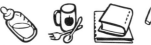

what you can do

You may find the most challenging part of treating your child's strep throat is completing the antibiotic course. To avoid rheumatic fever, it's important your child take antibiotics for the full period, usually 10 days. Of course you'll remember to give them while she has a fever and sore throat, but a week later when she's bouncing all over the house, it's easy to forget those last few doses. Put a note on your bathroom mirror, tie a string around your finger, or put the antibiotics in the fridge in front of the milk, but don't fail to finish the course.

You'll want to keep your child comfortable while she's recovering from strep. Pain relievers like acetaminophen (eg, Tylenol) and ibuprofen (eg, Advil, Motrin) help with sore throat and fever. She may tolerate warm fluids like chicken broth or apple juice, or she may prefer smoothies or milkshakes (go ahead and make a little extra for yourself). Keeping your child hydrated poses your greatest challenge when she feels like she's swallowing glass shards.

when to call the doctor

The pain and fever from strep throat normally resolve over 2 to 3 days. If they last longer, call the doctor back.

Strep remains contagious for the first 24 hours after the first dose of antibiotics. After that your child should again be fit for human companionship, including school.

strep tease: other causes of sore throat

Two medical terms describe inflammation in the throat, *tonsillitis* and *pharyngitis*. Pharyngitis refers to inflammation anywhere in the throat, an area doctors call the pharynx. Tonsillitis simply means inflammation of the tonsils, although in practice some doctors use it to mean, "I really feel like prescribing this child antibiotics even though she doesn't have strep." If the majority of such inflammation doesn't come from strep, what else might be going on back there?

Most often, pharyngitis and tonsillitis result from any of the thousands of viruses that cause colds. A scratchy throat is frequently the earliest symptom of a cold, and postnasal drip and coughing irritate the throat as well. Sore throats from cold viruses should get better on their own within 4 to 5 days.

Among the nastier non-strep causes of sore throat is hand-foot-and-mouth disease, also known as coxsackievirus A-16 infection. Despite the similar names, coxsackievirus is not at all related to the hoof-and-mouth disease that affects livestock. (If your child does have hooves, call a veterinarian stat!) In addition to fever and little blisters at the fingers and toes, coxsackie-virus causes shallow ulcers in the mouth, often on the soft palate and the tissue around the tonsils. These ulcers cause intense pain; children suffer-ing this infection often drool rather than swallow their own saliva. Usually hand-foot-and-mouth disease affects toddlers and preschoolers.

No medicines speed the resolution of hand-foot-and-mouth disease, but antacids like Maalox and Mylanta can relieve some of the pain if you can get your child to swish them around in her mouth. Some doctors prescribe a concoction called *magic mouthwash,* usually a mixture of an antacid, an antihistamine, and sometimes a steroid or ulcer medication. The most important thing to do if your child has hand-foot-and-mouth disease is to keep her hydrated, using small sips of cool, nonacidic fluid. Your child may return to school or child care when she feels better, usually 2 to 3 days after the infection starts. Ulcers may take a good week to go away completely.

when to call the doctor

If your child has a stiff neck or seems unable to swallow at all, she needs to see a doctor immediately.

Another cause of similarly painful mouth ulcers is herpes infection. The herpes that infects children's mouths is not a sexually transmitted infection. Herpes ulcers not only infect the throat, they often involve the gums and the lips as well, first producing blisters and progressing to crusted sores. In patients with healthy immune systems, the disease will go away on its own in 1 to 2 weeks, but a doctor may prescribe antiviral medicines so long as the diagnosis is made during the first 2 days of illness. After the first 48 hours, the medicines don't help. Otherwise, care of herpes mouth infections is similar to that for coxsackievirus infection, with a focus on keeping the child comfortable and hydrated.

When you're just sure your child has strep but the tests come back negative, she may in fact have mono. Mononucleosis causes fever, sore throat, swollen lymph nodes, abdominal pain, and fatigue, just like strep. To confuse matters more, kids with mono often develop exudate on their tonsils and even petechiae on their soft palates.

Because many people associate mono with kissing, parents are often surprised to learn it also affects preschoolers whose most intimate show of affection is to hold hands while playing "Ring Around the Rosie." While kissing is indeed an effective way to pass mono from one person to the next, so is sharing a cup of juice at snack time. Mono infections strike children at all ages, although they do peak during the teen years.

Mono always results from a viral infection, most often with Epstein-Barr virus (EBV). (No, that's not the same Epstein who named the pearls. What is it with these Epsteins and naming stuff?) Another virus, cytomegalovirus (CMV), also causes mono, along with a variety of other viruses that may result in similar syndromes.

One hallmark of mononucleosis is fatigue. Victims often feel exhausted by minimal exertion, and it may take weeks for them to resume full activity levels. Mono can also produce prolonged fevers, lasting from 1 to 3 weeks. Patients' spleens sometimes swell dramatically with mono infections, putting them at risk of rare but potentially fatal spleen rupture if they sustain a hard blow to the abdomen. If your child's doctor diagnoses her with mono, he may keep her out of high-risk sports like lacrosse, martial arts, or curling (brutal body checks in curling!) until her spleen shrinks back to its normal size.

Doctors may diagnose mono based on history and physical examination alone, especially if a child's spleen is enlarged. In some cases, a quick office test called a Monospot or heterophil antibody can identify mono-nucleosis using a drop of blood from a finger stick. A laboratory analysis of the child's blood might also identify the presence of EBV or CMV.

Most treatment for mono focuses on symptom relief, especially for fever and sore throat. No medicines help children recover faster from mono infections, but doctors may prescribe steroids in rare cases where the throat swelling is so severe that it threatens to block a child's airway. As you might imagine, these children are usually hospitalized until they improve. One reason not to prescribe antibiotics to every child with a sore throat is that children with mono tend to get a dramatic rash if they take amoxicillin while they're infected.

One other infectious cause of sore throat deserves special mention: gonorrhea (yes, *that* gonorrhea). Gonorrhea infection of the throat is always sexually transmitted, usually among teens who engage in oral sex. Gonorrhea shows up on special throat cultures and responds quickly to antibiotics, but the doctor has to think to look for it first. Doctors will often ask to speak with teenaged patients privately to ask about habits that may put their health at risk. Even if you have a very close and honest relationship with your teenager, you should encourage her to have this conversation with her doctor and to be frank in her answers. In many cases, her pediatrician can help her talk with you about topics she may be anxious to discuss.

Sometimes infections involve the deeper tissues of the throat, causing abscesses behind the tonsils *(peritonsillar abscess)* or at the very back of the oropharynx *(retropharyngeal abscess)*. Children with these infec-tions may find it very difficult to swallow, talk, or move their necks. They often have high temperatures, well above 102°F. Doctors identify abscesses by examining the throat, although they often need a computed tomography scan to determine just how bad they are. These infections are life-threatening, requiring hospitalization, intravenous antibiotic therapy, and often surgical drainage. Fortunately, they are also relatively rare.

what, these old things?

In prior decades the indication for removing a child's tonsils was that she still had them. Tonsils took all the blame for sore throats, so after a few bouts of pharyngitis it seemed to make sense to just get rid of them. Tonsillectomy remains a common procedure today, but pediatricians and otolaryngologists are now much more cautious about recommending the surgery. Today we recognize 3 reasons to remove a child's tonsils: severe recurrent pharyngitis, obstructive sleep apnea, and suspected tonsillar cancer.

A child can still contract strep throat without tonsils; in fact, taking them out makes only a marginal difference in how often children get sore throats. For any surgery, doctors like to know that the benefits outweigh the risks, and that seems to be the case for children who suffer 7 episodes of strep throat or severe throat infection in 1 year, 5 infections per year for 2 years in a row, or 3 infections per year for 3 years. Individual cases vary; for example, if your child is allergic to many different antibiotics, she may benefit from tonsillectomy after fewer infections.

Obstructive sleep apnea occurs when a child's airway closes periodically during sleep, causing the oxygen level in her bloodstream to fall. A child with obstructive sleep apnea often snores loudly, and you may hear her sputtering to catch her breath at night. Doctors diagnose obstructive sleep apnea by history and physical examination, but they may want to confirm the diagnosis with an overnight study in a sleep laboratory (polysomnography). There technicians can monitor the child's breathing, heart rhythm, sleep cycles, and blood oxygen level.

Children with obstructive sleep apnea may suffer behavioral problems, bed-wetting, and poor school performance. Not all children with obstructive sleep apnea have enlarged tonsils; obesity causes the condition as well. In cases in which tonsillar enlargement does seem to be the cause, tonsillectomy often provides a cure.

Cancer of the tonsils is rare, but in cases in which one tonsil seems abnormally large, an otolaryngologist may want to remove it for biopsy. In some cases, surgery not only diagnoses the cancer, it cures it.

You should now be in a better position to help your child endure the numerous sore throats she is likely to suffer over the years. If you're lucky, she will never catch strep or require a tonsillectomy. She may well make the *Guinness Book of World Records* one day, but hopefully it will be for something more fun than having the world's largest tonsils. There's always Most Snails on the Face, set in 2009 by 11-year-old Fin Keheler of Sandy, UT. But remember, the snails have to stay on for 10 seconds.

22

what's the heading?
headaches and when to worry

fatherhood is immensely rewarding, but like every big endeavor it comes with its share of headaches—and sometime's they're not even yours! Headaches rank among the most common medical complaints of childhood. The vast majority of childhood headaches are harmless and go away on their own or with simple interventions. A few of them represent life-threatening conditions like meningitis, encephalitis, or brain tumors. Figuring out what to do is enough to make your head hurt.

stuff that makes your head hurt

Headache features prominently in many common childhood illnesses. Strep throat, influenza, mononucleosis, the common cold, and sinus infections all make kids' heads hurt. Many children suffer headaches any time they get a fever, regardless of the cause. Tooth grinding and cavities sometimes contribute to headaches as well. More rarely, conditions like high blood pressure *(hypertension),* obstructive sleep apnea, or systemic lupus erythematosus announce themselves with headache.

when to call the doctor
If your child seems unusually ill or if he has a fever for more than 3 days or a temperature above 104°F that won't come down 2 hours after treatment, call his doctor for advice.

284

22. What's the Heading? Headaches and When to Worry

standing at a tension

The majority of childhood headaches fall into the grab-bag category we call tension headaches. These headaches derive their name from the way they feel, like someone has tightened a band around the sufferer's head. The discomfort involves both sides of the head, not just one. It may be worse in the front of the head, but it can also extend into the muscles of the neck and shoulders. Early theories of headache attributed this pain to actual muscle tension, but more recent studies suggest that this theory is oversimplified and probably inaccurate, proving yet again that in medicine pretty much any nice, simple concept is bound to be wrong.

Triggers of tension headache abound, including but not limited to lack of sleep, hunger or thirst, exposure to bright light, and prolonged time spent in an awkward posture. While parents are quick to suspect vision problems as a cause of headache, they're rarely to blame. Of course, if your child is complaining of difficulty seeing, it's always wise to have a professional screen his vision.

Among the most common causes of tension headache is, you guessed it, tension, or in other words, psychological stress. Sometimes the cause of the stress is as obvious as difficulty with a subject at school or anxiety over a divorce. Other times it helps to have a doctor, psychologist, or counselor explore causes of your child's anxiety. When stress causes headaches, a variety of relaxation techniques provide powerful, non-medicinal relief.

Massaging the muscles of the head and neck can help relieve the pain, as can a short nap or applying a cool compress. Children who haven't eaten in more than 4 hours might try a little snack. Often these headaches will respond to an over-the-counter pain reliever like acetaminophen (eg, Tylenol), ibuprofen (eg, Advil, Motrin), or naproxen (eg, Aleve). Ironically, these medicines can sometimes be the cause of pain as well. Children who take a pain reliever more than 2 or 3 times a week may suffer from rebound headaches on the days they don't medicate. In these cases, just limiting a child's use of pain relievers can reduce his headache frequency.

when to call the doctor
If your child starts complaining of tension headaches more than 3 or 4 times a month, you should consult a doctor about possible causes and solutions.

your grain? no, migraine

In the past people assumed migraines were a privilege of adulthood, like paying taxes or growing ear hair. In fact, migraines are among the more common causes of headache in childhood, even affecting infants. Rates do rise with age, with only 1% to 2% of preschoolers suffering migraines as opposed to 15% of teenaged girls. Migraines usually manifest as severe headaches, but some children experience bizarre variations of migraines that include dizzy spells, repeated stomachaches, or even temporary partial paralysis.

Migraine headaches tend to recur over time. The pain may involve the whole head, but compared with pain from tension headaches, it's more likely to be one-sided. Children often have a hard time describing their pain, but a more verbal child may tell you the pain is pounding, throbbing, or stabbing. Headaches often last from an hour or two to a couple of days; pain may improve or go away completely with a nap. Migraines sometimes interfere with a child's ability to concentrate or make him sleepy. Many children with migraines find that bright lights and loud noises worsen their pain. Migraine pain may be severe enough to cause nausea or even vomiting, although any headache that makes a child vomit deserves medical evaluation.

The feature that most distinguishes migraine headaches is aura. Not all children with migraines experience aura, but those who do may report a strange sensation that tells them a headache is coming before the pain actually starts. They may experience smells, sounds, flashing lights, wavy lines in their vision, or dark areas in their eyesight preceding or accompanying the headache. An extreme version of aura carries the colorful name Alice in Wonderland syndrome, in which objects appear abnormally small, large, far away, or distorted in shape. Lewis Carroll, the author of *Alice's Adventures in Wonderland,* did in fact suffer from migraines, and scholars suspect Alice's story arose in part from Carroll's experience with aura.

With careful attention you can often identify a trigger for your child's migraines. Some common triggers, like changes in the weather, menstrual cycles, and exposure to strong smells, are hard or impossible to avoid. Up to 44% of children, however, are sensitive to certain foods, especially cheese, chocolate, and citrus fruits. Caffeine is another common headache

286

22. What's the Heading? Headaches and When to Worry

trigger. If you can find and eliminate one of these triggers, you can often dramatically cut the frequency of the headaches.

In many cases, keeping a headache diary reveals a previously invisible headache trigger. The diary should include details of the timing and severity of headaches as well as notes on sleep, activity, and diet. It's up to your child whether to also include his deepest hopes, dreams, and fears.

Genetics play a huge role in migraines. Migraines result from mutations in the genes that code for calcium channels in the nerve cells of the brain. These mutations cause changes in the way chemicals move in and out of brain cells, leading to a painful cascade of nerve signals, blood vessel changes, and inflammation. For almost every child with migraines you'll find at least one close relative with a history of severe, recurrent headaches. That relative may not even be aware that her headaches are migraines; many people attribute such pain to "sinuses" or, alternately, to their spouses.

Migraines often respond well to conventional medicines and alternative or non-medicine interventions. Many children get relief from taking acetaminophen, ibuprofen, or naproxen. The sooner they take the medicine after the onset of pain, the better it works. Ergotamine tartrate, once a popular prescription migraine therapy, is now rarely used, but it may still have a role in treating some sufferers.

A newer class of medications, the triptans (sumatriptan, zolmitriptan, naratriptan, rizatriptan), are designed specifically to treat migraine pain. Of these, only sumatriptan (eg, Imitrex) is Food and Drug Administration–approved for adolescents, and none are approved for children younger than 12 years. Studies, however, have shown these medicines to be safe for children, and doctors often prescribe them off-label. Sometimes, after using one of these medicines a few times, children report a dramatic decrease in the frequency of their headaches. Whatever pain reliever your child uses, remember to give it no more than twice a week to avoid rebound headaches.

When migraines occur more than 2 or 3 times a month, children can take a daily medicine to prevent them. These medicines are not pain-relievers; instead they affect brain cells to keep migraines from starting. Preventive medicines can be life-transforming for children whose headaches limit their participation in school or activities. Choices come from a variety of medication classes including blood pressure medicines like beta-blockers (propranolol) and calcium channel blockers (verapamil), antihistamines (cyproheptadine), antidepressants (amitriptyline), and seizure medications (topiramate, valproic acid, gabapentin).

None of these medicines is without side effects; your child's doctor will tailor a therapy that works best with your child's lifestyle and medical history. Usually with time, your child will find a medicine that keeps headaches from interfering with his life without causing significant problems. Whatever medicine he uses, your child probably will not need to take it for life. After a few months on the medicine, his doctor may advise weaning it slowly to see if headaches return. Depending on how bad headaches are, you might want to time this trial off medicine with a school break.

what you can do

Migraines respond especially well to complementary and alternative therapies. Sometimes these are as simple as making sure your child gets a good night's sleep and encouraging him to exercise. A variety of stress management techniques have proven helpful in controlling migraines, including guided imagery relaxation, self-hypnosis, and even yoga. Biofeedback, autogenic training, meditation, acupuncture, and massage therapy also reduce the frequency and severity of migraines for many patients. Some dietary supplements, particularly calcium, magnesium, and riboflavin (vitamin B$_2$), cut the severity of migraines as well. If you try any of these supplements for your child, remember that with medicines more is not better; stick with the recommended daily dose.

the fear is all in your head

When parents bring a child to the doctor for headaches, they're often hoping to hear Arnold Schwarzenegger's tagline from the 1990 comedy *Kindergarten Cop*: "It's not a tumor!" Brain tumors are certainly among the most frightening causes of headache, but there are a few other particularly dangerous possibilities doctors want to rule out. Infections of the brain tissue itself *(encephalitis)* or of the fluid and membranes around the brain *(meningitis)* require rapid diagnosis and treatment to avoid permanent

288

22. What's the Heading? Headaches and When to Worry

disability or death. Abnormal blood vessels, such as arteriovenous malformations (AVMs), may bleed or expand, putting pressure on critical brain structures. A variety of processes may lead fluid to collect around the brain, causing pressure to build up in the skull.

when to call the doctor

Some signs of headache should prompt you to get your child immediate medical care. If he is difficult to arouse, unconscious, confused, having trouble speaking or walking, or complaining of blurred or double vision, call emergency medical services (911). Fever, neck stiffness, vomiting, and pain with light suggest infections like meningitis or encephalitis, which should be treated immediately. A headache that comes on suddenly or is the most severe a child has ever had deserves prompt evaluation. Call your child's doctor if he has an isolated headache that lasts longer than 24 hours or a recurrent headache for more than 3 days.

Headache associated with personality changes, worsening school performance, or intermittent difficulty with tasks like walking, talking, or writing may not be an emergency, but it warrants medical attention. Doctors also worry about recurring headaches that worsen progressively, becoming more frequent or severe over a period of weeks to months. Headaches that awaken children from sleep or appear early in the morning also tend to peak a doctor's interest. Headache pain that worsens with cough or bending over suggests increased pressure inside the skull. As a general rule, any headache that is worse than what the child usually experiences should have you on the phone with the doctor's office.

a checkup from the neck up

A good medical history and physical examination remain the most important tools a doctor has to figure out the cause of a child's headaches. Your child's doctor will want to know when the headaches started, how often they happen, what they feel like, how severe they are, and whether they're getting better or worse. She'll ask about symptoms like fever, runny nose, nasal congestion, and cough as well as about appetite, abdominal pain, vomiting, diarrhea, and joint or muscle pain. Be honest about any stresses in the household, even if you think your child hasn't been paying attention to them. Ask close family members whether they've ever suffered from recurrent headaches.

The physical examination for headache may look like more of a game than a medical examination. The doctor will look inside the child's eyes for evidence of increased pressure in the brain and check the nose, ears, and mouth for signs of infection. She may even listen to the skull with her stethoscope for the sounds of an AVM. In addition to the usual heart, lung, and belly check, she'll also test the nervous system, starting with assessments of vision and hearing, and progressing to examine perception, strength, reflexes, and coordination in every part of the body.

She will ask your child to squint, raise his eyebrows, grin, and blow his cheeks out like a frog. He'll shrug his shoulders, grab the doctor's fingers, raise his legs, and walk on his tiptoes. The doctor will tickle the soles of his feet and ask him to touch his nose, then reach out to touch her finger and go back again. He'll have to stand up straight with his eyes closed and pretend to walk a tightrope. The whole process takes several minutes, and it looks like a game of Simon Says—if Simon were deranged.

After going through all this, very few children need any imaging studies. Brain tumors usually produce abnormalities on the physical examination within 6 months, so if your child has been having headaches for a year and has a normal neurologic examination, you can feel comfortable it's not a tumor. If the doctor does find something that concerns her, she may order a computed tomography scan, magnetic resonance imaging, or a study of the blood vessels in the brain called an angiogram. She may perform a lumbar puncture (spinal tap) if she suspects meningitis or encephalitis. For a lumbar puncture, the doctor introduces a needle into the lower part of the spinal column to withdraw a sample of the fluid that surrounds the brain and spinal cord. This procedure remains the only accurate way to diagnose and treat infections of the brain and surrounding tissues.

hardheaded

There are really only 2 wrong ways to respond when your child hits his head—overreact and underreact. Avoid those and you'll do fine. But then I suppose you'll be wanting more details.

The only 2 things required for a child to sustain a head injury are a head and momentum. Often, gravity provides the momentum, but if your child

290

22. What's the Heading? Headaches and When to Worry

is moving in any direction at all, he is at risk for a head bonk. Toddlers, for example, are guaranteed to fall and hit their heads repeatedly while they're learning to walk. Their heads start so close to the ground, however, that they rarely pick up enough speed to injure themselves. Other types of head trauma warrant a bit more concern.

Scalp injuries seem designed to freak parents out. The scalp carries a rich blood supply, meaning that even minor cuts tend to produce a lot of bleeding. Just as with any other laceration, you'll want to apply pressure to stop the bleeding and do your best to clean the wound. Applying an ice pack may serve 2 purposes, relieving pain and slowing the bleeding at the same time.

when to call the doctor

Once you can see a scalp cut well, you can assess whether it looks deep enough to need closure with stitches, staples, or surgical glue. If you're in doubt, get your child to a doctor to have the wound examined as soon as possible.

Scalp bruises can look ugly, and they take weeks to heal. Over a few days the blood from the bruise may drain down into the tissues of the eyelids, causing a black eye. Blood from the bruise may also collect into a firm mass, a goose egg that shrinks over a matter of weeks to months. A goose egg on the forehead rarely signifies a serious injury.

Skull fractures are frightening, but fortunately they're also rare, complicating only 1% to 2% of pediatric head injuries. Fractures occur more commonly on the sides of the head, where the thinner parietal and temporal bones lie. The frontal bone of the forehead and the occipital bone in the back of the head are thicker and less likely to break. If you see a goose egg on the side of your child's head you should have a doctor evaluate him; he may have a fracture under the bruise. Likewise, if you feel a dent in the child's head or if he has swelling more than about an inch across, a doctor should see him.

Most skull fractures heal on their own without intervention, but if your child's doctor diagnoses a fracture, she may want to observe the child overnight in the hospital. Skull fractures that are depressed into the brain tissue or that break the skin require a neurosurgeon's attention.

when to call the doctor

Other reasons to get your child evaluated include a fall from a height of 3 feet (younger than 2 years) or 5 feet (older than 2). Any significant impact to an infant's head deserves a medical examination. You should also have your child seen if he's struck in the head by a hard object traveling at high speed like, say, a baseball bat. Watch for clear fluid dripping from the nose or ears; in fractures of the base of the skull, fluid may leak from around the brain.

A child who sustains a blow to the head risks concussion, a mild brain injury that alters brain function. Attitudes toward concussion have transformed in recent years as we've learned from studies of injured athletes and soldiers how serious these injuries can actually be. In past decades, for example, a football player who sustained a concussion might be sent right back into play so long as he could walk. We now know that repeated concussions can lead to permanent brain damage and even sudden death. Dozens of states have passed laws mandating that coaches remove athletes from play as soon as they sustain a concussion, keeping them out until they receive proper medical evaluation.

when to call the doctor

Some signs of concussion are obvious. If your child or teen loses consciousness after a blow to the head, even briefly, he should see a doctor. If he remains unconscious or is hard to wake up for more than a minute, call emergency medical services (EMS) (911). Other reasons to call EMS include seizures, any suspicion of neck injury (do not move the child or let him turn his head until EMS arrives), confusion, slurred speech, unsteady gait, or weakness or numbness in the arms or legs.

Vomiting is another hard-to-miss sign of concussion, although you don't necessarily need to call emergency medical services (911) unless the child vomits repeatedly. Other, more subtle symptoms of concussion include headache, confusion, dizziness, blurred vision, difficulty remembering

292

22. What's the Heading? Headaches and When to Worry

things, problems concentrating, and personality changes such as depression and aggression. While some kids recover quickly from concussion, others need weeks or longer to return to full function.

when to call the doctor

If you even suspect your child has had a concussion, he should see a doctor. Resuming mental or physical exercise too early prolongs the symptoms of the concussion and, if it exposes the child to another injury, may endanger his life. Don't let your child do homework, run around, or even play challenging video games until instructed by his doctor.

In addition to the neurologic examination described previously, the doctor will also put the child through a battery of tests to assess his mental function. Many of the problems children with concussions suffer are subtle, and formal tests of memory and concentration help identify them. If your child is going to participate in contact sports, consider having him complete one of these questionnaires beforehand so you'll know where he's starting. More teams are actually doing this as a preseason routine. You can download the most popular of these tools, the SCAT 2 test, at http://sportsconcussions.org/coaches.html.

You should keep your child home for 24 hours after the accident so you can keep an eye on him. You're watching for worsening headache, confusion, nausea, vomiting, dizziness, vision changes, or any other sign he's getting worse. If these occur, of course, you'll call his doctor.

You're prepared now to deal with any number of headaches your child might tell you about. While this chapter is not meant to be a comprehensive textbook of neurology, hopefully it has at least given you a… wait for it…heads-up.

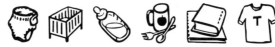

what you can do

Many people believe that if a child injures his head you must keep him awake all night. This is a false belief, popularized, I can only assume, by coffee manufacturers. You should observe your child closely for 2 hours after the initial injury, encouraging him to lie down and rest somewhere you can keep an eye on him. After the first 2 hours, do wake him up and make sure he can walk and talk normally. During that period, hold off on giving any pain medicines or food in case he vomits. Do have him sleep in the same room with you for the next couple of nights so you'll be nearby if he develops a bad headache, vomiting, or confusion. You might wake him up once in the middle of the first night to make sure he's OK.

23

making the grade:
when to worry about ADHD

when parents come to me worried about their child's behavior
or school performance, they often express concern that the child will be
"labeled" as having attention-deficit/hyperactivity disorder (ADHD). To
be honest, I've tried many times to label a kid with ADHD, but no matter
what I do it seems as soon as the child takes a bath, the label falls right off.
The fact is that ADHD is a real condition that affects between 4% and
12% of school-aged children. Whatever stigma may have attached itself
to the problem in past decades has fallen off as surely as a damp sticker.
Of course, I also have skin in this game—I am the father of a child
with ADHD.

where's my disorder?

When someone at a party asks me, "What is ADHD anyway?" I make
sure he has a full glass and a plate of hors d'oeuvres before I answer; we're
going to be there a while. The first thing to know is that ADHD is real, not
just a term used to medicalize normal childhood behavior or throw drugs
at kids who just need a little discipline. A description of the behaviors that
underlie ADHD first appeared in the medical literature in 1798. ADHD
medications came into use in 1937, although we've refined them a bit since

then. More recently, brain imaging technology has given researchers a window into the precise differences in brain anatomy and activity associated with the symptoms of ADHD.

At its heart, ADHD is a failure to inhibit impulses and attend to tasks. Attention is a complex process or, more accurately, a group of processes that demand coordination among several brain regions. Say, for example, you want to read a book. You have to remember where the book is, which depends on your keeping it in a predictable place or making note of where you last put it away. You have to shift your attention from whatever you were doing previously to focus on reading. As you read, you have to remember what the last sentence said to make sense of the next one. To get through a chapter you must not listen to the conversation of the couple next to you, watch boys throw a ball outside, or jump up every few seconds to add radishes to your grocery list. Each of these tasks requires a specific type of mental effort; a lapse in any one of them will prevent you from getting anything out of the book.

Kids with ADHD have changes in their brain chemicals and structures that make them less able than other children to attend to one task or control their impulses. These changes are often inherited. It's not unusual for a parent, on learning his child has ADHD, to realize he has it too. Close relatives of children with ADHD are about 5 times more likely than average to also have the condition. Other processes that affect brain development can increase a child's risk of having ADHD. Children who are born prematurely, even just a little, carry a higher risk for ADHD. Maternal alcohol and drug use during pregnancy also raises a child's risk for the condition, as do malnutrition, lead poisoning, and, rarely, head trauma or exposure to other environmental toxins. Studies suggest that even excessive television or video game use may affect brain development in ways that lead to ADHD.

Being common and complicated, ADHD has given rise to a number of harmful myths. My favorite is, "My child can spend hours playing video games, so he must not have ADHD." This misunderstanding keeps some kids from getting the help they need. In truth, video games seem designed to appeal most to children who have attention problems—they are full of constantly changing stimuli and frequent rewards. ADHD makes it difficult for kids to focus on things that might potentially be boring, like math problems or reading assignments, not exciting tasks like blasting aliens or racing cars.

Other myths harm children by labeling them with terms much worse than ADHD. People may accuse a child with ADHD of being "lazy," assuming that the spread between her obvious intelligence and lousy grades results from a lack of effort. The truth is that kids with ADHD can sometimes overcome their inability to focus with sheer intelligence during the first few years of school, but as schoolwork demands longer periods of concentration, it ultimately overwhelms even the most brilliant child.

People may attribute the problems of ADHD to a child's personality, saying the child is a "dreamer" or "wide open." When that dreaming keeps a child from passing math or the wide-open kid spends half his time in time-out for constantly breaking household rules, however, these children assume their problems are hopeless, rather than symptoms of a treatable condition. We don't treat ADHD to squelch a child's personality but to let that personality flourish in more productive avenues.

Blaming the parents inflicts similar harm. Children with ADHD often pose disciplinary challenges for parents, but imperfect parental discipline doesn't cause the condition. Parents often feel relieved to learn a child's behavior is caused by his ADHD and not just a sign that they're miserable failures. Inconsistent discipline can certainly worsen ADHD symptoms, and many children with ADHD benefit from being in a structured environment. Making an accurate diagnosis gives doctors an opportunity to help parents tailor their discipline techniques to their child's particular needs.

Another myth is that children take medicine to "cure" their ADHD. Over time some children do develop mechanisms to compensate for ADHD, but the condition is chronic, lifelong for many. ADHD is not like an infection for which you take 10 days' worth of antibiotics and it's gone. It's more like asthma or diabetes, conditions that usually respond very well to medical control but are unlikely to just go away one day.

A final myth is that if a child doesn't meet criteria for ADHD after an evaluation, she doesn't require any special help. Learning and concentration are complex processes, and many factors can make them more challenging for some children. If your child seems to have problems with behavior or schoolwork, continue working with appropriate professionals to help her reach the full potential you know she has.

how will i know?

The core symptoms of ADHD include *inattention, impulsivity,* and *hyperactivity.* One feature of ADHD that frustrates parents and doctors is that there is no single test to determine who has the condition and who doesn't. ADHD remains a descriptive diagnosis, which doesn't mean it can't be made accurately, just that it requires a lot of question-asking to make. To some extent the diagnosis of ADHD always remains subjective, depending in part on the judgment of observers.

How soon a child gets diagnosed with ADHD depends on how that child manifests the condition. That, in turn, often depends on the child's sex. Boys are 3 times more likely than girls to be diagnosed with ADHD, and they tend to be younger when they're diagnosed. Boys with ADHD are much more likely than girls to display poor impulse control. They may act out, disobey teachers and parents, have trouble getting along with other children, injure themselves, and break stuff. There's nothing like getting suspended from kindergarten to get you some medical attention. Girls, on the other hand, are more likely to manifest their ADHD with poor attention. They often do fine in school until the work starts to require prolonged periods of concentration, usually around third or fourth grade. Then, when their grades start to fall off, someone may bring up ADHD testing.

Technically the diagnosis of ADHD follows criteria laid out in the most recent edition of the *Diagnostic and Statistical Manual of Mental Disorders (DSM),* the book doctors and psychiatric professionals use to categorize the conditions they treat. Diagnosis begins when someone who interacts with a child regularly suspects she may have ADHD. Many times this person is a teacher because school is the environment most likely to make prolonged demands on the child's attention. Some parents worry that a teacher will "diagnose" their child with ADHD, but only a medical or psychological professional can make that diagnosis. A teacher's input is critical to the process, but some teachers identify up to 15% of students as possibly having ADHD; many fewer kids actually end up being treated for the condition.

You have to take a child's age into account when diagnosing ADHD. To pose a concern, her behavior should be unusual compared with her peers. Can your 3-year-old not sit still for 5 minutes? Neither can anyone else's! That's not ADHD. Does your 7-year-old have to pop up out of her chair every 20 seconds? Now you're talking. To have ADHD a child should display at least some symptoms before age 7. A child may end up being diagnosed with ADHD in preschool, but often the more structured demands of kindergarten or grade school alert teachers and parents a child may need evaluation. Symptoms also need to continue for at least 6 months. Any child is allowed a brief rough spot.

To count as significant, symptoms have to interfere with the child's function during daily life. Usually when a child has ADHD, her behavior will cause problems at school, at home, and with friends on a regular basis. If a child is doing well in all these arenas, it's hard to say that whatever inattention she may have deserves medical intervention. Problems from ADHD should be frequent and persistent. Even the best kids have bad days, but that doesn't mean they have ADHD.

The behavior also must occur in more than one environment. A child who does great at home, summer camp, and her friend's sleepover may be making poor grades, but it's probably not because she has ADHD. As part of the evaluation, her doctor will insist on collecting information from observers in at least 2 environments that demand attention and impulse control. One of those environments should always be school, although when children are homeschooled, defining what is home and what is school may require clarification.

To be ADHD the child's behavior should not be due to another cause. This rule seems kind of obvious, but in practice it's one of the higher hurdles to accurate diagnosis of ADHD. The evaluation of ADHD must include a search for other physical and social problems that may be contributing to the child's behavior. Kids' school performance can suffer for any number of reasons, including but not limited to poor vision or hearing; a learning disorder; depression; sleep deprivation; malnutrition; excessive time with computers, video games, or television; anxiety; bullying; an undiagnosed seizure disorder; a brain tumor; or drug use. Some children perform poorly in school not because they have ADHD but because they are cognitively challenged; IQ testing helps identify these children to make sure they get appropriate help. Children also vary in their normal development; some are just better at some stuff than others!

As you might imagine, a doctor evaluating a child for ADHD must collect a lot of information from a lot of people. To simplify the process, doctors usually rely on one of several questionnaires. The most popular include the American Academy of Pediatrics (AAP) National Initiative for Children's Healthcare Quality (NICHQ) Vanderbilt ADHD assessment scales, Conners parent and teacher rating scales, Child Behavior Checklist, Parents' Evaluation of Developmental Status (PEDS), and Barkley home and school situations questionnaires. These instruments vary by the age of child they're designed to assess and environment in which they are to be used, but they all are designed to rank children's behavior based on the *DSM* criteria for ADHD.

Questionnaires are only one part of making a diagnosis of ADHD. The visit also requires an extensive medical history, looking for risk factors for ADHD as well as other possible contributors to the child's behavioral problems. Preterm birth, a pending divorce, or a parent's history of ADHD all matter in making the diagnosis. The physical examination is also comprehensive, including measurements of height and weight, a vision and hearing screen, a routine medical examination, and a thorough neurologic examination. Your child doesn't need to display ADHD behavior during the examination any more than she has to cough during an evaluation for asthma. The doctor's office is a very different place from school or home, and the doctor knows that.

Blood tests, electroencephalograms, and imaging examinations still have no place in the routine diagnosis of ADHD unless the history and physical examination suggest another illness that deserves investigation. Recently, software developers have designed computerized systems that claim to make the diagnosis of ADHD using technology. While these systems may help clarify the diagnosis, nothing takes the place of a comprehensive history and examination.

A child with ADHD may fall into 1 of 3 different diagnostic categories based on whether inattention, hyperactivity, or impulsivity seem to dominate her behavior. *Inattentive-only* ADHD predominates in girls. These children seem to daydream rather than listen. They don't appear to attend well to details, and careless errors pull their grades down. They may fail to follow through, forget important facts, and avoid activities that require sustained concentration. If your child doesn't call to tell you she forgot her homework because she also forgot your phone number, she might fall into this category.

Children with *hyperactive/impulsive* ADHD actually pay attention well, but they have difficulty inhibiting their own behavior. They seem impatient, talk too much, act out, and have a tough time taking turns. These children seem full of more energy than they know what to do with. While this is actually the smallest group of kids with ADHD, they tend to come to medical attention earliest, as you might imagine. If you've resorted to using only plastic cups and plates in your house, this is probably your kid.

Children with *combined inattentive/hyperactive/impulsive* ADHD obviously display all of the previous traits. Many parents assume any child with ADHD must fall into this category, but it's useful to know whether your child truly displays all 3 symptom types or only 1 or 2. She will be able to leverage the areas where she's strongest to help her overcome difficulties stemming from areas she finds more challenging.

The diagnostic process doesn't stop just with identifying and categorizing ADHD. Many children with ADHD face more than one challenge to their function; having ADHD actually raises a child's risk of having other behavioral problems as well. We call these *coexisting conditions*. The questionnaires used for ADHD diagnosis include sections designed to screen for these problems as well.

One group of coexisting conditions, learning disabilities, make it harder for kids to master the skills required to perform their schoolwork. Even with perfect attention and impulse control, some children suffer from problems like dyslexia that make it difficult for them to read, write, or understand math. Psychologists, teachers, and guidance counselors use a variety of tests, including IQ tests, to identify these problems.

Mood disorders such as depression affect around 18% of children with ADHD. Sometimes depression results from the ADHD itself, as children start to feel their poor grades and propensity for getting in trouble make them less worthwhile. Mood disorders can also be inherited or arise from other life stressors. Affected children require separate counseling and medication to cope with these problems.

Anxiety plagues up to a quarter of children with ADHD. They may experience chest tightness, headaches, nausea, racing pulse, or irrational feelings of worry or panic. Just as with depression, separate counseling and medication can alleviate these sometimes crippling symptoms.

Oppositional-defiant disorder and conduct disorder represent 2 closely related and challenging problems that affect up to 35% of children with ADHD. The behaviors associated with these disorders may look a lot like uncontrolled ADHD, but they can persist after other symptoms of ADHD have come under good control. Kids with oppositional-defiant disorder treat authority figures with disdain and hostility well beyond the usual boundary testing expected of growing children. They may also exhibit uncontrolled anger outbursts and annoy others on purpose. These are normal behaviors for any child sometimes, but kids with the disorder take them to extremes. Conduct disorder can be summed up as doing unto others what you would not have them do unto you. Affected children break rules, destroy property, and violate others' rights. Either of these disorders can land children in trouble with the law and deserve intensive counseling for the child and family.

action figures

So once you've determined a child has ADHD and you've identified other coexisting conditions, what's next? ADHD is a complex condition that affects multiple aspects of a child's life. An appropriate treatment plan involves not just the doctor but a whole team including parents, teachers, other caregivers, counselors, and most importantly, your child.

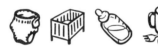

what you can do

The first step in therapy is to identify specific, measurable problems you and your child would like to see improve. "She should act better" is not a goal. "We would like her to remember to bring her homework folder to school every day this week" is. Goals don't have to be academic. They may involve family relationships, friendships, self-esteem, or even accidental injuries.

Team members should decide what sort of monitoring will be appropriate; if you don't know what you're watching for, how will you know she's doing better? Grades are an obvious measure of performance, but you could also keep track of other behaviors, like whether your child picks up her dirty clothes or how often she hits her brother. You'll also want to determine a follow-up schedule for your child. When you're starting therapy she may need to see the doctor or a counselor every couple of weeks. As a rule, your child should go no more than 6 months between evaluations.

Education plays a huge role in managing ADHD. Not only do you and your child need to learn as much as you can about the condition, but siblings, teachers, and friends may also need to be brought up to speed. Family counseling can help parents learn discipline techniques that are especially effective with ADHD. Siblings may feel like the affected child "gets away with everything" because she has ADHD, and they can learn what expectations are appropriate as well as work through any anger or discomfort they may feel about the condition.

Behavior therapy is a useful extension of this counseling. A variety of therapeutic techniques may help, but many therapists now favor an approach called *cognitive-behavioral therapy.* Cognitive-behavioral therapy focuses on constructive actions people can take to cope with situations as they arise, and it has proven effective in multiple well-conducted trials. Therapy, however, is only one component of effective ADHD management. Behavior therapy alone tends to achieve only marginal improvements in ADHD when not combined with medication.

Your child's school should participate actively in the treatment team. Children with ADHD may benefit from special accommodations like sitting in the front of the classroom or taking tests in an environment with minimal distractions. Children with ADHD often respond very well to one-on-one instruction. Depending on your child's diagnosis and

what you can do

There are several ways you as a parent can help your child with ADHD succeed. One is to provide a strong sense of structure in the household. Do your best to maintain a stable bedtime, wake-up time, and meal plan for your child. Your expectations of her behavior should be clear, and she should have no trouble understanding what positive and negative consequences to expect (see Chapter 16). Take every opportunity to focus on what she does well. If she cleans up her room, plays a game of cards with her brother, or makes a better than expected grade, be sure she knows how proud of her you are. The more she succeeds, the more she will envision herself as someone who succeeds.

coexisting conditions, she may qualify by federal law for an Individual Education Plan (IEP) that spells out what measures the school will take to help her. Make sure you sit down with her teacher and school guidance counselor after she is diagnosed to coordinate your efforts and make sure your child is getting the most out of her educational environment.

Focus, too, on her strengths. ADHD often frees children up to solve problems in less conventional, more creative ways than kids without the disorder. Let her know how much you appreciate the special skills and talents she brings to the world not just in spite of her ADHD, but because of it.

pharm hands

As a pediatrician and parent of a child with ADHD, I understand why many parents feel conflicted about using medication to treat the disorder. Some parents express immense relief that they finally have a way to help their children. Others flat-out reject the prospect of treating a behavioral disorder with medicine on philosophic or religious grounds. ADHD researchers have worked for decades exploring potential nonmedical approaches to treating the disorder. So far medications are the only treatments that have proven broadly successful in treating ADHD. Let's take a moment to review the very valid concerns parents may have about ADHD medication.

- *"I don't want to change my child's personality."* When doctors or psychiatric professionals talk about personality, we use the term emotional range to describe how far apart a person's highs and lows are. A child with a wide range may squeal with glee when she's happy and bawl with grief when she's sad. If a child's range includes uncontrollable and destructive behavior, the medicine is supposed to help her rein in those actions. But if your child's personality seems "flat" or she seems withdrawn when she's taking medicine, she may be on the wrong medicine or too high a dose. Her doctor will ask you about her personality and help you find a treatment regimen that helps your child focus without robbing her of the individualism you cherish.

  Some children grow moody or irritable when they're first starting medicine for ADHD, especially at night when the medicine is wearing off. This side effect usually fades after a week or two of regular dosing, although it may return with dosage increases and medication changes. Your child's doctor should be monitoring this symptom at follow-up visits. If it fails to go away, a dosage adjustment or medication change may be in order.

- *"I've heard that ADHD medications stunt children's growth."* Many ADHD medications can suppress a child's appetite. This effect often is strongest when a child is first starting the medicine or increasing her dose. Among the most important things your child's doctor will do at follow-up is plot her weight and height, making sure she's still eating all she needs to grow and develop normally.

- *"I've heard that the medicines cause headaches, abdominal pain, insomnia, or sleepiness."* You've heard right. Those are all potential side effects of ADHD medications. Most of these side effects fade over the course of a couple of weeks following the start of a new medication or dose adjustment, but they are all symptoms your child's doctor should be following and taking into account as you craft an effective treatment plan.

- *"If my child takes drugs for ADHD, she's more likely to drink, smoke, or take recreational drugs."* This fear is not only unfounded, it's actually backward. Teens and adults with ADHD do indeed face an increased risk of substance abuse compared with the general population. They're also more likely to experience unintended pregnancy, traffic accidents, and legal trouble. Avoiding all these consequences involves strong impulse control, attention, and appropriate understanding of the consequences of behavior. The better controlled a person's ADHD is, the better her chances are of making sound decisions.

- *"I don't want my child to be on this medicine forever."* Treating ADHD doesn't make it last any longer than not treating it. ADHD is a chronic condition that often continues to affect people's lives well into adulthood. The parts of the brain that handle impulse control and decision-making are the last to develop, still growing well into a person's late teens and early twenties. Some children with ADHD do ultimately develop good-enough focus to stop using medications. Others use the time they're on the medicine to develop coping strategies they can leverage when they're not taking it. The advantage of being an adult is that you have more choice about how you spend your day; rather than following a school curriculum, an adult with ADHD can enter a field where she can capitalize on the strengths the condition lends her, such as increased creativity or energy.

- *"I read that ADHD can be controlled with a gluten-free diet/sugar-free diet/organic diet/applied kinesiology/sensory integration therapy/visual training/chiropractic manipulation/megadoses of vitamins/sound therapy/ balance training...."* The search for nonmedical alternatives to ADHD management has been exhaustive, and alternative therapies all have their advocates, many well-meaning but some downright fraudulent. Of all the alternative treatments attempted so far for ADHD, only one has withstood any sort of rigorous scientific study, and that is eliminating certain dietary allergens. This approach, however, works for only a very small minority of ADHD patients, and it can involve radical lifestyle changes. Before you launch on such an endeavor, consider involving a licensed allergy specialist to discuss the pros and cons of elimination diets.

As for all the other stuff, the first question to ask of any therapy is, "Does solid science tell us this is safe and effective?" Anyone can show success at anything in a small, uncontrolled study or a handful of case reports. Your child's doctor should be willing to look over any literature you hand him and help you assess its validity. In the meantime, be aware that withholding effective ADHD therapy from an affected child is not without cost. Every day her symptoms continue unabated she is failing to learn, interact with her peers, and participate in her family life as fully as she might.

Most medications for ADHD fall into 1 of 2 classes of stimulants—those based on methylphenidate (eg, Ritalin, Methylin, Metadate, Focalin, Concerta) and those based on amphetamine (eg, Dexedrine, Dextrostat, Adderall). You might ask, "Why give a kid a stimulant when it seems like stimulation is the problem?" The answer has to do with what part of the brain these drugs stimulate. At the doses used for ADHD management, these drugs target the parts of the brain associated with concentration and behavior control. About 80% of children with ADHD show a dramatic positive response to stimulant medications.

Some children seem to respond better to methylphenidate-based drugs, while others do better on dextroamphetamine. Figuring out which kind works best for which child remains a matter of trial and error. The drugs in each category differ from each other mainly in duration of action. Some stimulants are designed to start working quickly and stick around for only around 4 hours. Others are engineered to last for 8, 10, even 14 hours. In tailoring a therapy for your child, her doctor will pay special attention to what times of day seem to be the best and worst for her. A child who does great all day at school and then tanks when it's time for her to do her homework may need a longer-acting medicine or a short-acting medicine to take at lunchtime, for example.

Non-stimulant medications for ADHD are also available, although it's not clear they are as useful for as many children. Atomoxetine (eg, Strattera) is a member of the antipsychotic class that has had some success in controlling ADHD symptoms. Another option is a long-acting version of the blood pressure medicine guanfacine (eg, Intuniv). Many doctors combine guanfacine with stimulant medications to better control symptoms of hyperactivity or help children who seem to have trouble sleeping when they take stimulants. Another blood pressure medicine, clonidine, has similar effects to guanfacine.

Children with ADHD have a real medical condition with very real consequences at school, among friends, within the family, and in life. A holistic approach to therapy involves a team of parents, teachers, health professionals, and especially the child, all focused on helping the child succeed in showing the world all she has to offer. If your child is to have a label it will probably be one of her own startlingly original design, applied with a novel, bath-resistant adhesive.

24

electronica: television, computers, video games, and mobile phones

I've often asked myself why we insist our children go play outside. Fresh air? Full of wasps. Sunshine? Can you say, "Skin cancer"? Grass between your toes? Sure, if you can feel it for all the splinters! Of course if you keep kids indoors, it's just one mess after another, what with all that playing and exploring they do. No, the only way to keep children quiet, happy, and clean is to sit them down with some good old-fashioned electronic entertainment. Between handheld gaming devices, Internet-enabled game consoles, laptop computers, DVD players, streaming video, mobile phones, and the thousand or so channels on television (TV), they need never scrape a single knee or suffer their first mosquito bite. Today's kids (and their parents) have it made!

Or do they? Used wisely, electronic media can teach our children lessons about social behavior, help them master some academic and motor skills, and even get them to exercise. Electronic media also can worsen every problem that plagues today's children—promiscuity, smoking, drug use, obesity, eating disorders, violence, depression, and poor school performance. Children absorb everything they experience, and media are incredibly powerful tools for shaping a child's thoughts and behavior. How you address media use may ultimately determine whether your child lives out his dreams or your nightmares. But hey, no pressure.

neither einstein nor mozart watched videos

Parents are often shocked when I tell them that pediatricians think it's a bad idea for children to watch TV before age 2. Surveys tell us about 40% of infants are watching some sort of video by age 5 months, and by age 2 the number rises to 90%. They seem to enjoy it, after all, so where's the harm? What if parents limit the viewing to educational shows? What don't pediatricians understand about "educational"?

To answer these questions we have to return briefly to the child's developing brain (for the full tour, see Chapter 2). Kids' brains grow profoundly during the first 3 years of life, with the brain tripling in mass in just the first 12 months. The stimuli children experience during this period profoundly influence brain development. Images on screens behave in ways that differ dramatically from those in the real world. Because we're all steeped in the visual language of screens, it's easy to forget those differences until we think about them.

Imagine a ball in real life and a ball on TV. Infants are developing 3-dimensional vision. The world of the screen exists in 2 dimensions, so the ball is just a flat, shaded circle. If you roll a ball across the floor it proceeds in a single motion, slowing gradually until it stops. The same action on TV is broken up—you see the ball leave someone's hand, then there's a shot of it in motion, then a picture of the ball at rest. If your infant wants to grab a ball in real life he'll lunge for it, grasp at it, or crawl after it. The stuff on the screen just disappears, to be replaced by other stuff; you can never get your hands (or mouth) on it. Infants may stare at the bright colors and motion on a screen, but their brains are incapable of making sense or meaning out of all those bizarre pictures. It takes 2 full years for a baby's brain to develop to the point where the symbols on a screen come to represent their equivalents in the real world.

Because of this confusion, children up to age 3 learn better from the real world than they do from any screen, especially when it comes to language. They do seem to learn a little more if they're watching in the company of a person who is talking to them about what they're seeing, in the same way you would while looking at a picture book.

So sure, babies and toddlers don't get anything out of watching TV, but if they seem to like it, where's the harm? If a little TV is what it takes for you to get dinner on the table, isn't it better for them than, say, starving? Yes, watching TV is better than starving, but it's worse than not watching TV. Good evidence suggests that screen viewing before age 2 has lasting negative effects on children's language development, reading skills, and short-term memory. It also contributes to problems with sleep and attention. If "you are what you eat," then the brain is what it experiences, and video entertainment is like mental junk food for babies and toddlers.

The problem lies not only with what toddlers are doing while they're watching TV; it's what they aren't doing. Specifically, children are programmed to learn from interacting with other people. The dance of facial expressions, tone of voice, and body language between a toddler and parent is not only beautiful, it's so complex that researchers have to record these interactions on video and slow them down just to see everything that's going on. Whenever one party in this dance, child or parent, is watching TV, the exchange comes to a halt. A toddler learns a lot more from banging pans on the floor while you cook dinner than he does from watching a screen for the same amount of time, because every now and then the 2 of you look at each other.

Just having the TV on in the background, even if "no one is watching it," is enough to delay language development. Normally a parent speaks about 940 words per hour when a toddler is around. With the television on, that number falls by 770! Fewer words means less learning.

Toddlers are also learning to pay attention for prolonged periods. Toddlers who watch more TV are more likely to have problems paying attention at age 7. Video programming is constantly changing, constantly interesting, and almost never forces a child to deal with anything more tedious than an infomercial.

After age 2 things change, at least somewhat. During the preschool years some children do learn some skills from educational TV. Well-designed shows can teach kids literacy, math, science, problem-solving, and pro-social behavior. Children get more out of interactive programs like *Dora the Explorer* and *Sesame Street* when they answer the characters' questions. Educational TV makes the biggest difference for children whose homes are the least intellectually stimulating.

what you can do

Naturally, children learn more when they watch TV with a parent than if they watch alone. Content matters, a lot. All programs educate kids about something, but stick with ones that are designed to teach children stuff they should actually know. Regardless of content, cap your child's TV time at 2 hours a day. Remember, too, TV is still TV whether you actually watch it on a TV screen or on a mobile phone or computer.

media, myself, and i

When thinking about the effect of media on school-aged children, it's easy for parents to underestimate just how intensely virtual experience shapes a child's world view. For one thing, even if you think you watched a lot of TV or played a lot of video games when you were growing up, today's kids are in a whole different league. According to the Kaiser Family Foundation, children's average media consumption rose from 7.5 hours a day in 1999 to 10.75 hours a day in 2010. That means media now take up more hours of a child's life than any other activity, including sleep. That sort of impact is bound to leave a mark.

Children are also more susceptible than adults to virtual experience. Their brains are growing, and their reality-testing skills are still developing. You can tell them the stuff on TV is make-believe all you want, and they may even understand it at some level, but at a deeper level our brains never evolved to cope with any experience more virtual than the village storyteller weaving a yarn by the campfire. To understand how media can so profoundly influence a child's world view, it helps to know a little about the mirror neuron system.

When we witness an action by another person, a certain portion of our brain dedicates itself to mimicking that action. If you ever find yourself echoing the last few words someone else just said or balling your fists up while watching a fight, you've seen the system at work. When we see another person's face express sadness or joy, our own face reflects that expression unconsciously, helping us grasp what that person is feeling.

The mirror neuron system plays an enormous role in learning and understanding others' emotions.

We can't turn our mirror neurons off when we turn the TV on. In fact, much of what we enjoy about entertainment is the sense of losing ourselves. For the duration of a movie we are the ones who battle the bad guys and get the girl, at least in our own minds. Video games traffic in an even more immersive experience. To some extent, you could define entertainment as the purposeful stimulation of the mirror neuron system to experience sensations our own lives don't necessarily provide.

Children's brains are remarkably plastic. They are wired to learn from everything, and learning involves rewiring neurons. When kids watch TV or play a video game, their brains are programming themselves based on these virtual experiences. That's not a process that just stops because the experience isn't "real." As far as the child's brain is concerned, it's real enough. Learning alters behavior, and behaviors have consequences. As we'll see later in the chapter, helping your child make healthy choices in media use makes a very real difference in outcomes that are not at all virtual.

vampire sex ed

I'm going to go out on a limb here and assume you want your child to grow up understanding that sex is a deeply emotional expression of love between 2 mature people who have taken time to build a relationship of trust and intimacy. You probably want him to wait to have sex until he's mature enough to understand the full implications of sexual activity, including the substantial risks of sexually transmitted infections (STIs), unintended pregnancy, and emotional trauma. If these are your goals, media can be your worst enemy or, if you use them right, a powerful ally.

Around 70% of TV shows US children and teens watch include sexual content—more, in fact, than programs targeted to adults. Fewer than 14% of these shows ever demonstrate the consequences of these encounters, although there are now at least a couple of reality shows about little else. Let's face it—few people want to watch the beautiful stars of their favorite prime-time dramas deal with chlamydia and pregnancy. Children who watch sexual content earlier are more likely to have sex at a younger age than children whose parents limit their access to such shows. Children and teens who watch more sexual content also suffer higher rates of unplanned pregnancies and STIs.

Television, of course, is just the start. Nearly half of Internet users between the ages of 10 and 17 have seen pornography online. Twenty percent of mobile phone users aged 13 to 19 have sent sexually explicit messages, and 40% have received them. Among older adolescents with social media profiles on sites like Facebook, nearly a quarter posted references to sex. Every parent fears that some sexual predator will use the Internet to victimize his child, but while real, those fears don't reflect the more common reality—we have to teach our children not to use the media to victimize themselves.

what you can do

In the same way that watching *Sesame Street* with your preschooler helps him learn to read, watching *True Blood* with your teen helps him make sense of the sex he sees on the screen. Take time during or after the show to ask your child to think beyond what the program presents. What does he think would happen if someone behaved that way in real life? How might the character feel the next day? What would he do if he were in a similar situation? Viewing sex in TV shows and movies can provide opportunities to have those conversations you might otherwise find too awkward to get around to. You may feel uncomfortable sitting in the den with your kid watching characters going at it on-screen, but it gives you a chance to explore your teen's thoughts and teach him values that can protect him in the real world.

If you want your child to understand what he's seeing, it helps to be around when he's seeing it. A majority of children in the United States have a TV in their bedroom, but that doesn't make it a good idea. Kids with their own TVs tend to watch more, and their parents have little control over what they watch. If there's still time, don't let your child have a TV or computer somewhere you can't keep an eye on what's going on. Otherwise it may be time to sell that TV on Craigslist and let your child spend the money on cool clothes.

You're smart; take some time to learn the parental control features of your TV, cable box, satellite system, or Internet browser. If you're unsure about a show or movie your child wants to watch, you can check a site like www.commonsensemedia.org for information. The Internet can be a source for accurate information about sexual health, too. Let your child know that sites like www.youngmenshealthsite.org and www.youngwomenshealth.org are places he can turn for answers to those questions he may find too embarrassing to ask face-to-face.

Make a rule that you can review your child's Web browsing history at any time; a child's right to privacy does not extend to watching pornography. Have a central location where your child's mobile phone goes to charge at night. Your kid may scream that none of his friends' parents have such rules, and he may be right, but there's nothing wrong with your child being just that much safer than his friends.

smoke screens

Assuming you're also one of those parents who doesn't want your child to start smoking, abusing alcohol, or using recreational drugs, you have yet another reason to guide your child's media use. If you guessed that children who watch more scenes of smoking and drinking in TV and movies are more likely to smoke and drink themselves, you guessed right. Thanks to the Internet many teens can now find alcohol, tobacco, and illegal drugs with just a few keystrokes and a credit card number.

Companies that sell tobacco and alcohol spend enormous amounts of money to advertise their products—$13 billion a year for tobacco, $5 billion a year for alcohol. While cigarettes companies no longer advertise on TV, tobacco use continues unchecked on-screen, which is in some ways better for them than paid advertising. Even if only the bad guys smoke, what teen doesn't want to be a rebel? Plus, tobacco companies have all those other media to exploit; who needs TV? Kids who are exposed to tobacco advertising and marketing are 50% more likely than their peers to take up smoking. Half of smokers start before age 13, and nearly all pick up the habit by age 19. Cigarette makers aren't stupid. When you kill your core market, recruiting new customers is the only way to maintain profits.

Young people view between 1,000 and 2,000 advertisements for alcohol products annually; alcohol advertisers tend to concentrate their commercials during teen-oriented shows and sporting events. Viewed another way, kids are 400 times more likely to see a commercial where beautiful, fun-loving people enjoy alcohol without any negative consequences than they are to see a public service announcement about the dangers of alcohol use. Beer marketers use online "advergames" to build brand loyalty among kids far too young to legally buy alcohol. In social media, 40% of older teens' profiles include references to substance abuse.

The same rules that protect kids from sexual influences in the media can help protect them from tobacco, alcohol, and drugs. As your child grows older you may feel like he doesn't listen to anything you say. Data, however, tell a different story. Parents' rules about media consumption strongly predict how much and what sort of media kids actually use.

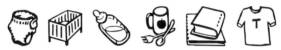

what you can do
Your willingness to talk openly about substance use and clarity about setting boundaries matter when it comes to your child's ultimate behavior.

it's only a game...or is it?

Other dads seem especially skeptical when I start talking about violence in TV shows, movies, and video games. We know, after all, that it's all pretend. Just because kids shoot dozens of people on a screen or watch as people are blown up, tortured, dismembered, or simply beaten senseless doesn't mean they're going to go out and do that stuff, right? After more than 3,000 studies of violent media and kids, the question is no longer whether violent entertainment leads to violent behavior, but how much and who is at the highest risk.

By age 18 the average American will have seen around 200,000 violent acts just on TV. If you've ever watched your kids turn off the TV and immediately start pummeling each other (if you haven't, mine can demonstrate), you get a sense of what their mirror neurons are up to. Children who watch violence in the media not only come away ready to try out some homemade karate kicks, they actually perceive the world as a much more dangerous place than it really is. They see over and over again that people routinely come under physical attack and violence is an effective solution to all sorts of problems. The more they participate in virtual violence, the less sensitized they become to the results of real-world violence.

Overall, about 10% of children's real-world violent behavior seems to arise from violence in the media. The effect varies widely from one child to the next. Kids who come from stable families enjoy some protection from this effect. Kids who already have impulse control problems or who have witnessed violent events in real life are more susceptible to violence in the media. Ironically, real-world experience in martial arts, boxing, wrestling, or contact sports teaches kids discipline, restraint, and sportsmanship in ways that are absent from the virtual realm. The cost of some gaming platforms would go a long way toward getting your kid his green belt!

the hard knocks of school

Researchers remain unclear on the extent to which watching TV and playing video games might cause ADHD (see Chapter 23). It is clear, however, that if you want your child to do better in school, getting him to spend more time with electronic entertainment is probably not the right way to go. While TV and video game use don't reduce exercise or reading time as much as you might imagine, they do track with poor sleep and problems working with words among school-aged children. Children and adolescents who play stimulating video games before bedtime have a harder time going to sleep and are more likely to wake up without the rest they need to get the most out of school. Mobile phones may now keep teens up all night texting as well, a good reason to have them charging somewhere besides the bedroom.

the weight of the problem

It's one thing to know that watching more TV increases a child's likelihood of being overweight. What's more interesting is that when children watch less TV, their weight tends to improve! Television is hardly the only cause of America's obesity epidemic, but it's an easy place to start.

Researchers propose a number of reasons that TV contributes to kids' weight gain, although none of them alone seems to tell the whole story. Kids move around less when they're watching TV, but it turns out that decrease in activity cannot explain much of the problem. Food marketing remains the top suspect. Watch TV with your child and you'll meet all sorts of colorful, friendly cartoon characters plugging equally colorful food. Remember Fred Flintstone and Barney Rubble? They haven't been on prime-time TV in 2 generations now, but they're still around to flog Flintstones and Fruity Pebbles cereals!

What Fred and Barney would do if they encountered Cheesasaurus Rex in his macaroni world is anyone's guess. It might get crowded in there if they were to invite Chester Cheeto (Cheetos make you run fast and wear sunglasses!), Cap'n Crunch (now senile), the Nabisco elves (confirmed bachelors), the Pepperidge Farm Goldfish (hiding under the bed but somehow never eaten by roaches), and the Cinnamon Toast Crunch flakes (they're cannibals!). American children and teens see up to 7,600 commercials per year for fast food and junk food just on TV. That doesn't begin to count the Web sites, banner ads, and online games that extend brands into kids' computers and mobile phones.

Media can also play an insidious role in eating disorders. Anorexia nervosa and bulimia were essentially unknown to the natives of Fiji until they got the gift of American TV programs, after which the conditions blossomed. Kids already affected with the disorders can turn to the Internet and find more than 100 Web sites with tips for purging, eating almost nothing, and hiding their behaviors.

Newer media, especially certain video games, also have the potential to help address the obesity problem. Active games like some for the Wii or the Kinect for Xbox don't usually provide vigorous exercise, but they can encourage kids to engage in mild to moderate levels of physical activity. Some days that's a lot more than they were going to do! Mobile phone apps can help kids log how far and fast they've run, biked, or swum, providing a source of pride as well as an incentive for them to do a little more each time.

network and netplay

There's nothing good or bad about childhood and adolescence your child can't amplify using social networks. Does your child like to make friends? He can have hundreds of them all over the world. Is he interested in a topic like geology, Revolutionary War history, or obscure blues musicians his friends aren't into? There's a group out there waiting for him. Does he draw pictures, compose music, or write poems? Now he can share his creations with the world and get instant feedback. Social networking allows kids to collaborate on homework, start charity projects, and express their creativity in ways members of my poster-board-and-landline generation never dreamed of.

At the same time, social media open up venues for the cruelty of kids to spread at the speed of a computer processor. Embarrassing photographs, insults, and closely held secrets can be broadcast instantly to everyone who matters in a kid's life. Cyberbullying, threatening or harassing a child through electronic communications, is a new and burgeoning problem. Cyberbullying removes the face-to-face part of the interaction, easing the way for other kids who might not be so cruel in the physical world to unleash some serious nastiness, often anonymously. Bullying can become so brutal it ends in suicide.

Many kids don't volunteer that they're victims of cyberbullying, so you'll want to be alert to sudden, unexplained personality changes, especially if your child seems upset after using a computer or mobile phone. You may have to play detective, asking your child directly if someone is making him feel bad or asking to see his message log.

what you can do

If you find that your child is being bullied, take it seriously. Save all messages and texts from the bully. In situations in which your child seems to face significant danger, the police can often trace the IP address to locate the bully so long as you save the messages.

As a parent you'll want to remind your child that his online activity leaves a digital footprint that may never be erased. Advise him never to give out personal information like his address or social security number. You can set limits on computer use so that it doesn't interfere with exercise, home-work, and sleep. Just as with TV, it's best to have the computer out in the open where you can see what your child is doing. Use the parental controls for your child's Web browser, although as a matter of courtesy let your child know you're doing so. You should always have access to your child's social media sites; chances are he'll feel proud teaching you how to navigate them.

cell biology

To call today's mobile devices "telephones" is like calling a car a "rolling air conditioning unit." How often does your child or teen even talk into the device? Mobile phones today are really Internet-capable texting devices that can also carry voice signals when needed. Once exclusively adult burdens, cell phones have migrated down the age brackets to the point that now 60% of tweens and 84% of teens own the devices. Even 22% of younger children now carry phones! I'm lucky my kids can't see me around 1995, brandishing my Motorola Flip like the President was about to call.

Because they are connected to the Internet, mobile phones can channel all the best and worst features of other media right into a child's hand. With a mobile phone your child can call you to let you know he's arrived safely at the park with a friend; he can also report an emergency almost anywhere.

Mobile phones' portability has opened up unique opportunities for health education and chronic disease management. Increasingly, phones are linking kids to their doctors' offices or medical centers to provide real-time advice and feedback for managing problems like diabetes and asthma. On the downside, mobile phones may keep kids awake all night or give them the power to make regrettable choices about sharing information or images before they've had a chance to think it through.

Just as with all other media, phones are all about how you use them. If the phone starts to interfere with sleep, homework, or healthy social interactions, you know what to do. Because they're so portable, mobile phones pose a special risk to the family dinner hour. Kids who eat dinner around a table with their parents enjoy not just a healthier diet but protection from harmful decision-making. You can only learn about your child's life and share your values, however, if everyone at the table isn't hunched over a phone returning texts. Of course, if you ask your kids to turn off their phones for dinner, you'll want to set an example.

Sexting, sending sexually explicit pictures or messages, is a problem that has garnered a lot of media attention. Fortunately, the best data suggest that only a small percentage of teens actually send such messages. That said, sexting puts teens at risk for major embarrassment, but sending them is against the law in many states, with very real repercussions.

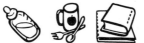

what you can do

When your child first gets a mobile phone, talk to him in an age-appropriate way about what sort of images and messages not to send. If he's younger, he should know that no one is ever supposed to send pictures of themselves unclothed and to tell you if he sees such images. With older children you can use the word sexting and remind them that courts consider it a form of pornography. You can even use stories in the media to reinforce what a bad idea sexting is, unless our politicians and celebrities become a lot smarter real soon.

Ensuring your child's media experiences inspire rather than harm him requires setting limits and examples, which will take some effort. You'll have to constantly educate yourself about technology. You'll need to spend some time watching what entertains your child instead of what's age-appropriate for you. Ideally you'll limit your child's TV time to 2 hours or less a day, which means you may have to help him figure out what to do once he turns it off. You'll need to put down your own cell phone, laptop, and TV remote long enough to have a technology-free family dinner.

In the process you're likely to have some conversations with him you never would have had, to learn things about your child that might otherwise have remained secrets. Of course, you can always send your child outdoors. Sunscreen is cheap, wasps rarely sting, and an occasional splinter may not be much of a price to pay for your child to feel the grass between his toes. Heck, you might even go out there yourself.

25

uh, so, it's like this: talking to your children about sexual development

my dad is a pediatrician, and like me he knows it's never too early
to start talking to children about sex. I remember the first time he saw my
oldest son, a week after he was born. Dad held him up, studying his dark,
expressive eyes, his long eyelashes like feathers from some exotic bird,
his strawberry lips pursed as though when they parted he might recite
a poem. Smiling, Dad spoke gently in my newborn son's still-soft ear:
"A condom every time, boy…every time."

Sexuality is an emotionally charged topic, presumably because sex is an
emotionally charged act. Seeing as how you're a dad, you may already be
aware that many people find sex enjoyable. In addition to stimulating the
brain's pleasure centers, sex also causes our brains to release oxytocin,
a hormone that engenders feelings of trust and bonding between people
(whether or not they intended to experience such emotions). In that
sense the words *making love* are quite literal—the fulfillment, joy, and
emotional attachment born of a sexual relationship are what many of
us imagine when we dream of romance.

At the same time, sex is among the riskiest activities a person can undertake, with possible outcomes that include the creation and loss of life. Depending on the situation, sex may be fraught with guilt, shame, fear, embarrassment, jealousy, or anger. As a parent it frightens me to imagine my own children one day falling under the sway of a force as powerful as human sexuality. That said, my kids already busted Santa Claus; what hope does the Stork really have?

Some parents worry that addressing sexual topics with their children will cause their kids to have sex earlier, like if they just don't mention sexuality, maybe their kids will forget about it and get distracted by some more interesting topic, like, say, the periodic table of elements. Not only are these parents wrong, they have it backward! Kids whose parents talk openly with them about sex are the most successful at delaying their first sexual encounter. As much as adults of every generation enjoy talking about "kids these days," national trends are promising: today's teens are less likely than those in previous decades to get pregnant, and their average age of first intercourse is actually later!

Your kids are going to learn about sex one way or another. They can learn about it from you, in a setting where you can help impart the values you hope they will share, or they can learn about it from their friends and the media, where the information may not always be so accurate. Think back to some of the "biology lessons" you heard in the locker room. Maybe you had smarter friends than mine, but remembering some of the stuff they said about sex, I can only assume they were not referring to any human species.

sex talk through the ages

We like to imagine childhood as a time without sexuality, but that's not quite right. A child's sense of gender, for example, begins when she discovers her genitals, usually around 8 to 10 months of life. I see parents in the office who worry their infants are exploring their nether parts with such vigor that they may injure themselves! I enjoy watching parents' relief when they hear that pretty much never happens.

By the second year of life, children become aware of physical differences between boys and girls. Your toddler will want to know what to call stuff. Your best bet is to go with words the rest of the world understands, like "vagina," "breasts," "penis," "scrotum," and "anus." That way she doesn't run to her teacher to report she was riding her tricycle and injured her "doohickey." Using proper terms also avoids branding body parts with a sense of shame.

By age 3 your child should be able to tell you whether she's a boy or a girl. It will take another year or so, however, before she fully understands that her gender will never change. You'll probably need to remind your preschooler more than once that certain parts of her body are private, specifically the parts normally covered by a bathing suit. Children this age may masturbate, which is perfectly normal unless it starts to interfere with daily activities. Don't freak out; just remind your child that this is a private activity and not something other people should see.

Around age 4 to 5, children grow eager to figure out pretty much everything, including stuff about bodies and basic sexuality. Expect some hard questions like, "How did I get into mommy's tummy?" and "How did I get out of mommy's tummy?" There is some risk these questions will be cute or funny, but don't laugh if you can help it. You don't want to embarrass your child and keep her from coming to you with questions.

You also don't want to get all serious like this is a *Big Deal*. It's not. It's just your child trying to figure some stuff out. That said, if you're not sure how to answer, "Let me get back to you on that" is a fair response. You can always do some reading or call your child's pediatrician for advice. You can try out your answer on another adult before you spring it on your kid. If the whole conversation makes you too queasy, look around the family for someone who feels more comfortable answering your child's questions until you feel ready.

Remember, too, that you don't have to reinvent the wheel here. Bookstores, libraries, and the Internet are full of age-appropriate resources to help you explain sexuality and sexual development to your children. Flip through some books and find one that seems right for your child and imparts the values you hope she'll learn.

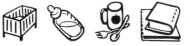

what you can do

Your answers at this age can be short and not terribly detailed. You don't have to pull out your old anatomy textbook, for example. Once you've given an answer, your child is usually satisfied for the time being. Like a good reporter, she'll be back later with follow-up questions if she feels the need. You might finish up by asking her, "Does that answer your question?" You might even check in with her after a few days and ask if she's thought of any more questions. Don't be surprised if you have to cover the same material over and over again. Kids, like adults, learn from repetition.

In the preschool years your child will also be trying to figure out the deal with genitals, like why boys have a penis and girls don't. Children may pull down their pants and touch each other's genitals out of curiosity. When this happens, it's another opportunity for you not to freak out. Instead, explain to your child that it's not appropriate for other people to touch her private parts. Let her know that the only people who should look at or touch her privates are her parents if they need to help bathe her or figure out what hurts, or a doctor or nurse when she is in a doctor's office and a parent is there.

Around the time your child starts kindergarten, you should also address the issue of secrets. As parents, we like to imagine child molesters as strangers; we may warn our children about "stranger danger" and tell them not to go anywhere with someone they don't know. This is all good advice, but the fact is that the vast majority of children who are sexually molested know their abusers. Molesters often work their way into positions of trust with children. Despite all evidence to the contrary, children tend to obey adults. Experts estimate that up to 80% of child molestation victims never report the abuse, or they do so long after the event.

By age 6 to 7 you'll find your child's questions grow more specific and complex. She is now interested in how relationships work, and she may want to know what it is that grown-ups do with each other. She's going to want to put together the puzzle of how the man and woman who love

what you can do
Remind your child that there are certain secrets she should never keep from her parents. Teach her that if someone asks to look at her or touch her in secret she should tell you immediately, and promise her she will not get in trouble for doing so.

each other very much end up having a baby. She might have her own ideas, or her friends might have shared their versions of the story with her.

Classic questions might concern just how it is that people have sex, what periods are, and why boys get erections. Before answering, start with a question of your own: "What have you heard about that?" It's not an accusation, just a way to understand the instructional challenge you're about to face. Besides, while your child is answering, you can be figuring out what you're going to say!

You're likely to find that questions come up in response to events in your child's life. If her teacher gets pregnant, for example, she may ask why it happened. She might see a newborn with an erection during a diaper change, or she might notice something during a television show that requires a little more explanation. Our family found that adopting a dog provided several unanticipated opportunities to discuss sexual behavior. If you don't make a big deal about answering your child's questions, she's likely to continue asking you questions, which means you get to keep giving her good answers.

By age 8 to 9 your child is likely to present you with some really big questions. If you're like most dads, you're probably thinking, "Isn't it a little early for this stuff?" but many girls are already experiencing the earliest changes of pubertal development at this age. At the same time, girls and boys have now developed a strong sense of right and wrong, and they have some basic concept of how babies are made.

Your child is likely to ask you some very personal questions: how did you and mom meet and fall in love? She may ask why some people fall in love with others of the same sex; she may worry that because she has friends of the same sex that means she'll be homosexual. You'll want to help her distinguish between "like" and *"like*-like." If she means that second one, don't worry; we'll talk more about gender identity and sexual orientation later in the chapter.

what you can do

The late elementary school years are a good time to help your child understand responsible sexual behavior. Start now discussing unintended pregnancy and birth control. Let her know that people can contract dangerous diseases from having sex, specifically HIV/AIDS. Tell her about waiting to have sex until she's older. Let her know that whenever she does become sexually active, condoms are the only reliable way to protect herself from disease.

If you feel awkward talking about this stuff with your fourth-grader, join the club. But then take a step back and think about how you've already prepared your child for other adult responsibilities she won't face for years. Does she know how you drive a car and follow the rules of the road? Has she asked what taxes are and why you pay every month to live in your house and turn on the lights? Have you told her about working for a living? At school her peers are already talking about who "likes" whom, and it will only be a few years before some of them begin kissing, petting, and more. You don't want to wait until then to start this conversation any more than you'd wait until her 15th birthday to talk about stop signs, speed limits, and double yellow lines.

As your child enters puberty, her interest in sexuality will ramp up considerably, as will your fear of what that interest might mean. It's important at this point to take a deep breath and remember that many teens do understand that they are not yet ready for intercourse. Especially in the early and middle teen years, their concerns reflect a desire to be attractive and a search for companionship and intimacy. Remember that today's teens are actually less likely to have sex than preceding generations. Now more than ever, you want to keep the door open to communication.

what you can do

Let your teen know that if she ever feels like she's in a threatening situation, she can call you and you'll come get her without questions or lectures. The 2 of you can even put that pledge in writing and sign it. Talk about the dangers of sexual pressure, of being a victim and a perpetrator. "No means no" should be an absolute for all parties in a relationship. Remind your child that anyone who doesn't respect her values does not deserve her affection. If your teen is in a relationship, be willing to talk frankly about ways your teen and her partner might pleasure each other without resorting to sexual intercourse.

Remind your teen that many young adults look back on their first sexual experience and wish they had waited longer. Help her visualize the life she hopes for, one that might be much more difficult to achieve with a baby or dangerous illness. Give her a chance to practice different scenarios and imagine how she might respond. "What would you say to a guy who tells you that if you really love him, you'll go all the way? What if he was drunk and groping you?" Kids who prepare for these situations are more likely to respond appropriately when the time comes.

Your actions will always speak more loudly than your words. If you are in a stable relationship with your child's mother, do you treat each other with affection and respect? If you are working on a new relationship, are you going about it in a way you hope your child will imitate? Can you fairly look at your child and say, "Don't do anything I wouldn't do?" If you don't walk the walk, then talking the talk isn't going to get you very far with your kid.

making change

There's comes a point in every father's life when he looks at his child and thinks, "Whoa! When did *that* happen?!" Sure, puberty struck you and all your friends, but it's possible you weren't taking notes at the time. It's natural for children and even their parents to wonder if the changes they're seeing are normal, if they're happening too soon or too late. The timing of puberty is often inherited, which means I can expect my kids to start maturing around age, say, 19. Let's look at when a variety of "that's" normally occur.

our daughters, ourselves?

Girls start developing a few years before boys on average. Breast buds are usually the first sign of development in girls, forming as early as age 7 or as late as age 13 depending on family history, ethnicity, and body composition. Within a year the first pubic hairs start to develop, usually around age 8 to 14. Around the same time the shape and texture of the vagina changes, with the opening lengthening and the labia (lips) growing darker and more pronounced. Girls hit a growth spurt between ages 9 and 14, a time when they are likely to be taller, faster, and stronger than many boys their age. They begin having periods any time between the ages of 9 and 16 years; periods are likely to be unpredictable during the first year or so after they start. Between the ages of 11 and 16 underarm hair and acne arrive to round out the whole puberty experience.

when to call the doctor

If you notice your daughter is developing earlier or later than you would expect based on these guidelines, bring it up with her doctor.

This is a good time to bring up a tricky subject: buying your daughter her first bra. Depending on your family situation you may find yourself as I did, standing in Justice, staring at a mysterious wall of undergarments, wondering how to proceed. I have been informed (too late) that you should not call out in front of her best friend, "So, uh, what looks good to you?" Let's review what you should do.

First, you have to pick your timing. Seeing as how you're a guy, your daughter may not necessarily approach you and say, "Dad, I think it's time we went and got me a bra." Instead you might have to broach the subject. Try something like, "I notice some of your friends are starting to wear bras. Have you thought about that?" If your daughter then faints with embarrassment, you might have to search for a female friend or family member to stand in for you. If, however, she is still standing, it's time to shop.

The venue matters. Your daughter probably does not want to run into one of her friends while standing next to her dad at Victoria's Secret. Consider going a bit out of your way, perhaps to another neighborhood, like, say, Australia. The Internet is another option, as long as you can insure free return shipping for whatever doesn't work out.

You'll want to learn some vocabulary. Your daughter's first bra will probably belong to a category that goes by several names. The old term *training bra* has fallen out of favor, replaced by *bralette* or *teen bra*. Other options are a *sports bra* and a *cami,* short for camisole. Many camisoles come with a Lycra or elastic inner shelf that functions as a bra. All of these items lack underwire or significant padding, making each a comfortable and age-appropriate first choice.

Sizing will be a matter of trial and error, but before you shop, invest in the sort of soft fabric tape measure tailors use. Your daughter can measure herself around her rib cage, which is one way bras are sized. The number in inches is likely to be in the high 20s to mid-30s. The other measurement, cup size, is noted in letters ranging from AA to F, going from smallest to largest. (If she ends up with something other than A, you may have waited too long.) The bra should be snug enough not to drift around but not tight enough to leave marks on her skin. Girls are likely to want to be like their friends. If your daughter is developing early, she may choose a bra that minimizes her body's changes. If she's lagging behind her peers, she may choose a little extra padding.

You'll also want to take into account some practical considerations. At this age most girls don't want to flaunt their bras. Go for subtle colors and patterns that are not likely to show through her clothing. Think about what she likes to wear, too. She may need a variety of styles of bra to accommodate different dresses or tops. Remember to buy enough of whatever you get to make it between laundry days, unless you plan on washing clothes every few nights.

Finally, remember that as conflicted as you may feel about your little girl reaching this new stage in her life, she is likely to feel equally strange. She may not want you to hug her the way you used to do, suddenly embarrassed at what you might feel or afraid her friends will see. Respect her autonomy by asking, "Can I give you a hug?" and don't take offense if her answer is "No." Let her know that she's still your little girl; if she enjoys playing catch with you or swinging together or showing you her dolls, invite her to do so. No one grows up all at once.

While we're on the subject of awkward shopping excursions, let's consider "feminine hygiene products." If you're a dad it's a fair bet you've never had a period yourself, and you may feel especially unprepared to help your daughter deal with her menstrual cycle. Periods, however, don't wait for everyone to feel ready to deal with them, or so I've heard. Your daughter's first period is likely to lag her breast development by a couple of years. She will know it's approaching because for about 6 months prior, she'll have some increased white, milky vaginal discharge.

This is another one of those conversations you're probably going to have to initiate. You might get some clues if you're the one who does laundry in your house, or you might just notice she's starting to look more mature. Start again with a question: "Have you thought about what we might do to get ready for your period when it begins?" She's likely to be embarrassed when you bring up the subject, but she'll also be relieved because she's probably already started worrying about that very scenario.

The first item on your shopping list should be *pads* (also called sanitary pads or sanitary napkins), absorbent liners that stick to the inside of a girl's underwear. Some have a strip of adhesive; others also have "wings" that fold over the sides of the underwear. Some are scented or treated with deodorant, but these chemicals can sometimes cause irritation or allergic reactions. Natural food stores sell reusable, washable pads made of cloth.

The thinnest pads, *panty liners,* will help with the discharge that precedes the onset of periods. Others are thicker for times when menstrual flow is heavier. Given that you may not be able to predict what your daughter's needs will be, it may be safest to keep a few different sizes on hand. A girl using pads should change them at least every 3 to 4 hours to prevent the buildup of bacteria. Pads will not flush down the toilet. You'll want to have a wastebasket for them in your daughter's bathroom; if you have a dog or cat, consider getting a trash can with a lid. Pads are also not the best choice for a trip to the pool because they will absorb water and swell.

Your daughter may also want to try using a *tampon,* a roll of absorbent material that fits inside the vagina. These, too, come in a variety of sizes and styles. Your best bet is to start with a "slender" tampon that has an applicator. "Super" and "ultra" tampons are made to be more absorbent. Manufacturers make your life easier here—they sell combination boxes of tampons so you don't have to pick just one style. Again, avoid perfumes and deodorants. Tampons are fine for use with swimming because they won't swell.

No matter how close your relationship, your daughter is going to have to figure out tampon insertion without your help. Every box of tampons includes clear instructions with illustrations. You can reassure your daughter that using a tampon will not disrupt her virginity, and there's no way to lose a tampon inside her body. It is important, however, that she change the tampon every 4 to 6 hours during the day. There's no danger in sleeping while using a tampon, but she should still change it after about 8 hours. Tampons that stay in too long can harbor bacteria that cause a dangerous illness called toxic shock syndrome. Never common, toxic shock syndrome is now very rare, but if your daughter has high fever, vomiting or diarrhea, severe muscle aches, a feeling of extreme weakness or dizziness, and a rash that looks like a sunburn, ask to make sure she hasn't had a tampon in for more than a few hours, and get her to a doctor quickly.

boyz II men

Being a dad is pretty much proof that you've experienced the male side of puberty, but you've probably suppressed some of the details. Boys' bodies start changing between ages 10 and 13 years, when the testicles begin to enlarge and the skin of the scrotum turns darker and coarser. Pubic hair grows starting between ages 10 and 15, and boys become taller and stronger around that time as well. Between ages 11 and 15 your son's voice deepens and his penis grows in length and width. Between ages 11 and 17 boys become able to ejaculate semen, meaning they're fertile. Facial hair, armpit hair, and acne are among the later pubertal changes to occur, arriving between ages 12 and 17.

when to call the doctor
Your son's doctor can help evaluate any concerns you might have that he might be developing too early or too late.

Puberty generates just as much embarrassment and anxiety for boys as it does for girls. Early in the process, for example, many boys will notice a lump under one or both of their nipples (*gynecomastia*). This is not cancer but a mass of breast tissue responding to the hormones floating around in the bloodstream. This lump is likely to go away on its own after a year or two, but if it becomes large enough to attract others' attention, you may want to address it with his doctor.

Involuntary erections are the bane of a teenaged boy's existence. Even without any stimulation or sexual thoughts, your son's penis may fill with blood, another response to hormonal stimulation. Your best bet for addressing this, aside from providing him a long-sleeved shirt to tie around his waist, is to remind him that all boys experience this and that it will become less frequent with time.

Wet dreams are another embarrassing aspect of male adolescence. What doctors call *nocturnal emissions* are spontaneous releases of semen that occur during sleep; they don't necessarily result from dreaming of erotic subjects. If your son seems eager to launder his own sheets suddenly, let him know it's something every male goes through, and it's not his fault.

what you can do

You might think to reassure your son about his voice cracking or changing, a result of his vocal cords assuming their larger, adult configuration. He may even get worried because one testicle hangs lower than the other. You might volunteer that guys are supposed to be made that way, letting him know that fine men's tailors take this fact into account by asking their gentlemen customers if they "dress left or dress right."

knock it before you try it

While puberty augments the differences between boys' and girls' bodies, there are some experiences of puberty that they share. One is an increased need for privacy. If you're not already doing it, knock before you barge into your child's room or bathroom. Respect her need to have a space of her own to dress, undress, and simply exist without your coming in unannounced. Remember, there's stuff you can't unsee.

Second, boys and girls will become interested in (some would say obsessed with) their appearance. Even if your family dynamic includes some good-natured teasing, leave your child's physical appearance out of it. As an adult you may be confident enough about yourself to laugh at your weight, nose, or hair, but these details are far too serious to your child to joke about. Puberty is hard enough already.

Third, be aware that boys and girls at this age both masturbate, stimulating their genitals for sexual enjoyment. This behavior is normal unless it's interfering with routine daily activity. Rather than address your child's masturbation directly, you might find a moment during a television show, movie, or relevant conversation to say something like, "I remember some of the crazy stuff other kids told me could happen to you if you masturbate. I hope you know that masturbating and not masturbating are both normal, and it's nothing bad or shameful." Don't expect your child to beam at you and say, "Thanks, Dad!" but be aware that your words may count more than you know.

unplanned parenthood

The best statistics suggest that at age 17 about half of American teens have had intercourse at least once. Some factors seem to help delay when this occurs; teens from intact families and girls with high self-esteem, for example, tend to start having sex at a later age. The best studies of adolescents who take a "virginity pledge" suggest that these kids have sex just as early as those who don't pledge, but that they are less likely to use birth control when they do have sex.

Some religious and cultural traditions consider birth control of any type to be immoral. As a pediatrician, my priority is minimizing adolescents' risks of unintended pregnancy and sexually transmitted infections (STIs) once they do become sexually active. While I respect all religious and cultural traditions, my profession obligates me to point out that condoms are the most effective means of preventing sexually active teens from contracting potentially deadly STIs.

Given that condoms are highly effective in preventing teen pregnancy and STIs, you'll want to talk frankly with your teen about these problems. First, remind her that many people don't even know they have an STI. Many teens believe they can look at a partner and "tell" if he has a disease, but you can explain that even if someone says he's been "tested," he may still have HIV, genital warts, or herpes. People carry and transmit all these infections, as well as chlamydia, gonorrhea, trichomonas, and syphilis, without symptoms or outward signs. The only safe assumption for your teen to make is that every sexual partner is potentially infectious.

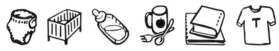

what you can do

You'll want to help your teen understand that she can become pregnant at any time, even if her partner "pulls out," she's having her period, or she jumps up and down or douches immediately afterward. There is no such thing as "just this once" because once is all it takes. It may help her to know that women often feel most like having sex (and are more attractive to men) at the time in their cycles when they are most likely to become pregnant. Don't be afraid to supply your teen with condoms and remind her that while it may still be years before she chooses to have sex, "no condom, no sex" should be an unbreakable rule.

Your teen should also know that there's a right way to use a condom (usually conveniently printed inside every box). To be effective, the guy has to put on a condom before sex begins. From that point on it may be too late to prevent pregnancy and disease transmission. He should leave a little space at the end by pinching about a quarter inch of the tip when he's rolling it on. The space should not be full of air, or it may pop like a balloon. Oil-based lubricants like Vaseline or massage oil can degrade latex; any lubricants should be water-based, like K-Y Jelly or Surgilube. As soon as the male ejaculates he should hold the condom at the base and pull out. If the couple has sex again, they need to use a fresh condom.

Having these conversations with your teen may not feel comfortable for either of you. Remember, however, that talking to kids about sex and even giving them condoms does not make them have sex any sooner. It does, however, lower the chances you'll become a grandfather before you're ready, as well as the chance you'll be talking to your child in a doctor's office about treating her infection.

what if my child is gay?

There are really 2 gender issues parents worry about, and it's important to clarify the differences. The most common is *homosexuality,* which describes people being sexually attracted to members of their same gender (we call this their *sexual orientation*). About 2% to 5% of the human population falls into this category. A second, much rarer condition involves confusion of gender identity, in which a child feels the gender of her body does not reflect her "real" gender.

The most important thing you can know as a dad is that you have little to no power to change your child's sexual orientation or identity. By age 3 kids tend to gravitate toward play and behaviors that they identify with their own gender, but they also cross over at times throughout early childhood. In other words, if you find your 5-year-old son wearing a dress and holding a baby doll, don't freak out; that's still normal.

By middle childhood children's sexual identities and orientation are more fixed. Children whose behavior seems unusual for their gender may suffer socially among their peers. This is important—don't make it worse by adding to the pressure! If you punish your daughter for running around in combat fatigues shooting Nerf guns or berate your son for showing you his latest sketches of dress designs, the only thing you're doing is pummeling your child's self-esteem.

when to call the doctor

A better approach is to ask your child a question: do you feel like you're a boy? A girl? If your child answers that she feels that she's a boy or wishes intently that she were one, you'll want to involve her pediatrician. He may recommend counseling to further explore her sense of gender identity and help her work through her sense of confusion.

Biologic and environmental factors contribute to a child's gender identity, and it's likely to take some time and work to determine the best approach to the issue. No matter what, make sure she knows you love her and value her for the person she is.

The more we learn about sexual orientation, the more it appears to be an almost completely innate property. In other words, you couldn't make your child gay if you tried, and you can't make her un-gay either. Many children have a solid sense of their sexual orientation by middle childhood, but teens may experiment with a variety of sexual behaviors before they solidify their sense of orientation.

what you can do

The most important thing you can do for a child or teen you think may be gay is to support her and let her know you love her. Homosexual kids often face enough fear and rejection from their peers; they're looking to their parents for security. You may still want to seek therapy for your child—not to change her sexual orientation, but to help her cope with what may be a challenging social landscape.

In surveys, 4 out of 5 parents say they have an obligation to provide their kids sex education. And what do they do with that obligation? Less than half of mothers tell their daughters much of anything; fathers talk even less. You, however, know better. You have a plan; you know what to do. If you get this right with your child, hopefully it will be an appropriately long time before you're gazing at your own newborn grandchild's face, reminding him to use a condom.

26

it's complicated: dealing with nontraditional parenting relationships

....

dad tip

During a separation or divorce, work with your children's mom to keep as many aspects of your kids' lives as possible consistent between the 2 homes. Be big enough to put aside whatever anger or pain you're feeling and work out some compromises you can both live with.

....

according to the 2010 US census, 66% of children lived with 2 married parents; another 4% lived with 2 unmarried parents. That leaves almost one-third of children living in some other arrangement. If, like me, you find yourself part of "some other arrangement," you may sometimes question what it means to be a "family" in a world that is in many ways geared to the traditional model. I mean, I ask myself questions like, "If we're not a traditional family, can we still shop at Family Dollar? Will they sell us discount tickets to the baseball game on Family Night? If Focus on the Family looks at us, will we be blurry?

Of course, nontraditional family arrangements present challenges well beyond buying baseball tickets. Children who grow up without both parents in the home face higher risks of poor school performance, depression, drug and alcohol use, and unplanned pregnancy than those from 2-parent homes. Viewed in isolation, the statistics can be frightening. But your children are not statistics; they're individuals. And they don't have a statistical father, they have you. If we know one thing, it's that fathers matter. Let's look at some of those "other arrangements" and see how much you can do to give your children the support, security, and love that will help them thrive.

long division: separation and divorce

Couples with children are less likely than couples without children to divorce, but the numbers are still discouraging: 40% of American couples with children ultimately divorce, as opposed to around 50% of childless couples. It's hard to overstate the emotional impact of divorce—children react much as they would to the death of a close family member. Men who experience divorce even have shorter life spans on average than those who don't, in part due to the toll stress takes on their health. Of course, no one has really compared the challenge of undergoing divorce with the stress of continuing to live in a dysfunctional family, so it's hard to tease out the effect of divorce itself from the factors that predispose people to ending a marriage.

How you handle this ordeal has an enormous effect on how your children will fare. Situations that end marriages tend to be emotional, and not the good kind of emotional—more like the angry, hurt, betrayed, guilty, bewildered kind. In the midst of all this anguish, attempting to cooperate with your spouse in making a plan for the kids may feel, shall we say, challenging. That said, no matter what happened in the course of your relationship, the 2 of you produced and raised one or more amazing, unique children, and they remain dependent on you to provide them a structure that feels safe and secure when their world is crashing down around them. Sure it's going to be hard, but you're a dad. You're going to man up and do what's right for your kids.

Each divorce comes with its own unique challenges, but for the most part they all proceed through the same phases. As you go through these phases it may you help to envision your support network of friends, family members, faith community, and mental health professionals as an army waiting to help you, like the US military responding to the 5-level defense readiness condition (DEFCON).

The first phase is the *pre-divorce* period, when stress and distance build between you and mom. Even if you've tried to keep your marital conflicts out of the kids' view, they have sensed there's a problem. Children often respond with "unexplained" behavior changes including fighting, crying, testing the limits of discipline, and having angry outbursts. This is a phase in which marital and family counseling may help you resolve your issues and restore function to the family. Even if you despair of keeping the marriage together, a counselor can help you and your spouse work out the next steps in a neutral environment. Right now your support network is at DEFCON 3—increased force readiness.

The next phase, *separation,* is a doozy. This is when one spouse (often but not always the father) leaves the household. The upside of this phase is that it relieves the constant stress of marital discord and replaces the fear of the unknown with the challenge of adapting to a new reality. The downside, of course, is the new reality, when a parent who used to take the kids to soccer practice, help them with their homework, or read them a bedtime story is no longer in the home to do so.

what you can do

Kids love predictability, so keep as many aspects of their lives as stable as you can. This is a good time to focus on everything in their lives that will stay the same, especially that both their parents will always still love them. The first time you have to leave your children and face an empty home, have your support network at DEFCON 1—you need them to mobilize, now.

Next comes what we call the *adjustment* period. Everyone starts to deal with the new patterns of life—moving between 2 households, negotiating discipline and expectations between 2 parents, dealing with substantial financial setbacks that often come with dividing a family. This phase will demand plenty of your emotional energy as you work with your spouse to help your children figure out their roles in this new life. Chances are you're all still grieving pretty hard at this point. You may drop your support network back to DEFCON 2, but continue to lean on your friends, your family, and even a professional counselor to help you find the reserves of energy you'll need to help your children embrace this new life.

With time you'll move into the next phase, the *reorganization* period, when life reaches a new and relatively stable equilibrium. The separation or divorce will be just another part of your world, and for the most part you, your (former) spouse, and your children will all be getting on with the business of your lives. It would be nice if you could skip over the whole adjustment period and just go straight to reorganization, but you're not allowed to skip steps in this game. The framework you establish during the adjustment period is what makes reorganization possible. After a period you may even experience a fifth phase, *remarriage*. This one, while generally happy, also comes with its own challenges; we'll touch on them a little later. Your support network should always remain at DEFCON 4 (above normal readiness); the challenges you face have lessened, but they may still arise in unpredictable ways.

breaking news

Telling children about a pending separation is among the hardest moments you can ever face as a father. Nothing in life prepares you to have a conversation this painful, but you can work with your spouse to keep the moment from being as bad as it might. The absolute worst thing you can do for your kids is to leave them in limbo, without a plan. "You mother and I are considering living apart" is not a sentence that engenders confidence. You're not asking your kids if they think it's OK. Chances are pretty good they don't.

If you're really going to do this thing, figure out as many details as possible ahead of time. When will the separation start? Who is staying in the home? Where will the children spend the first night of the separation? How often will they see each parent? What elements of their lives will remain the same? These are the questions your children will have, and you want to be ready with the answers.

In timing your announcement, you should also take into account your children's age. A preschooler or kindergartner, for example, has a very limited sense of future time, usually around a week. Telling him you're separating a month before the event just increases his anxiety. Older children may be able to use some extra time to consider what's about to happen and ask questions.

Be prepared for an emotional reaction from your child. He's probably not going to respond by giving you a hug and saying, "I know in the long run you'll both be happier." He may be sad, angry, frightened, or in many cases, some of all 3. He may cry, scream, act out, or lock himself in his room. If he needs some time alone give it to him, as long as you know he's safe. He may want to talk to you for hours or he may be so angry he has

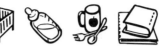

what you can do

If at all possible, make the separation announcement together with your spouse. Talk in advance about how and where you're going to tell the kids. At the mall or right before a birthday party, for example, is probably not the best choice. Talk to your child somewhere he has a nearby source of comfort, whether a teddy bear or special toy, a friend, or a close member of the extended family. Have tissues nearby; there's likely to be some crying. And for heaven's sake, if you and your spouse can only hold it together for 15 minutes, let it be these 15 minutes! Now is not the time to air out your grievances against each other or start fighting in front of the kids. "Your mom and I are having a hard time getting along, and we've decided that for now we cannot live together," works perfectly well. The details belong in the marriage counselor's office, not at the kitchen table.

nothing to say to you for the rest of the day. Just let him know you're there to talk when he's ready.

When the talking does begin, it's likely to involve a lot of questions. Children will want to know if this change in their lives is permanent or just temporary. It's OK to answer that you don't know; often you don't. Children will long for reconciliation even in situations in which one seems very unlikely. Expect to answer the same questions over and over again. "Are you and Mommy going to get back together?" is one you're likely to hear most often, as children hope perhaps next time they ask your answer will change.

Take this time to focus on everything that will remain the same. Will your child stay in the same house? Attend the same school? Get to keep all his toys? Still celebrate birthdays and major holidays? Most of all, make sure he knows both of his parents love him and always will. You really cannot stress that one enough.

Let your child know repeatedly that he didn't cause your separation. While it may be obvious to you that your child had nothing to do with the problems in your marriage, kids almost inevitably blame themselves, feeling like perhaps if they had just done something more they could have prevented this calamity. Some children will respond by redoubling their efforts to behave—making straight As, setting the table every night, raking the yard. Others may generate a crisis in hopes their parents will reunite to deal with it—acting out at school, running away from home, or flagrantly defying the rules of the household. Both types of behavior may signal a child's need for counseling.

Emphasize to your children whatever positives you can find in the situation. One nearly universal benefit is that you and mom won't always be fighting anymore, which should make everyone's life more pleasant. Your child may also get excited about furnishing a new room in your house or about enjoying 2 birthday celebrations.

At the same time, children are bound to have plenty of negative emotions, and the best thing you can do is to acknowledge them. Children want to know they've been heard, and simple statements of observation on your part can help them. "You sound like you're really sad about the divorce," "I hear that you're angry at us right now," or "You seem to be worried about what's going to happen," are all examples of active listening. Follow these statements with a pause and your child is likely to tell you more. What he says next may not make you happy, but he knows you're listening, which will help both of you heal.

You can be honest about your feelings as well, saying that you too are sad or angry things have turned out this way, but stop short of using your child as an ally, confidante, or spy. You have adults to talk to about what happened in your marriage or what angers you about your ex-wife. Your child is naturally going to feel love for both of his parents. No one should ever make him feel guilty for that. If he does happen to overhear you complaining about his mother, stop and explain that when people get upset they sometimes say hurtful things, but that his mother is a wonderful person who loves him very much.

Your child may ask some very pointed, even accusatory questions. "Why didn't you and mom work it out?" "Did you 2 ever love each other?" and "Why did you let her leave?" Each of these questions may make you angry; you may want to respond with a litany of everything your ex-wife did wrong. Don't. Relationships between human beings are complicated. People fall in love; their feelings change. Stuff happens. If you and mom can agree not to talk each other down to the kids, and you can both keep that promise, you will have taken a tremendous step toward helping your children embrace their new lives.

Be sure you and mom communicate directly with each other rather than through the kids. Between voice mail, e-mail, text messaging, and social media, there are plenty of ways the 2 of you can coordinate homework, doctors' visits, and sports schedules without having an emotional face-to-face conversation. Your child has enough to worry about without remembering to tell his mom you'll be picking him up early on Sunday.

In that same vein, your children are not spies. They may volunteer information about what's happening in their mom's household, but you may gently discourage them from reporting too much detail. You don't live there anymore. If you hear something that makes you fear for their safety or health, bring it up directly with their mom. If, on the other hand, you hear they had a great time with mom, be happy for them and her. That's how things are supposed to go.

Speaking of communication, your children will adjust better to living in 2 homes if as many things as possible remain consistent between them. Work with mom to keep things like bedtimes, chores, and household rules at least recognizable from one household to the other. You and mom are likely to disagree on some stuff, what with the divorce and all, but before you dig in your heels on something, talk it through and think about what's really best for the children. In most cases you can probably find a compromise that still gets the kids what they need to be safe and healthy.

You may feel guilty about the divorce and want to suspend all the rules for your kids, but remember what kids need to thrive—stable expectations, exercise, healthy food, intellectual stimulation, sleep, and love. Expect them to test you, even to use the divorce as a lever: "But Mommy lets us…" is a favorite. Often you'll find Mommy does not let them…or at least she doesn't do so regularly. At this point, stability is among the greatest gifts you have to offer.

In talking to your children about their new roles, let them know if you need them to do a little more. They may help pack lunches for school, pick up their clothes before leaving the house, or put away dishes. They may even have to be understanding if you have less spending money than before. At the same time, daughters especially may feel they must step into the mothering role now that you're alone. Let your daughter know that while you appreciate her trying to help, you're still the parent, and make sure your behavior reinforces the message.

what you can do

Try to stock each house with enough essentials that your children don't have to pack a steamer trunk for the weekend. In addition to toiletries and clothes, consider toys, games, and special stuffed animals. It's tempting at this time to try and make yours the "fun" house. You might go on a shopping spree, filling the place with video games, skateboards, and Pop-Tarts. But what's most important is that it be a comfortable house. You and mom are not in a bidding war for the kids, and no toy or treat is going to take the place of having an intact family. Look instead for things that bring you and your children together. Does your child like to read books with you? Build models? Ride bikes? As you work to make your house an enjoyable place for your kids, make sure you're sending the message, "I value the time we spend together," not just, "Here, have some stuff."

Extended family will also have an important role to play in your children's lives. Involvement by their grandparents, aunts, uncles, and cousins on both sides can help dampen the blow of the divorce. Look at all these people as your children's support network, and try to embrace their involvement in your kids' lives. You may have to build some flexibility into your schedule to help your children stay in touch with extended family members.

Pay attention to how you compare your child to his mother. You can say something positive like, "It looks like you have your mother's artistic talent!" But if you start telling your child he does something negative, "…just like your mother," he's going to wonder if maybe you'll divorce him next. At the same time, remember to let your child be a child. Your daughter may feel like she has to become your confidante or housekeeper now that her mom's not around. Make sure she knows it's still your job to take care of her and not the other way around.

a matter of time

As you move through the process of formal legal separation and divorce, you will be asked to settle on physical and legal custody. As you might imagine, *physical* custody describes where your children will live primarily. The parent with whom they spend the most nights is called the *custodial* or residential parent. Around 16% of the time, mothers and fathers share equal joint physical custody. Joint physical custody works best in situations in which the parents really do function together well. Unfortunately, these cases represent the minority of divorces. For the rest, mothers serve as physical custodian 72% of the time, fathers only 9%. Parents much more commonly share *legal* custody, meaning they both make decisions about education, medical care, and spiritual practices.

If you are the noncustodial parent, you'll need persistence and flexibility. Forty percent of children whose fathers live outside the home never see their dads at all. The remaining 60% see their fathers on average 69 days a year. With age, geographic mobility, and remarriage, many fathers drift away from their children's lives. Ten years after the end of a marriage, more than two-thirds of children report that they have not seen their fathers in more than a year.

Even when you are working hard to be an active part of your child's life, challenges may arrive. Custodial parents sometimes threaten to deny visitation to punish noncustodial parents for perceived wrongs. This is among many reasons to work hard at maintaining at least a functional relationship with your children's mother. Sometimes you'll need to be willing to make trades, for example, if your daughter has a sleepover she really wants to attend that happens to fall on one of your nights.

If your own schedule forces you to cancel a planned visit, try to explain it to your children in person well ahead of time. They want to know their dad is always there for them; failing to show up without warning does not reinforce that message. During the time you're not with your children, make sure you stay in touch as often as possible by phone, text message, e-mail, social network, or video call. Work out with mom how you'll share information about report cards, doctor's visits, and performances or games you might want to attend. Your presence and involvement don't matter less just because the custody arrangement gives you every other weekend.

Over time you're likely to find that you and mom establish a stable and even friendly working relationship. No matter what else has happened, the 2 of you have these children in common, and you both have their best interests at heart, even when you disagree about how those interests are served. Besides that, no one else is likely to understand the frustrations of dealing with a child's particular challenge or the joys of a child's special triumph quite as well as the one person who shared with you in that child's creation.

Divorce can lend holidays a particularly ironic sadness. Not that most holidays ever quite live up to the hype that surrounds them, but be prepared for your children to greet these "festive" occasions with mourning they seem to have moved past on other days of the year. No matter how generous they are, Santa Claus and the Easter Bunny cannot bring back the ideal family children wish for following a divorce. That doesn't mean you have to give up on having a good time, just that somewhere near the presents and cards you should also stash some tissues.

A variety of resources within and outside the family can help your child build resilience. You needed an army to get you through this, and your child should be able to mobilize some troops as well. Siblings often come together during a divorce. After all, no one else knows quite so well what it's like to live in this family. Siblings may also fight more when under stress.

when to call the doctor

If sibling fighting doesn't subside as life evens out again, talk to your kids' pediatrician about finding a counselor or therapist.

Different kids show different signs of stress when their parents' marriage falls apart. Younger children may regress, "forgetting" how to use the potty or becoming whiny and irritable. Be patient with this behavior at first, but if it persists you may want to talk to your child's pediatrician. Older children may respond to this family disruption with falling grades, unexplained aches and pains, poor behavior at school, and signs of depression like sleeplessness and irritability. Teens may display all these signs, or they may experiment with alcohol, drugs, or sexual activity. In any of these cases you're going to want to find your children and yourself professional help. This stuff is new to your family, but the pros deal with it all day long, and they're likely to have some useful ideas for all of you.

Given how common divorce is, your children will probably find that they have friends who have weathered similar ordeals. The school guidance counselor is often a great resource, performing individual therapy and convening groups of kids to talk about common challenges they face. Religious and community organizations often also host groups for kids dealing with divorce.

daddy's new friend

Following a divorce, you may not be able to face dating again for a long time, or you might be eager to experience a new relationship. Either way, if you have kids around you'll want to act with discretion. Remember that kids often imagine you and their mom will get back together, even after everything is legally finalized. They may view your dating as an effort to "replace" their mom. If the subject comes up, reassure them that no one can take the special place their mother has in their lives.

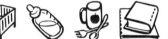

what you can do
You might be pretty excited about your new romantic life, but for a while share this excitement with your adult friends, not your kids. You're likely to experience a few false starts as you begin to date; your kids don't have to meet everyone you go out with. Instead, wait until you develop a serious, relatively stable relationship with someone before introducing that person to your children. They are likely to attach any number of hopes or resentments to anyone new who is the object of your attention and affection. Whether you see it that way or not, to them this is a very big deal.

Depending on their ages, you'll probably need to explain to your children the stages of romantic commitment, from dating, to a serious relationship, to engagement, to marriage. They may want to move you through the process faster than you're ready to go, so you'll want to be clear about where you are.

You'll want to make sure your children and your new romantic partner are both ready to meet each other. Don't forget to give your ex-wife a heads-up as well, out of courtesy. Tell your kids and partner a little about each other, and be ready to answer lots of questions. Decide with everyone on a good time and place. Don't expect your kids to instantly share your enthusiasm about this person. They may harbor fears about what this development means for their own lives, and they're going to need some time with your friend to make up their minds about what they think. Children may feel that showing your new partner too much affection represents some sort of disloyalty to their mother. With time, if things go well for everyone, your kids will hopefully build a positive relationship with this person on their own terms.

singles scene

What scares you? Poisonous snakes? Riding in small airplanes in rough weather? Riding in small airplanes full of poisonous snakes in rough weather? Once you've been a single parent, nothing else can shake you. There's nothing as frightening as looking around and realizing it's just the kids…and you. Many single dads arrive at the role through separation or divorce, but others find themselves in the position after mom loses a battle with drugs, alcohol, or mental illness; breaks the law; goes overseas on a military deployment; or dies. Regardless of the path that gets you there, single parenting presents one of life's most daunting challenges.

Meeting the challenge of single parenting requires discipline, flexibility, and a willingness to identify and mobilize sources of support. Start by reading about parenting, and not just this book, but ones devoted to how to be a better parent. Your child's pediatrician should have some ideas for you. There is no such thing as a "perfect" parent, but there are some approaches that consistently work better than others, and you're going to want to use those when appropriate.

Be willing to turn to family, friends, and professionals for help, too. One thing parents do in a family is to supply each other fresh perspectives when one of them gets stuck in a rut. If you're alone, someone may need to help you think of a new way to solve an old problem.

It's easy to forget to take care of yourself when kids are relying on you. Don't be one of those guys who never goes to the doctor or dentist. Now more than ever, maintaining your health is key. This includes your mental

what you can do

The demands on a single parent's time can be grueling. You're trying to make enough money to support your family, but then you also want to take time with your children and for yourself. You can start by looking at your budget and figuring out how you can live in a way that keeps you from having to work overtime and allows you a few dollars to invest in professional child care. Know that in studies of human happiness, doing stuff outranks having stuff every time. It's the experiences your children have with you that they'll remember, not what you bought them.

health. If tragedy has brought you to single parenthood, chances are good you're going to need some help getting back on an even keel so you can be emotionally available for your children. It may seem like a lot on top of everything else, but the basics of exercise, healthy eating, and getting enough sleep most nights will work wonders to supply you with the energy you'll need for the other stuff.

Whether you hire a professional sitter, rely on relatives, or trade nights with another parent, take some time to indulge yourself (seriously). Even if it's just to see a movie or take a walk in the park, time alone or with friends will help you quiet your head and get in touch with your own feelings. No matter how much you love your children, taking time for yourself will keep you from coming to resent the time you spend with them.

Structure in the family can save you. You don't have to be a drill sergeant, blowing a whistle to get the kids to take their baths, but the more your kids know what to expect, the better they'll be able to comply. Consistency in discipline will not ensure your children behave perfectly all the time, but it works a lot better than the alternative. If your children can eat their dinner, take their baths, and brush their teeth on time, you'll have the luxury of reading them a bedtime story.

Finally, in the push to get everything done, it can be hard to remember to listen to your kids. If one of them has something important to tell you, stop and look at his face while he's speaking. Make simple observations like, "You must have been really proud then," or, "Did that make you sad?" to let him know you're really attending to him. Kids who know they can get your attention in positive ways often feel less compelled to get it by more frustrating means.

don't be sad, be SAHD!

SAHD stands for stay-at-home dad. While the 2010 US Census counted only the 154,000 fathers who cared for children while earning no income outside the home, a more realistic figure includes those dads who provide primary care for their children while their wives work, even if the dads work at other times. This number is closer to 1.5 million, and these dads care for a quarter of children younger than 5 years in the United States.

I have put in time as a SAHD, and it's hard. While child care duties, cooking, cleaning, paying bills, and fixing the toilets leave little time for eating bonbons and watching soap operas, the real challenge is the sense of social isolation. Moms who work in the home can tap into a wide network of playgroups, neighborhood friends, and organized activities. But show up as the only guy at your local library's reading hour and you can actually see the moms scooting away from you in the imagination circle. The Internet or your local newspaper may help you find groups of dads to hang out with so you don't feel like a pariah on the park bench. Otherwise, start a group of your own! Check out www.daddyshome.org to see if there's already a group near you.

SAHDs also may suffer a crisis of identity. Many of us have been raised to equate our earning power with self-esteem. Doing a job that is unpaid, even if you doing that job is what enables your family to stay afloat, can threaten your sense of self-worth. Until you've shopped for groceries and gone to the dry cleaners with your toddler on a Tuesday morning, you don't realize how few working-aged men there are out there at those times! On the other hand, you can take pity on those men who don't get to watch their children's first steps or hear them learn their alphabets because they were working all day. What job really is more important than nurturing your child and creating a home? Here again, finding other men in your position will reinforce your sense that what you're doing is possibly the manliest job of all.

yes, my fathers are home

Between 6 and 9 million children in the United States have 1 or 2 gay or lesbian parents. Around 22% of gay male couples are raising children. The topic of gay parents inspires plenty of controversy in the media, but in the pediatric literature data grow clearer each year that kids in these households face no substantially increased risks in their educational, cognitive, emotional, or sexual development compared with children who grow up with heterosexual parents. They have the same interests and sorts of relationships as children from other families. It's clear that the structure of these families plays a much smaller role in kids' adjustment than how their families function and communicate. A variety of studies have found that gay fathers' parenting styles are similar to those of heterosexual dads.

The challenges children of gay fathers face tend to come more from outside the home. Biases toward traditional family structures populate everything from the picture books kids read to the permission slips for their field trips ("Mother:_____, Father:_____"). If you're a gay dad, you might want to address these issues ahead of time with your child's teacher and guidance counselor.

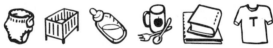

what you can do

The greatest unique challenge gay dads face within the family is answering children's questions about how their families are different. Your preschooler will want to know about how he was born and who his mother is. As always, provide clear, simple answers, knowing that once he digests those he'll be back later with more questions. School-aged children will seek more in-depth knowledge about their family backgrounds and will want to know how to reply to their peers' questions. Teens may become self-conscious and embarrassed about their parents, but this is usually the case no matter what the family structure! They may question their own sexual orientation and choices. You might take this opportunity to talk some about your own life.

Something as simple as including books in the class library that depict diverse families can make a big difference. Teachers may think ahead to Mother's Day and Father's Day to determine how your child can feel included. Some teachers even build a yearlong curriculum that includes family diversity as a theme. Depending on the sort of community you live in, you may have to prepare your child to face some biases and prejudices. Your child should let you and his teacher know early if he's being harassed.

Gay or straight, your family is not going to be perfect. There will be challenges that require listening, talking, and explaining. Your child will likely enjoy meeting other kids with families like his own as well as using online resources to learn about other kids' experiences. He may need a little extra help learning to deal with harassment when it occurs, but all kids get harassed about something at various times; this is just the thing that happens to make him different.

Is it hard to raise kids in a nontraditional family setting? Yes, it is. But then it's hard to raise kids, period. From experience I can tell you this much—they'll let you shop at the Family Dollar no matter who you are.

conclusion:
father time

this book started with a question: "Dad, what are you good for?" If you were to get all your information from greeting cards or commercials, you'd think we fathers are mainly around to hog remote controls, collect socket wrenches, and consume beer and chicken wings. Sitcom fans, on the other hand, know that dads leave up toilet seats, burn simple breakfast foods, and tell little white lies that spin wildly out of control, leading to a series of embarrassing but not life-threatening physical injuries. None of these stereotypes apply to real fathers, except maybe the one about the toilet seats.

Of course in reality, there are as many answers to the question of what dads are good for as there are fathers. I love a lot of things about practicing pediatrics, but I especially enjoy seeing how different dads nurture their kids. I meet some real drill sergeants…I mean, they wear uniforms and train military recruits. They also love to cradle their babies. I know a chef who makes his own baby food using vegetables whose names I can't spell. I see a jaded tech writer who can't wait to share new gadgets with his teenaged daughter. In fatherhood, as in the rest of life, each of us has our own unique gifts to share.

Despite recent demographic changes, many people still have low expectations for fathers' general competence; it's always fun to surprise these people. I hope that after reading this book you've grown even better at certain things, from treating diaper rash, to knowing when a cough might represent pneumonia, to buying your adolescent daughter sanitary napkins (remember, stand up straight and look the checkout lady in the eye; she knows they're not for you). There is no formula to guarantee any child won't end up doing poorly in school, experimenting with drugs and alcohol, or taking unwise sexual risks, but you should have a good tool kit to better protect your child from falling into these traps.

I used to think that if I could just get my kids past certain dangers, I might stop worrying about them. Once my son turned 1 year old, or my daughter got to kindergarten, or my youngest made it into college, I could relax. I now realize that the moment I became a dad I bought a lifetime of concern. Fatherhood is not a job from which one retires. But really, who would want to? Nothing motivates me to work harder, run faster, or think quicker than my kids. If you hoped for a life of excitement and adventure, you can stop dreaming. This is it. What are you good for as a father? Plenty today, but tomorrow you're guaranteed to add something else to the list.

congratulations! you're a dad.

index